SEVENTH EDITION

Medical Dosage Calculations

JUNE LOOBY OLSEN, RN, MS

Professor of Nursing (Emeritus)
The College of Staten Island
Staten Island, New York

ANTHONY PATRICK GIANGRASSO, PhD

Professor of Mathematics
La Guardia Community College
Long Island City, New York

Prentice Hall Health
Upper Saddle River, New Jersey, 07458

Library of Congress Cataloging-in-Publication Data

Olsen, June Looby.
    Medical dosage calculations   /   June Looby Olsen, Anthony Patrick
  Giangrasso.—7th ed.
       p. cm.
    ISBN 0-8053-9162-2
    1. Pharmaceutical arithmetic.   2. Pharmaceutical arithmetic
Problems, exercises, etc.   I. Giangrasso, Anthony Patrick.
II. Title
    [DNLM: 1. Pharmaceutical Preparations—administration & dosage
Nurses' Instruction.   2. Mathematics Nurses' Instruction.   QV 748
052m 2000]
RS57.M425   2000
615' . 14—dc21
DNLM/DLC
for Library of Congress   99-34128
                                                    CIP

Manager, Addison Wesley Nursing: Paul Blackburn
Senior Project Editor: Virginia Simione Jutson
Associate Editor: Stephanie Kellogg
Publishing Assistants: Susan Teahan, Peggy Hammett
Managing Editor: Wendy Earl
Production Supervisor: Sharon Montooth
Text and Cover Designer: Carolyn Deacy
Director of Manufacturing and Production: Bruce Johnson
Manufacturing Buyer: Ilene Sanford
Compositor: York Graphic Services, Inc.
Printer/Binder: Banta

Previously published by Addison Wesley Nursing
A Division of the Benjamin/Cummings Publishing Company, Inc.
Redwood City, California 94065

© 2000 by Prentice-Hall, Inc.
Upper Saddle River, New Jersey 07458

Printed in the United States of America

10 9 8 7 6 5 4 3

ISBN 0-8053-9162-2

Prentice Hall International (UK) Limited, London
Prentice Hall of Australia Pty. Limited, Sydney
Prentice Hall Canada, Inc., Toronto
Prentice Hall Hispanoamericana, S.A., Mexico
Prentice Hall of India Private Limited, New Delhi
Prentice Hall of Japan, Inc., Tokyo

DEDICATION

To my granddaughter, Taylor, who has brought so much joy to our family.

June Looby Olsen

In memory of my good friends, Anna and Adam Kowalski.

Anthony Patrick Giangrasso

Preface

In a growing range of health-care settings, nursing and allied health professionals are assuming increasing responsibilities in every aspect of drug administration. The first step in assuming this responsibility is learning to calculate drug dosages accurately. Dosage calculation is not just about math skills, it is an introduction into the **professional context** of drug administration. Calculation skills and the reason for their application—this is what *Medical Dosage Calculations* has taught thousands of students with unmatched success through six editions.

Medical Dosage Calculations is a combined text and workbook designed for the student of dosage calculations. Its consistent focus on safety, accuracy, and professionalism make it a valuable part of a dosage calculation course for nursing or allied health-care programs. It is also highly effective for independent study and may be used as a refresher to dosage calculation skills or as a professional reference.

Topics introduced and developed in *Medical Dosage Calculations* include:

- basic arithmetic skills
- systems of measurement
- dosage calculations for all common forms of drug preparations
- IV and specialized calculations

In addition to these topics, this edition includes substantially more information about basic drug administration. Readers will learn how to interpret actual drug labels, package inserts, and various forms of medication orders, as well as how to recognize a wide variety of syringes.

KEY FEATURES OF *MEDICAL DOSAGE CALCULATIONS*

We have built on the strengths of the previous editions by continuing to provide the thoroughness of a textbook with the practicality and convenience of a workbook. Here are the important features that have made *Medical Dosage Calculations* an effective and popular book through six editions.

- *Dimensional Analysis Calculation Method.* Dimensional analysis is a technique in which the units on the drug package are systematically converted to the units on the drug order. We were the first authors to employ dimensional analysis for drug calculation. Our method has become the primary dosage calculation technique among nursing and allied health educators. This method helps assure safety while eliminating the need to memorize formulas.

- *Learn by Example.* Each chapter unfolds basic concepts and skills through a series of examples:

▶ **EXAMPLE 6.3**

How many tablets should you give a patient if the order is for grain $\frac{1}{2}$ of codeine sulfate and each tablet contains grain $\frac{1}{4}$?

In this problem you want to convert the order grain $\frac{1}{2}$ to tablets.

$$\text{gr } \frac{1}{2} = ? \text{ tab}$$

You want to cancel the grain and determine the equivalent amount in tablets.

$$\text{gr } \frac{1}{2} \times \frac{? \text{ tab}}{? \text{ gr}} = ? \text{ tab}$$

Since 1 tab $=$ gr $\frac{1}{4}$ the fraction is $\dfrac{1 \text{ tab}}{\text{gr } \frac{1}{4}}$.

$$\cancel{\text{gr}} \frac{1}{2} \times \frac{1 \text{ tab}}{\cancel{\text{gr}} \frac{1}{4}} = \frac{1 \text{ tab}}{\frac{2}{4}} = 1 \text{ tab} \div \frac{2}{4} = 1 \text{ tab} \times \frac{4}{2} = 2 \text{ tab}$$

So grain $\frac{1}{2}$ is equivalent to 2 tablets, and you should give the patient 2 tablets of codeine sulfate.

This method teaches concepts by *showing* the application.

- *Case Studies.* Realistic case scenarios allow the student to apply concepts and techniques presented in the text to a clinical setting.

- *Problem Sets.* This text/workbook offers learners over 1000 practice opportunities. Each chapter's practice opportunities are grouped into four problem sets:
  - Try These for Practice
  - Exercises
  - Additional Exercises
  - Cumulative Review Exercises

When applicable, each problem set reinforces skills in interpreting drug labels and medication orders and in recognizing syringes.

- *Comprehensive Self-Tests.* Upon completion of this text/workbook, these Self-Tests quiz the students comprehensive knowledge. Answers to three of the Self-Tests can be found in the book.

Organization. The skills mastered in *Medical Dosage Calculations* are arranged into four basic learning units:

- **Unit 1: Basic Calculation and Administration Skills**

  After a review of basic number skills, this section introduces the essentials of drug administration. A separate chapter introduces dimensional analysis using a friendly, commonsense approach.

- **Unit 2: Systems of Measurement for Dosage Calculations**

  This section covers the three systems of measurement that nurses and other allied health professionals must understand to interpret medication orders and calculate dosages. Readers learn to convert measurements between and within measurement systems.

- **Unit 3: Common Medication Preparations**

  The heart of the book, the chapters in this unit prepare readers to calculate oral and parenteral medication dosages and introduce the preparation of solutions.

- **Unit 4: Specialized Medication Preparations**

  This important final section provides a solid base for calculating IV and enteral flow rates, intravenous piggyback infusions and duration of infusions, as well as pediatric dosages.

BENEFITS OF USING *MEDICAL DOSAGE CALCULATIONS*

- Constant skill reinforcement through frequent practice opportunities.
- Over 1000 problems for students to solve.
- Commonly used medications featured.
- Actual drug labels, syringes, drug package inserts, and medication orders are illustrated throughout the text.
- Ample work space on every page for note-taking and problem-solving.
- Answers to Try These For Practice, Exercises, and Cumulative Review Exercises are found in the text and at the end of the text.
- Detachable Pocketminder to be carried on the job as a quick reference for essential dosage calculation information.

SUPPLEMENTAL MATERIALS

Instructor's Guide

This combined *Instructor's Guide/Testbank* (0-8053-9174-6) provides extra test questions, answers to test questions, answers to Additional Exercises, answers to Comprehensive Self-Tests, a list of Key Terms, possible teaching approaches relevant to each chapter, an overview of chapter missions, and a comprehensive examination with answers. This guide helps instructors prepare lectures and examinations quickly.

Student Study Wizard CD-ROM

This CD-ROM is included free with the text. It contains 120 multiple choice questions.

REVIEWERS FOR THE SEVENTH EDITION

Jeannette May Anderson, RN, MSN
Tarrant County Junior College, Fort Worth, Texas
M&M Nurse Review Centre, Arlington, Texas

Deborah Dalrymple, RN, MSN, CRNI
Montgomery County Community College
Blue Bell, Pennsylvania

Patricia Graham, RN, BSN
Georgia School of Nursing
Augusta, Georgia

REVIEWERS FOR THE SIXTH EDITION

Deborah Dalrymple, RN, MSN, CRNI
Barbara Goodkin, MSN
Maxine Goos, RN, MSN
Ann Miller, MSN
Claire Mortensen, MSN

ACKNOWLEDGMENTS

Our special thanks to the faculty and students at the College of Staten Island and La Guardia Community College, especially Eugenia Borgia Murray, who have participated with support and suggestions for the past 28 years. Also, a thank you to our editor, Stephanie Kellogg, and publishing assistant, Peggy Hammett.

My loving thanks and warmest regards to my daughter, Michelle Olsen Keefe. With her assistance and research, this text developed into its seventh edition.

Special thanks also to our former coauthor, Leon J. Ablon, for his contributions to the previous six editions. To our friend and former coauthor, the late Helen Siner Weisman, we remember you. You honored our writing group by your professional attitude and knowledge. We miss you.

We are pleased to acknowledge the following pharmaceutical companies that granted us permission to reproduce their labels:

Abbott Laboratories
Astra Pharmaceutical Products Inc.
Baxter Incorporated
Bristol-Myers Squibb Company
Ciba-Geigy
DuPont Pharmaceuticals
Geneva Pharmaceuticals, Inc.
Glaxo-Wellcome Company
Eli Lilly and Company

Knoll Pharmaceuticals
Lederle Laboratories
Novartis Pharmaceuticals
  Corporation
Pfizer Incorporated
Pharmacia & Upjohn
Roerig Division, Pfizer Incorporated
Schein Pharmaceutical, Inc.
Smith Kline Beecham

Contents

UNIT TWO *Systems of Measurement for Dosage Calculations 61*

UNIT THREE *Common Medication Preparations 99*

Name: _____ **Date:** _____

Class: _____ **Instructor:** _____

Diagnostic Test of Arithmetic

The following Diagnostic Test illustrates all the arithmetic skills needed to do the computations in this text. Take the test and compare your answers with the answers found at the end of the test. If you discover areas of weakness, carefully review the relevant review materials in Chapter 1 so that you will be mathematically prepared for the rest of the test.

1. Write 0.625 as a fraction. _____

2. Write $\frac{2750}{1000}$ as a decimal number. _____

3. Round 4.781 to the nearest tenth. _____

4. Write $\frac{2}{3}$ as a decimal number rounded to the nearest hundredth.

   _____

5. $\frac{8.4}{0.21} =$ _____

6. $3.267 \times 100 =$ _____

7. $42.51 \div 10 =$ _____

8. $65 \div 0.05 =$ _____

9. $\frac{10}{21} \times 7 \times \frac{3}{5}$ _____

10. $4\frac{2}{3} \div 21 =$ _____

11. $\frac{3}{4} \div \frac{9}{16} =$ _____

12. $\frac{\frac{3}{4}}{12} =$ _____

13. Write 35% as a fraction. _____

14. Write 2.5% as a decimal number without using the % symbol.

   _____

15. Write $4\frac{3}{5}$ as an improper fraction. _____

Answers: **1.** $\frac{5}{8}$ **2.** 2.75 **3.** 4.8 **4.** 0.67 **5.** 40 **6.** 326.7 **7.** 4.251
8. 1300 **9.** 2 **10.** $\frac{2}{9}$ **11.** $\frac{4}{3}$ or $\frac{11}{3}$ **12.** $\frac{1}{16}$ **13.** $\frac{7}{20}$ **14.** 0.025 **15.** $\frac{23}{5}$

Basic Calculation and Administration Skills

CHAPTER ONE

Review of Arithmetic for Medical Dosage Calculations

▶ **Objectives**

After completing this chapter, you will be able to

- Convert decimal numbers to fractions.
- Convert fractions to decimal numbers.
- Round decimal numbers to a desired number of places.
- Multiply and divide decimal numbers.
- Multiply and divide fractions.
- Simplify complex fractions.
- Write percentages as decimal numbers.
- Write percentages as fractions.

Medical dosage calculations can involve whole numbers, fractions, decimal numbers, and percentages. Your results on the *Diagnostic Test of Arithmetic*, found on the previous page, will have identified your areas of strength and weakness. You can use Chapter 1 to improve your math skills or simply to review the kinds of calculations you will encounter in this text.

CHANGING DECIMAL NUMBERS AND WHOLE NUMBERS TO FRACTIONS

A decimal number represents a fraction with a denominator of 10, 100, 1000, and so on. Each decimal number has three parts: the whole-number part, the decimal point, and the fraction part. Table 1.1 shows the names of the decimal positions.

Reading a decimal number will help you to write it as a fraction.

Decimal Number	$\longrightarrow$	Read	$\longrightarrow$	Fraction
4.1	$\longrightarrow$	four and one tenth	$\longrightarrow$	$4\frac{1}{10}$
0.3	$\longrightarrow$	three tenths	$\longrightarrow$	$\frac{3}{10}$
0.07	$\longrightarrow$	seven hundredths	$\longrightarrow$	$\frac{7}{100}$
0.231	$\longrightarrow$	two hundred thirty-one thousandths	$\longrightarrow$	$\frac{231}{1000}$
0.0025	$\longrightarrow$	twenty-five ten thousandths	$\longrightarrow$	$\frac{25}{10,000}$

A number can be written in many different forms. For example, the decimal number 3.5 is read as *three and five tenths*. In fraction form, it is $3\frac{5}{10}$ or $3\frac{1}{2}$. You can also write $3\frac{1}{2}$ as an **improper fraction,** as follows:

$$3\frac{1}{2} = \frac{3 \times 2 + 1}{2} = \frac{7}{2}$$

▶ TABLE 1.1

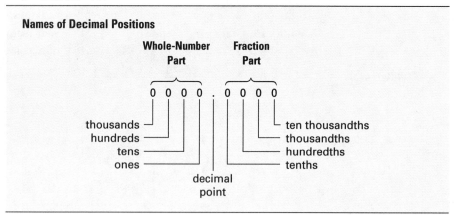

Names of Decimal Positions

▶ EXAMPLE 1.1

Write 2.25 as an improper fraction.

The number 2.25 is read *two and twenty-five hundredths* and written $2\frac{25}{100}$. You can simplify:

$$2\frac{25}{100} = 2\frac{\overset{1}{\cancel{25}}}{\underset{4}{\cancel{100}}} = 2\frac{1}{4} = \frac{2 \times 4 + 1}{4} = \frac{9}{4}$$

NOTE

Simplify $\frac{25}{100}$ to $\frac{1}{4}$ by dividing both numerator and denominator by the same number, 25. This is called *canceling*.

CHANGING FRACTIONS TO DECIMAL NUMBERS

To change a fraction to a decimal, think of the fraction as a division problem. For example:

$$\frac{2}{5} \quad \text{means} \quad 2 \div 5 \quad \text{or} \quad 5\overline{)2}$$

Here are the steps for this division.

Step 1   Replace 2 with 2.0 and then place a decimal point directly above the decimal point in 2.0.

$$5\overline{)2.0}^{\,.}$$

Step 2   Perform the division.

$$\begin{array}{r} 0.4 \\ 5\overline{)2.0} \\ \underline{2\ 0} \\ 0 \end{array}$$

So, $\frac{2}{5} = 0.4$.

▶ **E X A M P L E   1 . 2**

Write $\frac{5}{2}$ as a decimal number.

$$\frac{5}{2} \quad \text{means} \quad 2\overline{)5}$$

Step 1 $2\overline{)5.0}^{\,.}$

Step 2
$$\begin{array}{r} 2.5 \\ 2\overline{)5.0} \\ \underline{4} \\ 1\,0 \\ \underline{1\,0} \end{array}$$

So $\frac{5}{2} = 2.5$.

▶ **E X A M P L E 1 . 3**

Write $\frac{193}{10}$ as a decimal number.

$$\frac{193}{10} \quad \text{means} \quad 10\overline{)193}$$

Step 1 $10\overline{)193.0}^{\,\cdot}$

Step 2
$$\begin{array}{r} 19.3 \\ 10\overline{)193.0} \\ \underline{10} \\ 93 \\ \underline{90} \\ 30 \\ \underline{30} \\ 0 \end{array}$$

So, $\frac{193}{10} = 19.3$.

There is a quicker way to do this problem. To divide any decimal number by 10, you move the decimal point in the number one place to the left. Notice that there is one zero in 10.

$$\frac{193}{10} = \frac{193.}{10} = 19\,3. = 19.3$$

To divide a number by 100, move the decimal point in the number two places to the left, because there are two zeros in 100. So, the quick way to divide by 10, 100, 1000, and so on, is to count the zeros and then move the decimal point to the left the same number of places. The answer should always be a smaller number than the original. Check your answer to be sure.

▶ **E X A M P L E 1 . 4**

Write $\frac{9.25}{100}$ as a decimal number.

There are two zeros in 100, so move the decimal point in 9.25 two places to the left, and fill the empty position with a zero.

$$\frac{9.25}{100} = \underset{\frown}{9.25} = 0.0925$$

ROUNDING DECIMAL NUMBERS

Sometimes it's convenient to round answers—that is, to find an approximate answer rather than an exact one. To round 0.257 to the nearest tenth—that is, to round the answer to one decimal place—you do the following:

Look at the hundredths (second) decimal place digit. Because this digit is 5 or more, round 0.257 by adding 1 to the tenths (first) decimal place digit. Finally, drop all the digits after the tenths place. So 0.257 becomes 0.3 when rounded to the nearest tenth.

To round 6.4345 to the nearest hundredth—that is, to round the answer to two decimal places—you do the following:

Look at the thousandths (third) place digit. Since this digit is less than 5, round 6.4345 by leaving the hundredths digit alone. Finally, drop all the digits after the hundredths place. So 6.4345 becomes 6.43 when rounded to the nearest hundredth.

▶ **E X A M P L E 1.5**

Round 4.8075 to the nearest hundredth, tenth, and whole number.

4.8075 rounded to the nearest: hundredth = 4.81
tenth = 4.8
whole number = 5

MULTIPLYING AND DIVIDING DECIMAL NUMBERS

To multiply two decimal numbers, first multiply, ignoring the decimal points. Then count the total number of decimal places in the original two numbers. That sum equals the number of decimal places in the answer.

▶ **E X A M P L E 1.6**

$304.2 \times 0.16 = ?$

```
  304.2     ← 1 decimal place  ⎫ Total of 3
 ×0.16      ← 2 decimal places ⎭ decimal places
 18252
  3042
 48.672
```
↑
There are 3 decimal places in the answer.
Place the decimal point here.

So, $304.2 \times 0.16 = 48.672$.

▶ **E X A M P L E   1 . 7**

304.25 × 10 = ?

$$\begin{array}{r} 304.25 \\ \times 10 \\ \hline 3042.50 \end{array}$$ ← 2 decimal places ⎱ Total of 2
← 0 decimal places ⎰ decimal places

↑ There are 2 decimal places in the answer.
└── Place the decimal point here.

So, 304.25 × 10 = 3042.50 or 3042.5.

There is a quicker way to do this problem. To multiply any decimal number by 10, move the decimal point in the number being multiplied one place to the right. Notice that there is one zero in 10.

304.25 × 10 = 304.2‿5   or   3042.5

To multiply a number by 100, move the decimal point in the number two places to the right, because there are two zeros in 100. So, the quick way to multiply by 10, 100, 1000, and so on, is to count the zeros and then move the decimal point to the right the same number of places. The answer should always be a larger number than the original. Check your answer to be sure.

▶ **E X A M P L E   1 . 8**

23.597 × 1000 = ?

There are three zeros in 1000, so move the decimal point in 23.597 three places to the right.

23.597 × 1000 = 23.‿5‿9‿7   or   23,597

So, 23.597 × 1000 = 23,597.

▶ **E X A M P L E   1 . 9**

Write $\frac{106.8}{15}$ as a decimal number to the nearest tenth; that is, round the answer to one decimal place.

$$\frac{106.8}{15} \quad \text{means} \quad 15\overline{)106.8}$$

Step 1 $15\overline{)106.8}^{\,.}$

Step 2   Because you want the answer to the nearest tenth (one decimal place), do the division to two decimal places and then round the answer. Since the second place digit in the answer is *less than 5*, leave the first decimal place digit alone. Finally, drop the digit in the second (hundredths) decimal place.

$$
\begin{array}{r}
7.12 \\
15\overline{)106.80} \\
\underline{105} \\
18 \\
\underline{15} \\
30 \\
\underline{30} \\
0
\end{array}
$$

So, $\frac{106.8}{15}$ is 7.1 to the nearest tenth.

▶ **E X A M P L E   1 . 1 0**

$\frac{48}{0.002} = ?$

Note that there are three decimal places in 0.002, so move the decimal points in both numbers three places to the right.

$$\frac{48}{0.002} \quad \text{means} \quad 0.002\overline{)48.} \quad \text{or} \quad 0.002\,\overline{)48.000}$$

$$
\begin{array}{r}
24000. \\
2\overline{)48000.} \\
\underline{4} \\
8 \\
\underline{8} \\
0
\end{array}
$$

So, $\frac{48}{0.002} = 24,000$.

MULTIPLYING AND DIVIDING FRACTIONS

To *multiply* fractions, multiply the numerators to get the new numerator and multiply the denominators to get the new denominator.

▶ **E X A M P L E   1 . 1 1**

$\frac{3}{5} \times 6 \times \frac{1}{5} = ?$

A whole number can be written as a fraction with 1 in the denominator. In this example, write 6 as $\frac{6}{1}$.

$$\frac{3}{5} \times \frac{6}{1} \times \frac{1}{5} = \frac{3 \times 6 \times 1}{5 \times 1 \times 5} = \frac{18}{25}$$

▶ **E X A M P L E   1.12**

$\frac{4}{5} \times \frac{3}{10} \times \frac{20}{7} = ?$

It is often convenient to cancel before you multiply.

$$\frac{4}{5} \times \frac{3}{\overset{}{\underset{1}{10}}} \times \frac{\overset{2}{\cancel{20}}}{7} = \frac{24}{35}$$

To *divide* fractions, change the division problem to an equivalent multiplication problem by inverting the second fraction.

▶ **E X A M P L E   1.13**

$1\frac{2}{5} \div \frac{7}{9} = ?$

Write $1\frac{2}{5}$ as the fraction $\frac{7}{5}$. Division $\left(\frac{7}{5} \div \frac{7}{9}\right)$ becomes the multiplication $\left(\frac{7}{5} \times \frac{9}{7}\right)$.

$$\frac{\overset{1}{\cancel{7}}}{5} \times \frac{9}{\underset{1}{\cancel{7}}} = \frac{9}{5} = 1\frac{4}{5}$$

Sometimes you must deal with whole numbers, fractions, and decimal numbers in the same multiplication and division problems.

▶ **E X A M P L E   1.14**

$\frac{1}{300} \times 60 \times \frac{1}{0.4} = ?$

$$\frac{1}{\underset{5}{\cancel{300}}} \times \frac{\overset{1}{\cancel{60}}}{1} \times \frac{1}{0.4} = \frac{1}{5 \times 0.4} = \frac{1}{2}$$

NOTE

Avoid canceling decimal numbers. It is a possible source of error.

Sometimes you will need to simplify a fraction that contains decimal numbers.

► **E X A M P L E   1 . 1 5**

$0.35 \times \frac{1}{60} = ?$

$$\frac{0.35}{1} \times \frac{1}{60} = \frac{0.35}{60}$$

The numerator of this fraction is 0.35, a decimal number. You can write an equivalent form of the fraction by multiplying the numerator and denominator by 100.

$$\frac{0.35}{60} \times \frac{100}{100} = \frac{0.35}{60.00} = \frac{35}{6000} = \frac{7}{1200}$$

► **E X A M P L E   1 . 1 6**

Give the answer to the following problem in a fractional form containing no decimal numbers.

$0.88 \times \frac{1}{2.2} = ?$

$$\frac{0.88}{1} \times \frac{1}{2.2} = \frac{0.88}{2.2}$$

Multiply the numerator and the denominator of this fraction by 100 to eliminate both decimal numbers.

$$\frac{0.88}{2.2} \times \frac{100}{100} = \frac{0.88}{2.2} = \frac{88}{220} = \frac{2}{5}$$

You can do this problem a different way by dividing 0.88 by 2.2.

$$2.2\overline{)0.88}^{\,0.4} \quad \text{and} \quad 0.4 = \frac{2}{5}$$

COMPLEX FRACTIONS

Fractions that have numerators or denominators that are fractions are called *complex fractions.* The longer fraction line separates the numerator from the denominator and indicates division.

$$\frac{1}{\frac{2}{5}} \quad \text{means} \quad 1 \div \frac{2}{5} \quad \text{or} \quad 1 \times \frac{5}{2} \quad \text{which is} \quad \frac{5}{2}$$

$$\frac{\frac{1}{2}}{5} \quad \text{means} \quad \frac{1}{2} \div 5 \quad \text{or} \quad \frac{1}{2} \times \frac{1}{5} \quad \text{which is} \quad \frac{1}{10}$$

$\dfrac{\frac{3}{5}}{\frac{2}{5}}$ means $\dfrac{3}{5} \div \dfrac{2}{5}$ or $\dfrac{3}{\underset{1}{5}} \times \dfrac{\overset{1}{5}}{2}$ which is $\dfrac{3}{2}$

▶ **E X A M P L E   1 . 1 7**

$\dfrac{\frac{1}{25} \times 500}{\frac{1}{4}} = ?$

Convert to a simpler form.

$$\left(\dfrac{1}{25} \times \dfrac{500}{1} \right) \div \dfrac{1}{4} = ?$$

$$\left(\dfrac{1}{\underset{1}{25}} \times \dfrac{\overset{20}{500}}{1} \right) \div \dfrac{1}{4} =$$

$$\dfrac{20}{1} \div \dfrac{1}{4} =$$

$$\dfrac{20}{1} \times \dfrac{4}{1} = 80$$

▶ **E X A M P L E   1.18**

$\dfrac{2}{3} \times \dfrac{1}{\frac{3}{4}} = ?$

Convert to a simpler form.

$$\dfrac{\frac{2 \times 1}{3 \times 1}}{\frac{3}{1} \times \frac{3}{4}} = ?$$

$$\dfrac{\frac{2}{9}}{\frac{9}{4}} =$$

$$\dfrac{2}{1} \div \dfrac{9}{4} = \dfrac{2}{1} \times \dfrac{4}{9} = \dfrac{8}{9}$$

This problem could be done another way:

$$\frac{2}{3} \times \frac{1}{\frac{3}{4}} = ?$$

$$\frac{2}{3} \times \left(1 \div \frac{3}{4}\right) =$$

$$\frac{2}{3} \times \left(\frac{1}{1} \times \frac{4}{3}\right) =$$

$$\frac{2}{3} \times \frac{4}{3} = \frac{8}{9}$$

PERCENTAGES

Percent (%) means *parts per 100* or *divided by 100*. In calculations dealing with a percentage, you drop the % symbol, divide the number by 100, and write it as a fraction or a decimal number.

$$13\% \quad \text{means} \quad \frac{13}{100} \quad \text{or} \quad 0.13$$

$$100\% \quad \text{means} \quad \frac{100}{100} \quad \text{or} \quad 1$$

$$12.3\% \quad \text{means} \quad \frac{12.3}{100} \quad \text{or} \quad 0.123$$

$$6\frac{1}{2}\% \quad \text{means} \quad 6.5\% \quad \text{or} \quad \frac{6.5}{100} \quad \text{or} \quad 0.065$$

▶ **EXAMPLE 1.19**

Write 0.5% as a fraction.

$$0.5\% = \frac{0.5}{100} = \frac{5}{1000} = \frac{1}{200}$$

There is another way to get the answer. You know that $0.5 = \frac{1}{2}$. So,

$$0.5\% = \frac{1}{2}\% = \frac{1}{2} \div 100 = \frac{1}{2} \times \frac{1}{100} = \frac{1}{200}$$

You will find the answers to *Try These for Practice* after the questions and the answers to *Exercises* in Appendix A at the back of the book. Your instructor has the answers to the *Additional Exercises*.

Try These for Practice

Test your comprehension after reading the chapter. *The answers follow the questions.*

1. Write $\dfrac{7}{8}$ as a decimal number. _____

2. $\left(\dfrac{5}{12} \times \dfrac{8}{25} \right) \times \dfrac{2}{5} =$ _____

3. $\dfrac{3.46 \times 4.5}{0.3} =$ _____

4. $\dfrac{\dfrac{2}{5}}{\dfrac{6}{15}} =$ _____

5. Write 7.5% as a decimal number. _____

Answers: 1. 0.875 *2.* $\dfrac{4}{75}$ *3.* 51.9 *4.* 1 *5.* 0.075

Exercises

Reinforce your understanding in class or at home. *Check your answers in Appendix A at the back of the book.*

Convert the decimals to fractions.

1. 0.24 = _____   2. 3.24 = _____

Convert the fractions to decimals.

3. $\dfrac{5}{8} =$ _____   4. $\dfrac{4}{25} =$ _____

5. $\dfrac{1}{10} =$ _____

6. $\dfrac{1}{200} =$ _____

7. $\dfrac{1}{300} =$ _____
(nearest thousandth)

8. $\dfrac{4500}{100} =$ _____

9. $\dfrac{6.25}{1000} =$ _____

10. $\dfrac{142.6}{7} =$ _____
(nearest tenth)

Convert to decimals.

11. $\dfrac{7.2}{0.06} =$ _____

12. $\dfrac{72}{0.006} =$ _____

Multiply the decimals.

13. $123.4 \times 100 =$ _____

14. $5.125 \times 1.3 =$ _____

15. $36.42 \times 1000 =$ _____

Divide the decimals.

16. $85 \div 0.05 =$ _____

17. $8.5 \div 0.5 =$ _____

Write the answers to Problems 18 through 22 in fractional form.

18. $\dfrac{4}{15} \times 30 \times \dfrac{1}{2} =$ _____

19. $6\dfrac{1}{2} \div 3 =$ _____

20. $26 \div 3\dfrac{1}{4} =$ _____

21. $4.25 \times \dfrac{1}{5} =$ _____

22. $\dfrac{1}{250} \times 125 \times \dfrac{1}{0.5} =$ _____

Write the answers to Problems 23 through 26 in fractional form and in decimal form to the nearest tenth.

23. $4.75 \times \dfrac{1}{1.5} =$ _____

24. $\dfrac{3}{\frac{5}{10}} =$ _____

25. $\dfrac{\dfrac{1}{4}}{6} \times 8 =$ _____

26. $\dfrac{\dfrac{1}{4} \times 160}{\dfrac{5}{8}} =$ _____

Write the percentages as decimals.

27. $38\dfrac{2}{5}\% =$ _____

28. $35\% =$ _____

Write the percentages as fractions.

29. $6.75\% =$ _____

30. $1.5\% =$ _____

Additional Exercises

Now, on your own, test yourself! *Ask your instructor to check your answers.*

Write the decimals as fractions.

1. $0.015 =$ _____

2. $1.06 = 1\dfrac{3}{50}$

Write the fractions as decimals.

3. $\dfrac{6}{15} = 0.4$

4. $\dfrac{9}{50} = 0.18$

5. $\dfrac{3}{200} =$ _____

6. $\dfrac{1}{150} = 0.007$
   (nearest thousandth)

7. $\dfrac{1}{240} = 0.004$
   (nearest thousandth)

8. $\dfrac{264}{1000} =$ _____

Convert the following to decimals.

9. $\dfrac{43.5}{100} =$ _____

10. $\dfrac{503.8}{15} =$ _____
    (nearest tenth)

11. $\dfrac{6.3}{0.07} = 90$

Multiply the decimals.

12. $630 \times 0.007 =$ _4.41_

13. $56.18 \times 7.2 =$ _____

14. $8.277 \times 100 =$ _____

15. $63.2 \times 10 =$ _____

Divide the decimals.

16. $2.61 \div 0.3 =$ _____

17. $261 \div 0.003 =$ _____

Write the answers to Problems 18 through 23 in fractional form.

18. $\dfrac{5}{12} \times 10 \times \dfrac{1}{15} =$ _____

19. $8\dfrac{1}{2} \div 6 =$ _____

20. $39 \div 3\dfrac{1}{4} =$ _____

21. $9.45 \times \dfrac{1}{15} =$ _0.63 $= \dfrac{63}{100}$_

22. $\dfrac{4}{200} \times 50 \times \dfrac{1}{0.2} =$ _5 $= \dfrac{50}{10}$_

23. $8.35 \times \dfrac{0.25}{0.5} =$ _4.2 $= \dfrac{420}{100}$_

Write the answers to Problems 24 through 26 in fractional form and in decimal form to the nearest tenth.

24. $\dfrac{\frac{1}{3}}{2} =$ _0.2_

25. $\dfrac{\frac{4}{5}}{3} \times \dfrac{2}{9} =$ _0.9_

26. $\dfrac{\frac{7}{10} \times 150}{2} =$ _52.5_

Write the percentages as decimals.

27. $20.5\% =$ _0.205_

28. $42\% =$ _0.42_

Write the percentages as fractions.

29. $20.5\% =$ _$\dfrac{20.5}{100}$_

30. $24\% =$ _$\dfrac{24}{100}$_

CHAPTER TWO

Drug Administration

▶ Objectives

After completing this chapter, you will be able to

- Identify the parts of a medication order.

- Describe the information listed on a physician's order sheet and a medication administration record.

- Identify the routes of drug administration.

- Describe the forms in which medication is supplied.

- Interpret information found on medication labels and package inserts.

- Understand the "five rights" concerning medication administration.

- Identify the trade name and the generic name of a drug.

- Understand the legal implications involved in the administration of drugs.

This chapter presents the components of the drug order, drug label, drug package insert, physician's order sheet, and medication administration record. Each is discussed in the context of their use in an institutional health care setting, such as a hospital or extended-care facility.

WHO ADMINISTERS DRUGS?

To a patient, drugs can be life saving, therapeutic, or life threatening. Physicians and dentists can legally prescribe medications. In many states, physician's assistants and nurse practitioners can also prescribe a range of medications related to their areas of practice.

The registered professional nurse (RN), licensed practical nurse (LPN), and the vocational nurse (VN) are responsible for administering drugs ordered by the prescriber. Of course, physicians can also administer drugs to patients.

In most cases, however, drug administration is a process involving a chain of health care professionals. The prescriber **writes** the drug order, the pharmacist **fills** the order, and the nurse **administers** the drug to the patient. Everyone involved is equally responsible for the accuracy of the order and the safety of the patient.

In order to ensure patients' safety, health care professionals who administer medications must understand how drugs act. This knowledge helps them determine when a drug should not be administered or when it should be used cautiously. Understanding drug actions is also important in determining whether a prescribed drug will interact with another drug that the patient is receiving. Drug actions are discussed in pharmacology textbooks and drug handbooks.

THE DRUG ADMINISTRATION PROCESS

As someone who will be responsible for administering drugs to clients, you must know how to administer them safely. In particular, you must know the classic **Five "Rights" of Medication Administration:**

- right drug
- right dose
- right route
- right time
- right patient

The Right Drug

A drug is a substance that acts therapeutically on the physiologic processes of the human body. For example, the drug insulin is given to patients whose bodies do not manufacture sufficient insulin for the metabolism of food. Some drugs have more than one therapeutic property. Aspirin, for example, is an antipyretic (fever-reducing), analgesic (pain-relieving), and anti-inflammatory drug and has anticoagulant properties (decreases the viscosity of blood). A drug may be taken for any one, or all, of its therapeutic properties.

A drug can be prescribed using either its *generic name* or its *trade name.* For example, many companies manufacture the anti-inflammatory drug diclofenac sodium (Figure 2.1). Diclofenac sodium is the drug's generic name. As the drug label in the figure shows, the manufacturer calls this drug Voltaren.

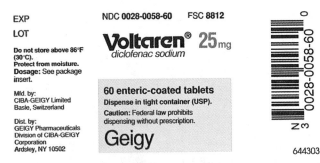

> **FIGURE 2.1** A drug's trade name and generic name. The trade name (Voltaren) can be identified by the raised ® to the right of the name. The drug's generic name (diclofenac sodium) usually appears in lowercase letters. The manufacturer (Geigy) chose the name Voltaren for its version of this anti-inflammatory drug.

So, in this case, Voltaren is the drug's trade name. A drug has only one generic name but can have many trade names. Each trade name is patented by the particular manufacturer of the drug.

The drug's trade name usually has the symbol ™ or ® printed to the right of the name (for example, Voltaren®). This is the drug's trademark or registration symbol. In addition, the trade name usually begins with an uppercase letter, whereas the generic name is printed in lowercase letters (see Figure 2.1). If the prescriber writes an order for Voltaren, then the brand Voltaren **must** be used, and no substitutions are allowed. But if the order uses the drug's generic name (for example, diclofenac sodium) or if the order indicates a trade name but states "substitution permitted," then diclofenac sodium made by any manufacturer may be administered. Each drug has a unique identification number which is assigned by the Drug Enforcement Agency (DEA). This number is called the **National Drug Code (NDC) number.** The NDC number for Voltaren (0028005860) is printed in two places on the label and is also encoded in the bar code.

> **WARNING**
>
> Read drug names carefully! Many drugs have similar looking names. For example, digoxin is *not* digitoxin, and cefotetan is *not* cefoxitin.

The Right Dose

There are many drug references available. They indicate the correct dose for a specific patient. These resources include pharmacology texts and drug handbooks, the *United States Pharmacopeia,* the *Physicians' Desk Reference,* and manufacturers' package inserts. Those prescribing and administering medications must learn the correct dose. It is their **legal responsibility** to know this information.

The right dose can be affected by the patient's weight or body surface area (BSA). Many drug doses administered to children or for cancer therapy are calculated based on BSA.

Body surface area is the actual measurement of the total skin area of a person measured in meters squared (m^2). Body surface area is determined by formulas or by the use of a BSA nomogram. You can measure the BSA of a child or an adult if you know his or her height and weight.

The Right Route

Medications must be administered in the form and via the route specified by the prescriber. Medications are manufactured in a variety of forms: liquids, vapors, and solids. Each drug can be administered by one or more routes: by injections (parenteral), by absorption through the skin or mucous membranes (cutaneous), or by mouth (oral).

Parenteral medications are administered by inserting a hypodermic needle attached to a syringe into a body part. The syringe contains the drug that is to be administered. The most common parenteral drug administration sites are listed in Table 2.1. Learn these abbreviations for the major routes of drug administration.

▶ TABLE 2.1

Major Parenteral Drug Administration Routes

Route	Abbreviation	Meaning
Intramuscular	IM	into the muscle
Subcutaneous	sc	into the subcutaneous tissue
Intravenous	IV	into the vein
Intracardiac	IC	into the cardiac muscle
Intradermal	ID	beneath the skin

Medications can also be administered **cutaneously**—that is, through the skin or mucous membrane. This route includes topical administration on the skin surface; inhalation through the nose or mouth; and application of solutions and ointments to the mucosa of the eyes, nose, ears, and mouth. A nitroglycerin patch and the now-familiar nicotine patch, which are applied to the skin, are examples of cutaneously administered drugs. Suppositories containing medications are inserted into the appropriate orifice (vagina, rectum, or urethra).

Oral drugs are administered **by mouth** (po). Oral drugs are supplied in both solid and liquid form. The most common forms are *tablets, capsules,* and *caplets* (Figure 2.2). Some tablets and capsules are manufactured in *sustained-release* (SR) or *extended-release* (XL) form. These slowly release a controlled amount of medication over a period of time (usually 24 hours). There are also tablets for *buccal administration* (absorbed by the mucosa of the oral cavity) and tablets for *sublingual administration* (absorbed under the tongue). Oral drugs also come in liquid form: *oral suspensions* and *elixirs.*

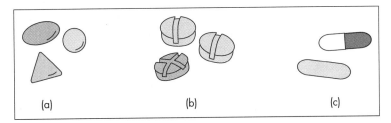

▶ **FIGURE 2.2** **Tablets, capsules, and caplets are manufactured in various shapes and forms: (a) unscored and enteric-coated tablets (should not be broken); (b) scored tablets, usually in halves (may be broken); (c) capsules and caplets (should not be broken).**

> **NOTE**
>
> The prescriber specifies the drug's route of administration. You cannot substitute one route of administration for another.

The Right Time

The prescriber will indicate when and how often a medication should be administered. For example, po medications can be given either before or after meals, depending on the action of the drug. A drug's frequency of administration may be stated specifically; for example, once a day (qd), twice a day (bid), three times a day (tid), and four times a day (qid). Also, medications can be ordered at varying times in a 24-hour day; for example, q4h (every four hours), q6h, q8h, q12h.

The Right Patient

In a hospital setting, the identification bracelet identifies the patient. The name on the drug order form and the name on the patient's identification bracelet *must* match. Some patients are allergic to certain drugs or have an idiosyncratic (unusual) reaction to a drug. Therefore, the person administering the drug must question the patient concerning allergies and record this information on the appropriate form.

> **WARNING**
>
> Anticipate side effects! A side effect is an undesired physiologic response to a drug. For example, codeine relieves pain. But its side effects include constipation, nausea, drowsiness, and itching. Record any side effects noted and discuss them with the prescriber.

DRUG ORDERS

A drug order (prescription) includes the patient's name, name of the drug, the dose, route of administration, and frequency of administration. This order must be written by a health professional licensed by the state to practice as a physician, dentist, advanced nurse practitioner, or a physician's assistant. This book uses the title "prescriber" to designate anyone with the authority to write a prescription. The pharmacist who fills the order by providing the medication ordered by the prescriber is also licensed by the state. A pharmacist cannot write an order or administer medications to patients.

A drug order can take various forms. Figure 2.3 is an example of a *physician's order sheet*. The essential components of a correctly written physician's order include the following information:

Date order written:	1/12/01
Time order written:	9:30 A.M.
Name of drug:	Xanax
Dose:	0.25 mg (milligram)
Route of administration:	po (by mouth)
Frequency of administration:	bid (twice a day)
Name of prescriber:	J. Olsen, MD

In addition, the physician's order sheet provides basic patient information:

Name of patient:	John Camden
Patient's registration number:	602412
Address:	23 Jones Ave., New York, NY 10024
Physician:	J. Olsen
Birthdate:	2/11/55

☩ GENERAL HOSPITAL ☩

PRESS HARD WITH BALLPOINT PEN. WRITE DATE & TIME AND SIGN EACH ORDER

DATE	TIME	A.M.
1/12/01	9:30	P.M.

xanax 0.25 mg po bid

IMPRINT
602412   1/11/01
John Camden   2/11/55
23 Jones Ave.   RC
New York, NY 10024   BCBS

J. Olsen, M.D.

ORDERS NOTED   A.M.
DATE 1/12/01 TIME 10   P.M.

❑ MEDEX   ❑ KARDEX

NURSE'S SIG. A. Giangrasso

SIGNATURE   J. Olsen   M.D.

FILLED BY   DATE

PHYSICIAN'S ORDERS

▶ **FIGURE 2.3 Physician's order sheet.**

Date of admission:	1/11/01
Religion:	Roman Catholic
Insurance:	Blue Cross, Blue Shield

You will find a list of the most common abbreviations that might appear on a drug order in Appendix B. Now, try interpreting the physician's order sheet in Figure 2.4. Record the following information:

Date order written: _____

Time order written: _____

Name of drug: _____

Dose: _____

Route of administration: _____

Frequency of administration: _____

Name of prescriber: _____

Name of patient: _____

Patient's registration number: _____

Address: _____

Physician: _____

Birthdate: _____

Date of admission: _____

Religion: _____

Insurance: _____

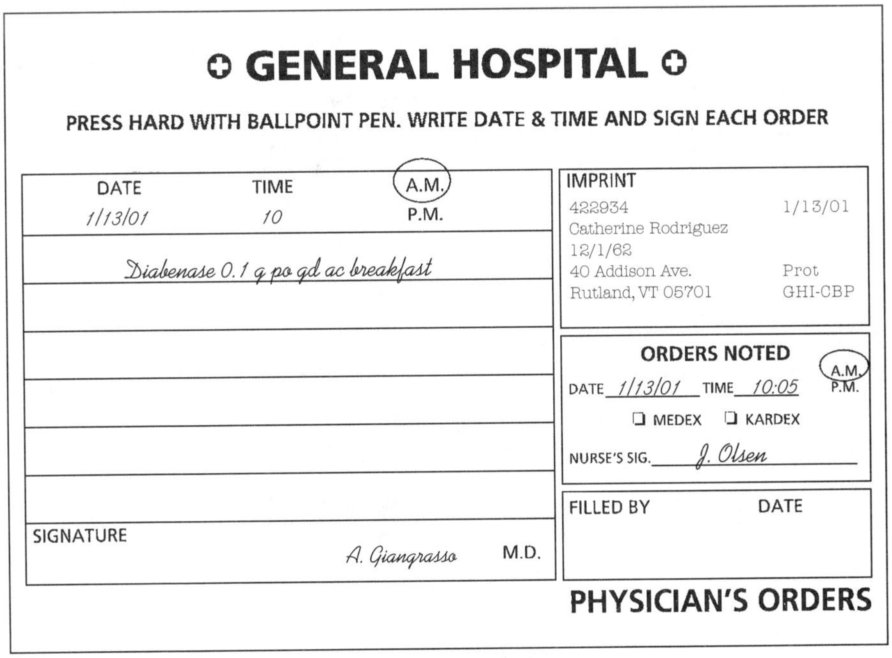

✚ GENERAL HOSPITAL ✚

PRESS HARD WITH BALLPOINT PEN. WRITE DATE & TIME AND SIGN EACH ORDER

DATE	TIME	A.M. / P.M.
1/13/01	10	(A.M.) P.M.

Diabenase 0.1 g po qd ac breakfast

IMPRINT

```
422934                    1/13/01
Catherine Rodriguez
12/1/62
40 Addison Ave.           Prot
Rutland, VT 05701         GHI-CBP
```

ORDERS NOTED

DATE _1/13/01_ TIME _10:05_ (A.M.) P.M.

❑ MEDEX ❑ KARDEX

NURSE'S SIG. _J. Olsen_

SIGNATURE

A. Giangrasso   M.D.

FILLED BY   DATE

PHYSICIAN'S ORDERS

▶ **FIGURE 2.4 Physician's order sheet.**

Here is what you should have found:

Date order written: _1/13/01_

Time order written: _10 A.M._

Name of drug: _Diabenase_

Dose: _0.1 g_

Route of administration: _po (by mouth)_

Frequency of administration: _qd ac breakfast (every day before breakfast)_

Name of prescriber: _A. Giangrasso M.D._

Name of patient: _Catherine Rodrigues_

Patient's registration number: _422934_

Address: _40 Addison Ave, Rutland, VT 05701_

Physician: _A. Giangrasso_

Birthdate: _12/1/62_

Date of admission: _1/13/01_

Religion: _Protestant_

Insurance: _GHI-CBP_

Note that just under the patient "imprint" there is a small section entitled "Orders Noted." This section indicates the date and time that the order was transcribed to the medication administration record (discussed later in this chapter). The signature belongs to the nurse who transcribed this order from the physician's order sheet to the medication administration record.

DRUG LABELS

You will need to understand the information found on drug labels in order to calculate drug dosages and to ensure that a drug is prepared and administered safely. Every drug label provides the same kinds of information. Study the parts of the label in Figure 2.5 for Ceclor, a drug that has bacteriostatic action. Follow the numbers on the label.

1. The manufacturer:
   The company that made the drug is Lilly.

2. National drug code (NDC) number:
   An identifying number assigned to this drug by the Drug Enforcement Agency: 0002-5130-87.

3. Name and form of drug:
   Ceclor is the trade name, indicated by the ® following the name. The generic name is cefaclor. The drug is in the form of a dry powder, which, when diluted with water, will become an oral suspension.

4. Directions for mixing:
   Add 31 mL of water in two portions to the dry mixture in the bottle. Shake well after each addition.

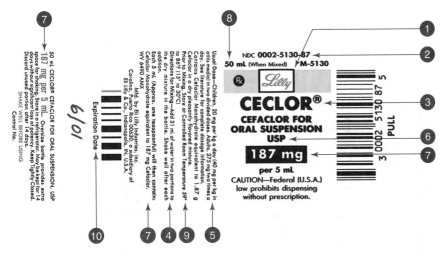

▶ FIGURE 2.5 Drug label for Ceclor; see text for explanation.

5. Dosage recommendations:
   Children, 20 mg per kg per day (40 mg per kg in otitis media) in two divided doses. Adults, 375 mg two times a day. See literature for complete dosage information.

6. USP:
   This means that the drug is prepared according to the standards set by the *United States Pharmacopeia*, which specifies the accepted formulations of drugs available in the United States.

7. Amount of drug per dose (shown in three places):
   Each dose contains 187 milligrams per 5 milliliters.

8. Volume of the reconstituted drug:
   When the drug is mixed according to the directions, there will be 50 mL of the oral suspension.

9. Storage directions:
   Some drugs have to be stored under controlled conditions if they are to retain their effectiveness. This drug should be stored at 59F to 86F (15C to 30C).

10. Expiration date:
    The expiration date specifies when the drug should be discarded. For example, 6/01 indicates that after June 30, 2001, the drug cannot be dispensed and should be discarded.

WARNING

Always read the expiration date! After the expiration date, the drug may lose its potency or act differently in the patient's body. Discard expired drugs. *Never* give them to patients!

Study the major kinds of information provided in Figure 2.6 for valsartan (Diovan).

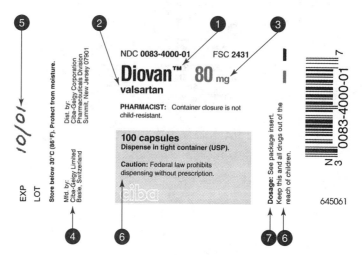

▶ FIGURE 2.6 **Drug label for Diovan: 1. Trade name: Diovan. 2. Generic name: valsartan. 3. Drug form: 80-milligram capsules. 4. Manufacturer: Ciba-Geigy Ltd. 5. Expiration date: October 2001. 6. Caution: Federal law prohibits dispensing without prescription. Warning: Keep out of reach of children. 7. Dose: See package insert.**

Study the kinds of information provided by the label for the antibiotic Augmentin in Figure 2.7.

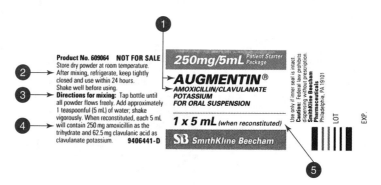

▶ FIGURE 2.7 **Drug label for Augmentin; see text for explanation.**

1. Trade name and generic name:
   The trade name is Augmentin, and the generic name is amoxicillin/clavulanate potassium.

2. Storage:
   Prior to mixing, the drug should be stored at room temperature. After mixing, it should be stored in a refrigerator and kept tightly closed and must be used within 24 hours.

3. Directions for mixing:
   Augmentin is packaged as a powder within the bottle. Before administering this medication, you need to add 5 milliliters of water and shake the mixture.

4. Amount of drug per dose after mixing:

Five milliliters of the prepared solution will contain 250 milligrams of Augmentin.

5. Volume of drug after mixing:

When mixed as directed, the bottle will contain 5 milliliters of Augmentin solution.

You will learn more about preparing drug solutions in Chapter 8.

▶ **E X A M P L E   2 . 1**

Examine the label shown in Figure 2.8 and record the following information:

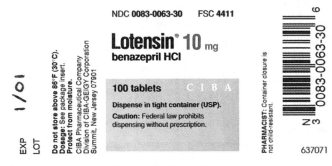

▶ **F I G U R E   2 . 8 Drug label for Lotensin.**

Trade name: _____

Generic name: _____

Form: _____

Dosage or strength: _____

Amount of drug in container: _____

Usual dosage: _____

Expiration date: _____

Storage temperature: _____

Here is what you should have found:

Trade name: *Lotensin* _____

Generic name: *benazepril HCl* _____

Form: *tablets* _____

Dosage or strength: *10 mg per tablet* _____

Amount of drug in container: *100 tablets* _____

Usual dosage: *See package insert* _____

Expiration date: *2001, January* _____

Storage temperature: *Not above 86°F (30°C), and protect from moisture* ____

► **EXAMPLE 2.2**

Examine the label shown in Figure 2.9 and record the information below:

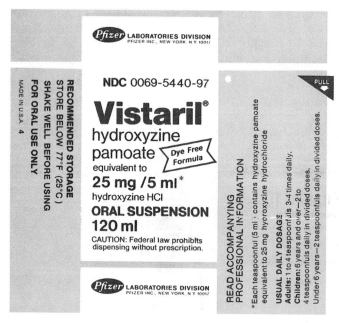

► **FIGURE 2.9 Drug label for Vistaril.**

Trade name: _____

Generic name: _____

Form: _____

Dosage or strength: _____

Amount in the bottle: _____

Usual dosage: _____

Here is what you should have found:

Trade name: *Vistaril* _____

Generic name: *hydroxyzine pamoate* _____

Form: *oral suspension* _____

Dosage or strength: *25 mg per 5 mL* _____

Amount in the bottle: *120 mL* _____

Usual dosage: *Adults: 1 to 4 teaspoons three to four times daily.*

Children: 6 years and over—2 to 4 teaspoons daily in divided doses.

Under 6 years—2 teaspoons daily in divided doses.

DRUG PACKAGE INSERTS

Sometimes information you need to safely prepare, administer, and store medications is not located on the drug label. In such cases, you may need to read the *package insert.* The pharmaceutical manufacturer includes a package insert with each container of a prescription drug.

The information on a drug package insert is intended for the physician, pharmacist, or drug administrator. It contains complex descriptions of a drug's chemistry and how it acts in the body. Figure 2.10 shows an example of two pages from a drug package insert for nitroglycerin transdermal system. Despite the complexity of the description, always consult the package insert when you need detailed information about

- mixing and storing a drug
- preparing a drug dose
- when the drug should *not* be used
- side effects and adverse reactions

The categories of information usually listed on a package insert are described in Table 2.2 on page 33.

NITROGLYCERIN TRANSDERMAL SYSTEM

Prescribing Information

DESCRIPTION

Nitroglycerin is 1,2,3-propanetriol trinitrate, an organic nitrate whose structural formula is:

$$H_2CONO_2$$
$$HCONO_2$$
$$H_2CONO_2$$

and whose molecular weight is 227.09. The organic nitrates are vasodilators, active on both arteries and veins.

The Nitroglycerin Transdermal System is a flat unit designed to provide continuous controlled release of nitroglycerin through intact skin. The rate of release of nitroglycerin is linearly dependent upon the area of the applied system; each cm^2 of applied system delivers approximately 0.02 mg of nitroglycerin per hour. Thus, the 10-, 20-, and 30-cm^2 systems deliver approximately 0.2, 0.4 and 0.6 mg of nitroglycerin per hour, respectively.

The remainder of the nitroglycerin in each system serves as a reservoir and is not delivered in normal use. After 12 hours, for example, each system has delivered 4% of its original content of nitroglycerin.

The Nitroglycerin Transdermal System contains nitroglycerin in a laminated matrix composed of polyvinyl chloride/polyvinyl acetate copolymer, di-(2-ethylhexyl) phthalate, isopropyl palmitate, colloidal silicon dioxide, aluminum foil laminate, polyethylene foam and acrylic adhesive. The 10-, 20- and 30-cm^2 systems contain 62.5 mg, 125.0 mg and 187.5 mg of nitroglycerin, respectively.

Cross section of the system:

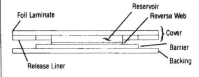

CLINICAL PHARMACOLOGY

The principal pharmacological action of nitroglycerin is relaxation of vascular smooth muscle and consequent dilatation of peripheral arteries and veins, especially the latter. Dilatation of the veins promotes peripheral pooling of blood and decreases venous return to the heart, thereby reducing left ventricular end-diastolic pressure and pulmonary capillary wedge pressure (preload). Arteriolar relaxation reduces systemic vascular resistance, systolic arterial pressure, and mean arterial pressure (afterload). Dilatation of the coronary arteries also occurs. The relative importance of preload reduction, afterload reduction, and coronary dilatation remains undefined.

Dosing regimens for most chronically used drugs are designed to provide plasma concentrations that are continuously greater than a minimally effective concentration. This strategy is inappropriate for organic nitrates. Several well-controlled clinical trials have used exercise testing to assess the anti-anginal efficacy of continuously-delivered nitrates. In the large majority of these trials, active agents were indistinguishable from placebo after 24 hours (or less) of continuous therapy. Attempts to overcome nitrate tolerance by dose escalation, even to doses far in excess of those used acutely, have consistently failed. Only after nitrates have been absent from the body for several hours has their antianginal efficacy been restored.

Pharmacokinetics: The volume of distribution of nitroglycerin is about 3 L/kg, and nitroglycerin is cleared from this volume at extremely rapid rates, with a resulting serum half-life of about 3 minutes. The observed clearance rates (close to 1 L/kg/min) greatly exceed hepatic blood flow; known sites of extrahepatic metabolism include red blood cells and vascular walls.

The first products in the metabolism of nitroglycerin are inorganic nitrate and the 1,2- and 1,3-dinitroglycerols. The dinitrates are less effective vasodilators than nitroglycerin, but they are longer-lived in the serum, and their net contribution to the overall effect of chronic nitroglycerin regimens is not known. The dinitrates are further metabolized to (non-vasoactive) mononitrates and, ultimately, to glycerol and carbon dioxide.

To avoid development of tolerance to nitroglycerin, drug-free intervals of 10-12 hours are known to be sufficient; shorter intervals have not been well studied. In one well-controlled clinical trial, subjects receiving nitroglycerin appeared to exhibit a rebound or withdrawal effect, so that their exercise tolerance at the end of the daily drug-free interval was *less* than that exhibited by the parallel group receiving placebo.

In healthy volunteers, steady-state plasma concentrations of nitroglycerin are reached by about two hours after application of a patch and are maintained for the duration of wearing the system (observations have been limited to 24 hours). Upon removal of the patch, the plasma concentration declines with a half-life of about an hour.

Clinical trials: Regimens in which nitroglycerin patches were worn for 12 hours daily have been studied in well-controlled trials up to 4 weeks in duration. Starting about 2 hours after application and continuing until 10-12 hours after application, patches that deliver at least 0.4 mg of nitroglycerin per hour have consistently demonstrated greater anti-anginal activity than placebo. Lower-dose patches have not been as well studied, but in one large, well-controlled trial in which higher-dose patches were also studied, patches delivering 0.2 mg/hr had significantly *less* anti-anginal activity than placebo.

It is reasonable to believe that the rate of nitroglycerin absorption from patches may vary with the site of application, but this relationship has not been adequately studied.

The onset of action of transdermal nitroglycerin is not sufficiently rapid for this product to be useful in aborting an acute anginal episode.

INDICATIONS AND USAGE

Transdermal nitroglycerin is indicated for the prevention of angina pectoris due to coronary artery disease. The onset of action of transdermal nitroglycerin is not sufficiently rapid for this product to be useful in aborting an acute attack.

CONTRAINDICATIONS

Allergic reactions to organic nitrates are extremely rare, but they do occur. Nitroglycerin is contraindicated in patients who are allergic to it. Allergy to the adhesives used in nitroglycerin patches has also been reported, and it similarly constitutes a contraindication to the use of this product.

WARNINGS

The benefits of transdermal nitroglycerin in patients with acute myocardial infarction or congestive heart failure have not been established. If one elects to use nitroglycerin in these conditions, careful clinical or hemodynamic monitoring must be used to avoid the hazards of hypotension and tachycardia.

A cardioverter/defibrillator should not be discharged through a paddle electrode that overlies a nitroglycerin transdermal patch. The arcing that may be seen in this situation is harmless itself, but it may be associated with local current concentration that can cause damage to the paddles and burns to the patient.

PRECAUTIONS

General: Severe hypotension, particularly with upright posture, may occur with even small doses of nitroglycerin. This drug should therefore be used with caution in patients who may be volume depleted or who, for whatever reason, are already hypotensive. Hypotension induced by nitroglycerin may be accompanied by paradoxical bradycardia and increased angina pectoris.

Nitrate therapy may aggravate the angina caused by hypertrophic cardiomyopathy.

▶ **FIGURE 2.10** A typical drug package insert.

As tolerance to other forms of nitroglycerin develops, the effect of sublingual nitroglycerin on exercise tolerance, although still observable, is somewhat blunted.

In industrial workers who have had long-term exposure to unknown (presumably high) doses of organic nitrates, tolerance clearly occurs. Chest pain, acute myocardial infarction, and even sudden death have occurred during temporary withdrawal of nitrates from these workers, demonstrating the existence of true physical dependence.

Several clinical trials in patients with angina pectoris have evaluated nitroglycerin regimens which incorporated a 10-12 hour nitrate-free interval. In some of these trials, an increase in the frequency of anginal attacks during the nitrate-free interval was observed in a small number of patients. In one trial, patients demonstrated decreased exercise tolerance at the end of the nitrate-free interval. Hemodynamic rebound has been observed only rarely; on the other hand, few studies were so designed that rebound, if it had occurred, would have been detected. The importance of these observations to the routine, clinical use of transdermal nitroglycerin is unknown.

Information for Patients: Daily headaches sometimes accompany treatment with nitroglycerin. In patients who get these headaches, the headaches may be a marker of the activity of the drug. Patients should resist the temptation to avoid headaches by altering the schedule of their treatment with nitroglycerin, since loss of headache may be associated with simultaneous loss of antianginal efficacy.

Treatment with nitroglycerin may be associated with lightheadedness on standing, especially just after rising from a recumbent or seated position. This effect may be more frequent in patients who have also consumed alcohol.

After normal use, there is enough residual nitroglycerin in discarded patches that they are a potential hazard to children and pets.

A patient leaflet is supplied with the systems.

Drug Interactions: The vasodilating effects of nitroglycerin may be additive with those of other vasodilators. Alcohol, in particular, has been found to exhibit additive effects of this variety.

Carcinogenesis, Mutagenesis, and Impairment of Fertility: Studies to evaluate the carcinogenic or mutagenic potential of nitroglycerin have not been performed. Nitroglycerin's effect upon reproductive capacity is similarly unknown.

Pregnancy category C: Animal reproduction studies have not been conducted with nitroglycerin. It is also not known whether nitroglycerin can cause fetal harm when administered to a pregnant woman or whether it can affect reproductive capacity. Nitroglycerin should be given to a pregnant woman only if clearly needed.

Nursing Mothers: It is not known whether nitroglycerin is excreted in human milk. Because many drugs are excreted in human milk, caution should be exercised when nitroglycerin is administered to a nursing woman.

Pediatric Use: Safety and effectiveness in children have not been established.

ADVERSE REACTIONS

Adverse reactions to nitroglycerin are generally dose-related, and almost all of these reactions are the result of nitroglycerin's activity as a vasodilator. Headache, which may be severe, is the most commonly reported side effect. Headache may be recurrent with each daily dose, especially at higher doses. Transient episodes of lightheadedness, occasionally related to blood pressure changes, may also occur. Hypotension occurs infrequently, but in some patients it may be severe enough to warrant discontinuation of therapy. Syncope, crescendo angina, and rebound hypertension have been reported but are uncommon.

Extremely rarely, ordinary doses of organic nitrates have caused methemoglobinemia in normal-seeming patients; for further discussion of its diagnosis and treatment see **Overdosage**.

Allergic reactions to nitroglycerin are also uncommon, and the great majority of those reported have been cases of contact dermatitis or fixed drug eruptions in patients receiving nitroglycerin in ointments or patches. There have been a few reports of genuine anaphylactoid reactions, and these reactions can probably occur in patients receiving nitroglycerin by any route.

In two placebo-controlled trials of intermittent therapy with nitroglycerin patches at 0.2 to 0.8 mg/hr, the most frequent adverse reactions among 307 subjects were as follows:

	placebo	patch
headache	18%	63%
lightheadedness	4%	6%
hypotension and/or syncope	0%	4%
increased angina	2%	2%

OVERDOSAGE

Hemodynamic Effects: The ill effects of nitroglycerin overdose are generally the results of nitroglycerin's capacity to induce vasodilatation, venous pooling, reduced cardiac output, and hypotension. These hemodynamic changes may have protean manifestations, including increased intracranial pressure, with any or all of persistent throbbing headache, confusion, and moderate fever, vertigo; palpitations; visual disturbances; nausea and vomiting (possibly with colic and even bloody diarrhea); syncope (especially in the upright posture); air hunger and dyspnea, later followed by reduced ventilatory effort; diaphoresis, with the skin either flushed or cold and clammy; heart block and bradycardia; paralysis; coma; seizures; and death.

Laboratory determinations of serum levels of nitroglycerin and its metabolites are not widely available, and such determinations have, in any event, no established role in the management of nitroglycerin overdose.

No data are available to suggest physiological maneuvers (e.g., maneuvers to change the pH of the urine) that might accelerate elimination of nitroglycerin and its active metabolites. Similarly, it is not known which — if any — of these substances can usefully be removed from the body by hemodialysis.

No specific antagonist to the vasodilator effects of nitroglycerin is known, and no intervention has been subject to controlled study as a therapy of nitroglycerin overdose. Because the hypotension associated with nitroglycerin overdose is the result of venodilatation and arterial hypovolemia, prudent therapy in this situation should be directed toward increase in central fluid volume. Passive elevation of the patient's legs may be sufficient, but intravenous infusion of normal saline or similar fluid may also be necessary.

The use of epinephrine or other arterial vasoconstrictors in this setting is likely to do more harm than good.

In patients with renal disease or congestive heart failure, therapy resulting in central volume expansion is not without hazard. Treatment of nitroglycerin overdose in these patients may be subtle and difficult, and invasive monitoring may be required.

Methemoglobinemia: Nitrate ions liberated during metabolism of nitroglycerin can oxidize hemoglobin into methemoglobin. Even in patients totally without cytochrome b_5 reductase activity, however, and even assuming that the nitrate moieties of nitroglycerin are quantitatively applied to oxidation of hemoglobin, about 1mg/kg of nitroglycerin should be required before any of these patients manifests clinically significant ($\geq$10%) methemoglobinemia. In patients with normal reductase function, significant production of methemoglobin should require even larger doses of nitroglycerin. In one study in which 36 patients received 2-4 weeks of continuous

nitroglycerin therapy at 3.1 to 4.4 mg/hr, the average methemoglobin level measured was 0.2%; this was comparable to that observed in parallel patients who received placebo.

Notwithstanding these observations, there are case reports of significant methemoglobinemia in association with moderate overdoses of organic nitrates. None of the affected patients had been thought to be unusually susceptible.

Methemoglobin levels are available from most clinical laboratories. The diagnosis should be suspected in patients who exhibit signs of impaired oxygen delivery despite adequate cardiac output and adequate arterial pO_2. Classically, methemoglobinemic blood is described as chocolate brown, without color change on exposure to air.

When methemoglobinemia is diagnosed, the treatment of choice is methylene blue, 1-2 mg/kg intravenously.

DOSAGE AND ADMINISTRATION

The suggested starting dose is between 0.2 mg/hr and 0.4 mg/hr. Doses between 0.4 mg/hr and 0.8 mg/hr have shown continued effectiveness for 10-12 hours daily for at least one month (the longest period studied) of intermittent administration. Although the minimum nitrate-free interval has not been defined, data show that a nitrate-free interval of 10-12 hours is sufficient (see **Clinical Pharmacology**). Thus, an appropriate dosing schedule for nitroglycerin patches would include a daily patch-on period of 12-14 hours and a daily patch-off period of 10-12 hours.

Although some well controlled clinical trials using exercise tolerance testing have shown maintenance of effectiveness when patches are worn continuously, the large majority of such controlled trials have shown the development of tolerance (i.e., complete loss of effect) within the first 24 hours after therapy was initiated. Dose adjustment, even to levels much higher than generally used, did not restore efficacy.

HOW SUPPLIED

Nitroglycerin Transdermal Therapeutic System.

Nitroglycerin transdermal Rated Release in vivo	Total Nitroglycerin in system	System Size	Carton Size
0.2 mg/hour	62.5 mg	10 cm²	30 units
0.4 mg/hour	125.0 mg	20 cm²	30 units
0.6 mg/hour	187.5 mg	30 cm²	30 units

STORAGE CONDITIONS:
Store at controlled room temperature 15°-30°C (59°-86°F).
Do not refrigerate.
CAUTION:
Federal law prohibits dispensing without prescription.
REVISION DATE: July 1993
HCS-075 (7/93)
HERCON LABORATORIES CORPORATION
EMIGSVILLE, PA 17318

▶ **F I G U R E   2 . 1 0** *(continued)*

▶ **E X A M P L E   2 . 3**

Read the excerpts provided from the package inserts in Figures 2.11 through 2.14, and fill in the requested information.

NITROGLYCERIN TRANSDERMAL SYSTEM

Prescribing Information
DESCRIPTION
Nitroglycerin is 1,2,3-propanetriol trinitrate, an organic nitrate whose structural formula is:

$$H_2CONO_2$$
$$HCONO_2$$
$$H_2CONO_2$$

▶ **F I G U R E   2 . 1 1 Description of Nitroglycerin Transdermal System.**

Types of Information on Drug Package Inserts

Information	Comments
Name of pharmaceutical company	
Name of the drug (trade/generic)	
Strength of drug and clinical formulation	
Clinical pharmacology	How the drug acts in the body.
Indications for using the drug	The conditions the drug is approved to treat.
Contraindications	Conditions under which the drug must *not* be given.
Warning information	Relative to the safety of the patient. For example, a potent diuretic drug that can deplete the body of electrolytes and fluid can cause a state of dehydration. Therefore, *close* medical supervision would be required for the patient.
Precautions	Indicate the assessments that must be done by a nurse to identify untoward results that could occur when a patient is given a medication. Serum diagnostic tests also identify changes in the patient's overall condition.
Adverse reactions	Drug reactions that could affect patient comfort and safety but that don't necessarily deter the prescriber from prescribing the drug.

1. What is the name of the drug (Figure 2.11)? _____

2. What is the most commonly reported side effect of this drug (Figure 2.12)?

_____

ADVERSE REACTIONS

Adverse reactions to nitroglycerin are generally dose-related, and almost all of these reactions are the result of nitroglycerin's activity as a vasodilator. Headache, which may be severe, is the most commonly reported side effect. Headache may be recurrent with each daily dose, especially at higher doses. Transient episodes of lightheadedness, occasionally related to blood pressure changes, may also occur. Hypotension occurs infrequently, but in some patients it may be severe enough to warrant discontinuation of therapy. Syncope, crescendo angina, and rebound hypertension have been reported but are uncommon.

► **FIGURE 2.12 Adverse reactions to Nitroglycerin Transdermal System.**

3. According to the information in Figure 2.13, how is this drug administered?

_____

The Nitroglycerin Transdermal System is a flat unit designed to provide continuous controlled release of nitroglycerin through intact skin. The rate of release of nitroglycerin is linearly dependent upon the area of the applied system; each cm² of applied system delivers approximately 0.02 mg of nitroglycerin per hour. Thus, the 10-, 20-, and 30-cm² systems deliver approximately 0.2, 0.4 and 0.6 mg of nitroglycerin per hour, respectively. The remainder of the nitroglycerin in each system serves as a reservoir and is not delivered in normal use. After 12 hours, for example, each system has delivered 4% of its original content of nitroglycerin.

► **FIGURE 2.13 Administration of Nitroglycerin Transdermal System.**

4. According to Figure 2.14, would this drug be ordered for a patient who is allergic to the adhesives used in nitroglycerin patches?

_____

CONTRAINDICATIONS
Allergic reactions to organic nitrates are extremely rare, but they do occur. Nitroglycerin is contraindicated in patients who are allergic to it. Allergy to the adhesives used in nitroglycerin patches has also been reported, and it similarly constitutes a contraindication to the use of this product. ,

▶ **FIGURE 2.14 Contraindications to Nitroglycerin Transdermal System.**

5. According to Figure 2.15, what is an appropriate dosing schedule for Nitroglycerin Transdermal System?

_____

DOSAGE AND ADMINISTRATION
The suggested starting dose is between 0.2 mg/hr and 0.4 mg/hr. Doses between 0.4 mg/hr and 0.8 mg/hr have shown continued effectiveness for 10-12 hours daily for at least one month (the longest period studied) of intermittent administration. Although the minimum nitrate-free interval has not been defined, data show that a nitrate-free interval of 10-12 hours is sufficient (see **Clinical Pharmacology**). Thus, an appropriate dosing schedule for nitroglycerin patches would include a daily patch-on period of 12-14 hours and a daily patch-off period of 10-12 hours.

▶ **FIGURE 2.15 Dosage of Nitroglycerin Transdermal System.**

Here is what you should have found:

1. Nitroglycerin.

2. Headaches.

3. Through the skin surface.

4. No.

5. Daily patch-on period of 12 to 14 hours and a daily patch-off period of 10 to 12 hours.

_____

MEDICATION ADMINISTRATION RECORDS

Medication administration records (MARs) are used to record information about the drugs a patient receives under a prescriber's orders. The following list indicates the kinds of information recorded on a MAR.

- Person receiving the medications:
  Name
  Date of birth
  Patient registration number
  Allergies
- Medication:
  Name
  Dosage

Time of administration
Route of administration
Date started
Date discontinued

■ Staff member administering medications:
Initials of those administering medications
Signatures of staff members administering medications

Although the type of information appearing on a MAR is fairly standard, the appearance of these records varies from one health care provider to another. For example, some MARs record the time of drug administration using the military clock. This system of recording time does not use A.M. or P.M. after the hour designation. Instead, the hours past 12 noon are designated by higher numbers. For example, 2:00 P.M. according to the standard clock is written 1400 (pronounced "fourteen hundred hours"). Figure 2.16 compares military and standard clock hours.

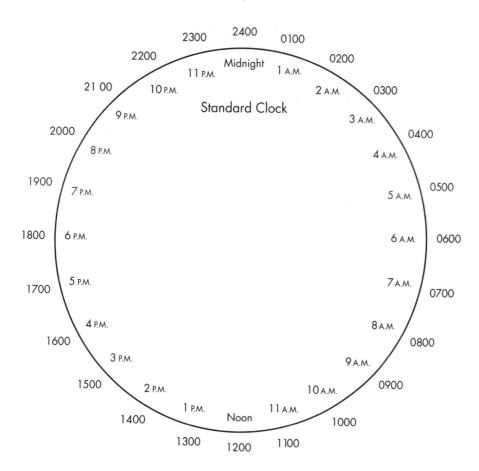

▶ FIGURE 2.16 **A comparison of the military (outer) and standard (inner) clock. 10 P.M. on a standard clock is 2200 (twenty-two hundred hours) on a military clock.**

789652
Wendy Kim
44 Chester Ave.
N.Y., N.Y. 10003

Dr. Leon Ablon

7/12/01
8/24/54
Christian
Aetna

UNIVERSITY HOSPITAL

DAILY MEDICATION ADMINISTRATION RECORD

PATIENT NAME *Wendy Kim*

ROOM # *422*

IF ANOTHER RECORD IS IN USE ☐

ALLERGIC TO (RECORD IN RED): *tomatoes, codeine, penicillin*

DATES GIVEN ↓   DATE DISCHARGED:

RED CHECK INITIAL	ORDER DATE	INITIAL	EXP DATE	MEDICATION, DOSAGE, FREQUENCY AND ROUTE	HOURS	12	13	14	15	16	17										
	9/12	JO	9/17	Augmentin 250 mg	0600	LA	LA	LA													
				po q 12 h	1800	MS	SG	SG													
	9/12	JO	9/17	Digoxin 0.125 mg qd po	0900	JO	JO	JO	LA												
	9/12	JO	9/17	Inderal 40 mg BID po	0900	JO	JO	JO	LA												
					1900	JO	JO	JO	JO												
	9/12	JO	9/17	Coumadin 2.5 mg daily po	1900	JO	JO	SG	SG												
	9/12	JO	9/17	Xanax 0.5 mg hs po	2100	MS	MS	SG	SG												
	9/15	JO	9/17	Augmentin 500 mg q 12 h po	✕	✕	✕	✕	LA												
					0600				LA												
					1800				SG												

INT.	NURSES' FULL SIGNATURE AND TITLE	INT.	NURSES' FULL SIGNATURE AND TITLE
MS	Mary Smith R.N.		
SG	Susan Green R.N.		
LA	Louise Alvarez R.N.		
JO	Jane Olsen L.P.N.		

39171 (10/91)

▶ **FIGURE 2.17 Medication administration record.**

In some health care facilities, the MAR is computerized. Hard copy of a MAR can be readily printed from the computerized patient data base. Each time a medication is administered to a patient, the MAR is updated at a computer terminal by the staff member who administered the drug.

Let's look at a MAR in detail (Figure 2.17). This MAR reveals the following information:

NOTES/WORKSPACE

Drug administered at 6 A.M. (0600) on 9/12/01: Augmentin 250 mg

Drugs administered between 12 noon and 11 P.M. (1200–2300) on 9/15/01: Inderal 40 mg, Coumadin 2.5 mg, Xanax 0.5 mg, and Augmentin 500 mg

Did Ms. Kim receive Augmentin 250 mg on 9/12/01, at 6 A.M. (0600)?

Yes.

When did Ms. Kim receive the last dose of Xanax?

9 P.M. (2100) on 9/15/01.

▶ E X A M P L E 2.4

Study the MAR in Figure 2.18; then fill in the following chart and answer the questions.

1. Which drugs were administered at 9 A.M. on 7/15? _____

2. Identify the drug administered IV at 6 P.M. on 7/14. _____

3. Which drug was administered subcutaneously on 7/16? _____

4. Who administered the ferrous gluconate on 7/16? _____

5. When was the thioguanine given on 7/15? _____

Name of Drug	Dose	Route of Administration	Time of Administration

UNIVERSITY HOSPITAL

DAILY MEDICATION ADMINISTRATION RECORD

12481632
David Samuels
378-12 Horida Ave.
Stocie, Il. 63642

Dr. June Olsen

7/3/01
12/20/60
RC
Medicaid

PATIENT NAME _David Samuels_

ROOM # _5421_

IF ANOTHER RECORD IS IN USE ☐

ALLERGIC TO (RECORD IN RED): _penicillin_

DATES GIVEN ↓   DATE DISCHARGED:

RED CHECK INITIAL	ORDER DATE	INITIAL	EXP DATE	MEDICATION, DOSAGE, FREQUENCY AND ROUTE	HOURS	14	15	16												
	7/14	Jo	7/19	Theragran 1 Tab Q.D. po	0900	LA	LA	LA												
				—																
	7/14	Jo	7/19	Ferrous Gluconate 300 mg qd po	0900	LA	LA	LA												
				—																
	7/14	Jo	7/18	Cytarabine 150 mg IV	0600	AG	AG	AG												
				q 12 h in 250 ml 5% D/w	1800	SG	SG	SG												
				for 5 days																
				—																
	7/12	Jo	7/21	thioguanine 150 mg po																
				bid for 5 days	0900	LA	LA	LA												
					1700	SG	SG	SG												
	7/14	Jo	7/20	Erythropoietin 3000 u s/c	0900	X	X	LA												
				TIW (MWF) only																

INT.	NURSES' FULL SIGNATURE AND TITLE	INT.	NURSES' FULL SIGNATURE AND TITLE
LA	Leon Ablon R.N.		
AG	Anthony Georgrosso R.N.		
SG	Suson Green R.N.		

39171 (10/91)

▶ **F I G U R E 2.18 Medication administration record.**

Here is what you should have found:

Name of Drug	Dose	Route of Administration	Time of Administration
Theragran	1 tablet	po	0900 (9 A.M.)
ferrous gluconate	300 mg	po	0900 (9 A.M.)
cytarabine	150 mg	IV	0600 (6 A.M.) 1800 (6 P.M.)
thioguanine	150 mg	po	0900 (9 A.M.) 1700 (5 P.M.)
erythropoietin	3000 u	sc	0900 (9 A.M.) tiw (Monday, Wednesday, Friday only)

1. Theragran 1 tablet, ferrous gluconate 300 mg, thioguanine 150 mg
2. cytarabine 150 mg
3. erythropoietin 3000 u
4. Leon Ablon
5. 9:00 A.M. and 5:00 P.M.

You will find the answers to *Try These for Practice* after the questions and the answers to *Exercises* in Appendix A at the back of the book. Your instructor has the answers to the *Additional Exercises*.

Try These for Practice

Test your comprehension after reading the chapter. Study the drug labels in Figure 2.19, and supply the following information. *The answers follow the questions.*

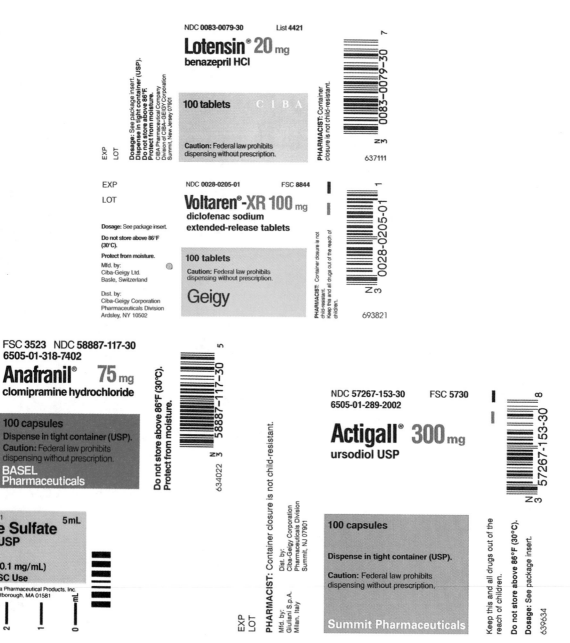

▶ FIGURE 2.19 Drug labels.

1. What is the route of administration for Voltaren?

_____

2. How many capsules are in the container of Actigall?

_____

3. What is the quantity of drug in each capsule of clomipramine hydrochloride?

_____

4. Write the trade name for the drug benazepril HCl.

_____

5. What is the quantity of drug in each milliliter of atropine sulfate?

_____

1. po   2. 100   3. 75 mg   4. Lotensin   5. 0.1 mg

Exercises

Reinforce your understanding in class or at home. Study the drug labels shown in Figure 2.19, and supply the following information. *Check your answers in Appendix A at the back of the book.*

1. Write the generic name for Anafranil.

_____

2. Write the trade name for diclofenac sodium.

_____

3. Which drug can be administered sc?

_____

4. What is the route of administration for ursodiol?

_____

5. Write a trade name for the drug whose NDC number is 0083-0079-30.

_____

6. Study the MAR in Figure 2.20. Fill in the following chart and answer the questions.

Name of Drug	Dose	Route of Administration	Time of Administration	Date Started	Date Discontinued
Isoproterenol					
Procardia					
indomethacin					
digoxin					
Diuril					
Carafate					

a. Identify the drugs administered on July 18, 2001.

_____

b. Identify the drugs administered po on July 20, 2001.

_____

c. How many drugs were administered at 9 P.M. on July 20, 2001?

_____

d. Which drugs were administered daily for 6 consecutive days?

_____

e. Who administered the indomethacin at 5:00 P.M. on July 20?

_____

f. Identify the drug for which the patient received 0.25 mg.

_____

g. How many doses of Carafate were received by Mr. Johnson on July 22?

_____

GENERAL HOSPITAL

YEAR 2001 · MONTH July		DAY	18		19		20		21		22		23	
SOLUTION MEDICATION ADDED DOSAGE AND INTERVAL			INITIALS* AND HOURS		INITIALS AND HOURS		INITIALS AND HOURS		INITIALS AND HOURS		INITIALS AND HOURS		INITIALS AND HOURS	
Date Started 7/18/01		I	JO		JO		JO		JO					
Isoproterenol 15 mg SL tid		AM	9		9		9		9					
		I	LA	LA	LA	LA	LA	LA	LA	LA				
Discontinued 7/21/01		PM	1	5	1	5	1	5	1	5				
Date Started 7/18/01		I	JO		JO		JO		JO					
Procardia 20 mg po bid		AM	9		9		9		9					
		I	LA		LA		LA		LA					
Discontinued 7/21/01		PM	5		5		5		5					
Date Started 7/18/01		I	JO		JO		JO		JO					
indomethacin 25 mg bid po		AM	9		9		9		9					
		I	LA		LA		LA		LA					
Discontinued 7/21/01		PM	5		5		5		5					
Date Started 7/18/01		I	JO		JO		JO		JO		JO		JO	
digoxin 0.25 mg qd po		AM	9		9		9		9		9		9	
		I												
Discontinued 7/23/01		PM												
Date Started 7/18/01		I	JO		JO		JO		JO		JO		JO	
Diuril 500 mg qd po		AM	9		9		9		9		9		9	
		I												
Discontinued 7/23/01		PM												
Date Started 7/20/01		I					JO		JO		JO			
Carofate 1g qid po ac & hs		AM					9		9		9			
		I					LA	LA	LA	LA	LA	LA	LA	LA	LA		
Discontinued 7/22/01		PM					1	5	9	1	5	9	1	5	9		
Date Started		I												
		AM												
		I												
Discontinued		PM												

ALLERGIES: (Specify) None

Init.	Signature
JO	Jane Olsen
LA	Leon Ablon
SG	Susan Green

*INITIALS – Nurses must sign name & title

PATIENT IDENTIFICATION

7286531   7/18/01

TYRELL JOHNSON   3/12/34
755 Bay Ridge Ave
Brooklyn, NY   Jewish
11209   Blue Cross

Dr. Anthony Giangrasso

▶ FIGURE 2.20 Medication administration record.

7. Study the physician's order sheet in Figure 2.21; then answer the following questions.

⊕ GENERAL HOSPITAL ⊕

PRESS HARD WITH BALLPOINT PEN. WRITE DATE & TIME AND SIGN EACH ORDER

DATE	TIME	A.M.
Oct 12, 2001	6	P.M.

Declomycin 300 mg po q6h

vitamin C 2 g po bid

Inderal 120 mg po qd

Esmolol 500 mg in

500 ml of 0.9% NS

infuse at rate of 15 mL/hr

SIGNATURE

l. Ablon   M.D.

IMPRINT

731122   10/12/01
Jose Sanchez   3/2/45
24 Third Ave.
Chicago, IL 54312   Medicaid

Dr. Leon Ablon

ORDERS NOTED   A.M.
DATE _10/12/01_ TIME _6:30_   P.M.
❑ MEDEX   ❑ KARDEX
NURSE'S SIG. _June Olsen_

FILLED BY	DATE

PHYSICIAN'S ORDERS

▶ **F I G U R E 2 . 2 1 Physician's order sheet.**

a. What is the dose of Declomycin?

_____

b. How many times a day do you administer vitamin C to Mr. Sanchez?

_____

c. If the last dose of Declomycin was given at 12 noon, at what time would you administer the next dose?

_____

d. How many milliliters of Esmolol will Mr. Sanchez receive in 60 minutes?

_____

e. What was the patient's date of admission?

_____

8. Use the package excerpt shown in Figure 2.22 to answer the following questions.

```
8:12.24
DECLOMYCIN®
DEMECLOCYCLINE HYDROCHLORIDE
FOR ORAL USE

Adults: Usual daily dose - Four divided doses of 150 mg each or two divided
doses of 300 mg each.
For children above eight years of age: Usual daily dose, 3-6 mg per pound
body weight per day, depending upon the severity of the disease, divided into
two to four doses

Gonorrhea patients sensitive to penicillin may be treated with demeclocycline
administered as an initial oral dose of 600 mg followed by 300 mg every 12
hours for four days to a total of 3 grams.

HOW SUPPLIED
DECLOMYCIN® demeclocycline hydrochloride Capsules. 150 mg are two-tone,
coral colored, soft gelatin capsules, printed with LL followed by D9 on the
light side in blue ink. are supplied as follows:
    NDC 0005-9208-23 - Bottle of 100
```

▶ **FIGURE 2.22 Package insert (excerpt) for Declomycin.**

    a. What is the generic name of the drug?

    _____

    b. What is the usual dose for an adult?

    _____

    c. What is the initial oral dose of Declomycin for patients with gonorrhea?

    _____

    d. How is this drug supplied?

    _____

Additional Exercises

Now, on your own, test yourself! *Ask your instructor to check your answers.*

1. Study the MAR in Figure 2.23; then fill in the chart that follows and answer the questions.

GENERAL HOSPITAL

YEAR 2001	MONTH May		DAY	3	4	5	6	7	8
				INITIALS* AND HOURS	INITIALS AND HOURS	INITIALS AND HOURS	INITIALS AND HOURS	INITIALS AND HOURS	INITIALS AND HOURS
Date Started 5/3/01	heparin 5000 units sc q 12 h		I	KO	KO	KO			
			AM	12	12	12			
			I	TW	TW	TW			
Discontinued 5/9/01			PM	12	12	12			
Date Started 5/3/01	Dilantin 100 mg BID po		I	TW	TW	TW			
			AM	9	9	9			
			I	SG	SG	SG			
Discontinued 5/9/01			PM	9	9	9			
Date Started 5/3/01	valproate sodium 600 mg qd po		I	SG	SG	SG			
			AM	9	9	9			
			I						
Discontinued 5/9/01			PM						
Date Started 5/3/01	Cipro 500 mg q8h po		I	KO	KO	KO			
			AM	6	6	6			
			I	TW KO	TW KO	TW KO			
Discontinued 5/9/01			PM	2 10	2 10	2 10			
Date Started 5/3/01	phenobarbital 20 mg po TID		I						
			AM	9	9	9			
			I	TW KO	TW KO	TW KO			
Discontinued 5/9/01			PM	2 6	2 6	2 6			
Date Started 5/3/01	regular insulin 20 units oc sc dinner		I						
			AM						
			I	KO	KO	KO			
Discontinued 5/9/01			PM	5:45	5:45	5:45			
Date Started 5/3/01	NPH insulin 62 units sc ac breakfast		I	MK	MK	MK			
			AM	7:45	7:45	7:45			
			I						
Discontinued 5/9/01			PM						

ALLERGIES: (Specify) Keflex

Init.	Signature
SG	Susan Geonne
MK	Michelle Keefe
KO	Keith Olsen
TW	Taylor West

*INITIALS – Nurses must sign name & title

PATIENT IDENTIFICATION

1317654   5/3/01
SALLY JOHNSON   5/30/34
100 River St
Rutland, Vt   RC
05701   BCBS
Anthony Giangrasso M.D.

▶ FIGURE 2.23 Medication administration record.

Name of Drug	Dose	Route of Administration	Time of Administration	Date Started	Date Discontinued
heparin					
Dilantin					
Valproate sodium					
Cipro					
phenobarbital					
regular insulin					
NPH insulin					

a. Which drug was administered at 12 noon on 5/4/01?

_____

b. Name the drugs administered at 10 P.M. on 5/3/01.

_____

c. Which drugs are to be administered by mouth?

_____

d. How many drugs were administered on May 4, 2001?

_____

e. How many units of regular insulin were administered on May 5, 2001?

_____

f. Identify the drug that was administered every 8 hours.

_____

g. Name the types of insulin administered on May 3, 2001.

_____

h. How many different drugs were administered subcutaneously on May 4, 2001?

_____

2. Study the physician's order sheet in Figure 2.24, and answer the following questions.

⊕ GENERAL HOSPITAL ⊕

PRESS HARD WITH BALLPOINT PEN. WRITE DATE & TIME AND SIGN EACH ORDER

DATE	TIME	A.M.
5/3/01	12 noon	P.M.

Bumex 2 mg po qd

digoxin 0.125 mg po bid for 3 days

spectrobid 400 mg po bid

Quibron 300 mg po bid

Reglan 5 mg po hs

heparin 5000 u sc qd

SIGNATURE

J. Olsen   M.D.

IMPRINT
678123   05/3/01
Jennifer Dodson   06/6/60
333 West North Street   Prot
Clearview, VT 06071   Aetna

J. Olsen, M.D.

ORDERS NOTED
DATE _5/3/01_ TIME _12:15_ A.M. / P.M.
☒ MEDEX ☐ KARDEX
NURSE'S SIG. _Leon Ablon_

FILLED BY   DATE

PHYSICIAN'S ORDERS

▶ **FIGURE 2.24 Physician's order sheet.**

a. What is the route of administration for Reglan?

_____

b. Which drugs should be administered at 10 P.M.?

_____

c. Identify the date digoxin is to be discontinued.

_____

d. Identify the route of administration for heparin.

_____

Study the drug labels in Figure 2.25, and supply the following information.

3. Write the generic name for Ritalin SR.

_____

4. What is the route of administration for terbutaline sulfate?

_____

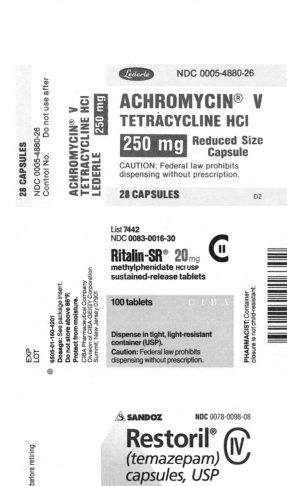
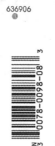

28 CAPSULES

NDC 0005-4880-26
Control No.   Do not use after

Lederle   NDC 0005-4880-26

ACHROMYCIN® V
TETRACYCLINE HCI

ACHROMYCIN® V
TETRACYCLINE HCI
LEDERLE   250 mg

250 mg   Reduced Size
Capsule

CAUTION: Federal law prohibits
dispensing without prescription.

28 CAPSULES   D2

USUAL DAILY DOSE
FOR ADULTS:
1 - 2 Grams divided in
two or four equal doses.
See accompanying circular.

Store at Controlled Room
Temperature 15-30° C (59-86° F).

Made in U.S.A.   17841

LEDERLE LABORATORIES DIVISION
American Cyanamid Company.
Pearl River, N.Y. 10965

List 7442
NDC 0083-0016-30   **C II**

Ritalin-SR® 20 mg
methylphenidate HCI USP
sustained-release tablets

100 tablets   CIBA

**Dispense in tight, light-resistant
container (USP).**
Caution: Federal law prohibits
dispensing without prescription.

EXP
LOT

6505-01-160-4201
Dosage: See package insert.
Do not store above 86°F.
Protect from moisture.

CIBA Pharmaceutical Company
Division of CIBA-GEIGY Corporation
Summit, New Jersey 07901

PHARMACIST: Container
closure is not child-resistant.

0083-0016-30

636906

Product No. 609064   **NOT FOR SALE**
Store dry powder at room temperature.
After mixing, refrigerate, keep tightly
closed and use within 24 hours.
Shake well before using.
Directions for mixing: Tap bottle until
all powder flows freely. Add approximately
1 teaspoonful (5 mL) of water; shake
vigorously. When reconstituted, each 5 mL
will contain 250 mg amoxicillin as the
trihydrate and 62.5 mg clavulanic acid as
clavulanate potassium.   **9406441-D**

250mg/5mL *Patient Starter Package*

AUGMENTIN®
AMOXICILLIN/CLAVULANATE
POTASSIUM
FOR ORAL SUSPENSION

1 x 5 mL (when reconstituted)

SB SmithKline Beecham

Use only if inner seal is intact.
Caution: Federal law prohibits
dispensing without prescription.
**SmithKline Beecham
Pharmaceuticals**
Philadelphia, PA 19101

LOT   EXP

SANDOZ   NDC 0078-0098-08

Restoril® **IV**
(temazepam)
capsules, USP

15 mg   500 Capsules

6505-01-116-0481
CAUTION: Federal law prohibits dispensing
without prescription.
20782101

Usual adult dosage: One or two capsules before retiring.

Store and dispense: Below 86°F (30°C);
tight, light-resistant container.

Sandoz Pharmaceuticals Corporation
East Hanover, New Jersey 07936

0078-0098-08

SAMPLE
LABEL

LOT
EXP.

20518003
Usual adult dosage: See package insert
for dosage information.
Store and dispense: Below 86°F (30°C);
tight container.
It is recommended that drug dispensing
should not exceed a weekly supply.
Dispensing should be contingent upon
the results of a WBC count.

NDC 0078-0126-05

100 TABLETS

CLOZARIL®
(clozapine)

25 mg

CAUTION: Federal law prohibits
dispensing without prescription.

Novartis Pharmaceuticals Corporation
East Hanover, New Jersey 07936

0078-0126-05

SAMPLE

LOT
EXP.

NDC 0078-0149-23

MIACALCIN®

(calcitonin-salmon)
INJECTION, SYNTHETIC

200 I.U. per mL
2 mL Multi-dose vial

For IM or SC injection
CAUTION: Federal law
prohibits dispensing
without prescription.
Store in refrigerator –
Between 2°-8°C
(36°-46°F)

Mkt. for **SANDOZ**
East Hanover, NJ 07936
6505-01-079-2655
22267502
3 920 408   3 920 410

NDC 0028-0105-01   FSC **2301**
6505-01-039-2808

Brethine® 5 mg
terbutaline sulfate tablets USP

100 tablets

**Dispense in tight, light-resistant
container (USP).**
Caution: Federal law prohibits
dispensing without prescription.

Geigy

EXP
LOT

Store between 59°-86°F (15°-30°C).
Dosage: See package insert.

Ciba-Geigy Corporation
Pharmaceuticals Division
Summit, NJ 07901

PHARMACIST: Container closure is
not child-resistant.

Keep this and all drugs out of the
reach of children.

0028-0105-01

644393

CLOZARIL®
(clozapine)
Tablets
100 mg

SANDOZ
East Hanover, NJ 07936

CLO-83

143 T 1415 EXP. JAN 96

▶ **FIGURE 2.25 Drug labels.**

5. What is the trade name of clozapine?

_____

6. How many milligrams of Augmentin are contained in 5 milliliters?

_____

7. How many milliliters are in the Miacalcin vial?

_____

8. Write a trade name for temazepam.

_____

9. What is the route of administration for Restoril?

_____

10. Write the generic name for Achromycin.

_____

11. How many international units of calcitonin-salmon are in 1 milliliter?

_____

12. Which drug is in the form of sustained-release tablets?

_____

13. Which drug expired in January 1996?

_____

CHAPTER THREE

Dimensional Analysis

▷ **Objectives**

After completing this chapter, you will be able to

- Solve a calculation problem using **dimensional analysis.**
- Identify some common units of measurement.
- Recognize the abbreviations for these units.
- State the equivalents for these units of measurement.
- Convert from one unit of measurement to another.

In this chapter you will learn to use dimensional analysis to calculate drug dosages. Dimensional analysis is a common sense approach to drug calculations that largely frees you from the need to memorize formulas. It is the method most commonly accepted in the physical sciences. Once you master this technique, you will be able to calculate drug dosages quickly and safely.

GETTING STARTED

One of the best ways to learn dimensional analysis is to convert units of measurement. Some common equivalent measurements are listed in Table 3.1.

▶ **TABLE 3.1**

Equivalents for Common Units
12 inches (in) = 1 foot (ft)
3 feet (ft) = 1 yard (yd)
16 ounces (oz) = 1 pound (lb)
60 seconds (sec) = 1 minute (min)
60 minutes (min) = 1 hour (h or hr)
24 hours (h or hr) = 1 day (d)
12 months (mon) = 1 year (yr)

You can use this information and dimensional analysis to solve problems. Suppose that you want to change 3 years into an equivalent number of months. The relationship is written as follows:

$$3 \text{ yr} = ? \text{ mon}$$

Whenever you divide something by itself, you get 1. Because 12 months is the same as 1 year, when you divide 12 months by 1 year, you get 1.

$$\frac{12 \text{ mon}}{1 \text{ yr}} = 1$$

Now see what happens when you multiply 3 years by $\frac{12 \text{ mon}}{1 \text{ yr}}$. The amount of time will not change, because you are really multiplying the time by 1.

$$3 \text{ yr} = \frac{3 \cancel{\text{ yr}}}{1} \times \frac{12 \text{ mon}}{1 \cancel{\text{ yr}}} = \frac{(3 \times 12) \text{ mon}}{1} = 36 \text{ mon}$$

So, 3 years is the same amount of time as 36 months.

> **NOTE**
>
> Cancel units just as you cancel numbers and letters in arithmetic and algebra.

Here is another problem. If a storm lasts for 72 hours, how many days does it last? You want to change 72 hours to days. The relationship is written as follows:

$$72 \text{ h} = ? \text{ d}$$

Notice that $\frac{1 \text{ d}}{24 \text{ h}} = 1$, since 1 day is the same as 24 hours. Now you multiply 72 hours by $\frac{1 \text{ d}}{24 \text{ h}}$. The amount of time will not change, because you are really multiplying it by 1.

$$72 \text{ h} \times \frac{1 \text{ d}}{24 \text{ h}} = ?$$

$$\frac{\overset{3}{\cancel{72}} \text{ h}}{1} \times \frac{1 \text{ d}}{\underset{1}{\cancel{24}} \text{ h}} = \frac{(3 \times 1) \text{ d}}{1} = 3 \text{ d}$$

So, the 72-hour storm lasts for 3 days.

In both problems you canceled the original units and ended up with the desired units. You did this by multiplying a fraction that was equal to 1. The fraction had the old units on the bottom and the new units on the top.

▶ E X A M P L E 3.1

Change 2 feet to an equivalent number of inches.

   2 ft = ? in

You want to cancel the feet and get the answer in inches. Therefore, multiply 2 feet by a fraction that has feet on the bottom (in the denominator) and inches on the top (in the numerator).

$$2 \text{ ft} \times \frac{? \text{ in}}{? \text{ ft}} = ? \text{ in}$$

Next, put in numbers that will make the fraction $\frac{? \text{ in}}{? \text{ ft}}$ equal to 1. Because 12 in = 1 ft, the fraction you want is $\frac{12 \text{ in}}{1 \text{ ft}}$. Now, multiply 2 feet by $\frac{12 \text{ in}}{1 \text{ ft}}$.

$$\frac{2 \cancel{\text{ ft}}}{1} \times \frac{12 \text{ in}}{1 \cancel{\text{ ft}}} = \frac{(2 \times 12) \text{ in}}{1} = 24 \text{ in}$$

So, 2 feet is the same as 24 inches.

▶ E X A M P L E 3.2

Change 36 inches to an equivalent number of feet.

   36 in = ? ft

You want to cancel the inches and get the answer in feet. So you must multiply 36 inches by a fraction that has inches on the bottom (in the denominator) and feet on the top (in the numerator).

$$36 \text{ in} \times \frac{? \text{ ft}}{? \text{ in}} = ?$$

Note $\frac{1 \text{ ft}}{12 \text{ in}} = 1$, because 1 foot is the same as 12 inches. Now, multiply 36 inches by $\frac{1 \text{ ft}}{12 \text{ in}}$.

$$\overset{3}{\cancel{36 \text{ in}}} \times \frac{1 \text{ ft}}{\cancel{12 \text{ in}}} = \frac{3 \times 1 \text{ ft}}{1} = 3 \text{ ft}$$

So, 36 inches is the same as 3 feet.

EXAMPLE 3.3

Change 15 yards to an equivalent length in feet.

15 yd = ? ft

You want to cancel the yards and get the answer in feet. So, multiply 15 yards by a fraction that has yards on the bottom (denominator). The answer must be in feet, so the fraction must have feet on the top (numerator).

$$15 \text{ yd} \times \frac{? \text{ ft}}{? \text{ yd}} = ? \text{ ft}$$

We must put in numbers that will make $\frac{? \text{ ft}}{? \text{ yd}}$ equal to 1. Because 3 ft = 1 yd, the fraction we want is $\frac{3 \text{ ft}}{1 \text{ yd}}$. Now multiply 15 yards by $\frac{3 \text{ ft}}{1 \text{ yd}}$.

$$15 \cancel{\text{ yd}} \times \frac{3 \text{ ft}}{1 \cancel{\text{ yd}}} = \frac{15 \times 3 \text{ ft}}{1} = 45 \text{ ft}$$

So, 15 yards is the same as 45 feet.

EXAMPLE 3.4

Change 0.25 feet to an equivalent length in inches.

0.25 ft = ? in

You want to cancel feet and get the answer in inches. So, multiply 0.25 feet by a fraction that looks like $\frac{? \text{ in}}{? \text{ ft}}$.

$$0.25 \text{ ft} \times \frac{? \text{ in}}{? \text{ ft}} = ? \text{ in}$$

Because 12 in = 1 ft, the fraction we want is $\frac{12 \text{ in}}{1 \text{ ft}}$.

$$0.25 \cancel{\text{ ft}} \times \frac{12 \text{ in}}{1 \cancel{\text{ ft}}} = \frac{0.25 \times 12 \text{ in}}{1} = 3 \text{ in}$$

So, 0.25 feet is the same as 3 inches.

Change 64 ounces to pounds.

64 oz = ? lb

You want to cancel ounces and get the answer in pounds. So, multiply 64 ounces by a fraction that looks like $\frac{?\ lb}{?\ oz}$.

$$64\ oz \times \frac{?\ lb}{?\ oz} = ?$$

Because 16 oz = 1 lb, the fraction we want is $\frac{1\ lb}{16\ oz}$.

$$\overset{4}{\cancel{64\ oz}} \times \frac{1\ lb}{\underset{1}{\cancel{16\ oz}}} = 4\ lb$$

So, 64 ounces is the same as 4 pounds.

You will find the answers to *Try These for Practice* below. Answers to *Exercises* appear in Appendix A at the back of the book. Your instructor has the answers to the *Additional Exercises*.

Try These for Practice

Test your comprehension after reading the chapter.

1. An infant weighs 8 pounds. What is its weight in ounces? _____

2. A woman is 60 inches tall. How tall is she in feet? _____

3. It takes 36 months to pay off an automobile loan. How many years is that? _____

4. How many seconds are in $4\frac{1}{2}$ minutes? _____

5. How many yards does 30 feet equal? _____

Answers: 1. 128 ounces   2. 5 feet   3. 3 years   4. 270 seconds   5. 10 yards

Exercises

Reinforce your understanding in class or at home.

1. 2.5 yr = _____ mon   **2.** 7 d = _____ h

3. 3 lb = _____ oz   **4.** 360 sec = _____ min

5. 240 in = _____ ft

6. 9 ft = _____ yd

7. 4 oz = _____ lb

8. $1\frac{1}{2}$ yd = _____ ft

9. $1\frac{3}{4}$ yr = _____ mon

10. $\frac{1}{2}$ min = _____ sec

11. What is the height of a 6-foot-tall patient in inches? _____

12. An IV solution has been infusing for 5 minutes. How many seconds is that? _____

13. Change 3.75 hours to minutes. _____

14. How many years are there in 18 months? _____

15. What part of an hour is 45 minutes? _____

16. If your patient measures 66 inches in height, what does the patient measure in feet? _____

17. Convert 80 hours to days. _____

18. An infant weighs 6 pounds at birth. What is its weight in ounces? _____

19. A person is 5 feet 8 inches tall. Express this height in inches. ___68___

20. If an infant weighs $7\frac{1}{2}$ pounds, what is the equivalent in ounces? _____

Additional Exercises

Now, on your own, test yourself! Ask your instructor to check your answers.

1. 720 mon = _____ yr

2. 36 h = _____ d

3. 32 oz = _____ lb

4. 6.5 min = _____ sec

5. $3\frac{1}{2}$ ft = _____ in

6. 4 yd = _____ ft

7. $6\frac{1}{4}$ lb = _____ oz

8. 1.25 ft = _____ in

9. 6 mon = _____ yr

10. 30 sec = _____ min

11. What is the height in feet of a child who is 36 inches tall? _____

12. Change 300 seconds to minutes. _____

13. What part of a pound is 4 ounces? _____

14. How many months are in 5 years? _____

15. Change $2\frac{1}{2}$ hours to minutes. _____

16. Convert 7 days to hours. _____

17. An infant weighs 88 ounces. What is its weight in pounds? _____

18. What is the weight in ounces of an infant who weighs 6 pounds 3 ounces? _____

19. What is the height in inches of a girl who is 5 feet 6 inches tall? _____

20. Change 150 seconds to minutes. _____

Systems of Measurement for Dosage Calculations

The Apothecary, Household, and Metric Systems

At present, there are three systems used to measure drugs: the *apothecary system,* the **household system,** and the ***International System of Units (SI).*** The SI, commonly known as the *metric system,* is replacing the other systems of measurement. However, the other systems are still in use, so you must understand all three systems and learn how to convert from one to another. In this chapter you will be introduced to the three systems. You will notice that the apothecary and household systems use fractions, such as $\frac{1}{2}$ and $2\frac{3}{4}$, whereas the metric system uses decimal numbers, such as 0.5 and 2.75.

THE APOTHECARY SYSTEM

The apothecary system is one of the oldest systems of drug measurement. Although it is infrequently used, you must nevertheless understand the apothecary system in order to administer medications safely.

Liquid Volume in the Apothecary System

Drugs in liquid form are measured by volume. The volume of a liquid is the amount of space it occupies. The equivalents for the units of measurement for liquid volume in the apothecary system are shown in Table 4.1 along with their abbreviations.

▶ **TABLE 4.1**

Common Equivalents for Apothecary Liquid Volume Units

quart (qt) 1 = pints (pt) 2
quart (qt) 1 = ounces (℥ or oz) 32
pint (pt) 1 = ounces (℥ or oz) 16
ounce (℥ or oz) 1 = drams (ℨ) 8
dram (ℨ) 1 = minims (♏) 60

NOTE

In the apothecary system, the abbreviation or symbol for the unit is placed before the quantity (as in pt 2). However, it is sometimes written the other way (2 pt) as well.

You can use dimensional analysis to convert from one unit to an equivalent unit within the apothecary system the same way you converted units in Chapter 3. You multiply the old measurement by a fraction that is equal to 1; the fraction has the old units on the bottom (the denominator) and the new units on top (the numerator) as the following examples show.

▶ **EXAMPLE 4.1**

The order reads minims 180 of guaifenesin (Robitussin). How many drams of this expectorant would you administer?

$$♏\ 180 = dr\ ?$$

You want to cancel the minims and obtain the equivalent amount in drams.

$$♏\ 180 \times \frac{dr\ ?}{♏\ ?} = dr\ ?$$

Because ♏ 60 = dr 1, the fraction you want is $\frac{dr\ 1}{♏\ 60}$.

$$\cancel{\text{m}\,180}^{3} \times \frac{\text{dr } 1}{\cancel{\text{m}\,60}_{1}} = \text{dr } 3$$

So, minims 180 is the same as drams 3, and you would administer drams 3 of guaifenesin.

▶ EXAMPLE 4.2

The patient is to receive drams 4 of magaldrate (Riopan). How many ounces of this antacid would you administer?

$$\text{ʒ } 4 = \text{ʒ} \, ?$$

You want to cancel the drams and get the answer in ounces.

$$\text{ʒ } 4 \times \frac{\text{ʒ } ?}{\text{ʒ } ?} = \text{ʒ } ?$$

Because ʒ 8 = ʒ 1, the fraction you want is $\frac{\text{ʒ } 1}{\text{ʒ } 8}$

$$\cancel{\text{ʒ } 4}^{1} \times \frac{\text{ʒ } 1}{\cancel{\text{ʒ } 8}_{2}} = \text{ʒ } \frac{1}{2}$$

So, drams 4 is the same as ounce $\frac{1}{2}$, and you would administer ounce $\frac{1}{2}$ of Riopan.

Weight in the Apothecary System

The grain (gr) is the only unit of weight in the apothecary system that is used in administering medications. You will be converting this unit to its equivalent in other systems of measurement in Chapter 5.

Roman Numerals

Dosages in the apothecary system are sometimes written using Roman numerals. Table 4.2 shows Roman numerals.

▶ TABLE 4.2

Roman Numerals					
1	I	7	VII	$\frac{1}{2}$	ss
2	II	8	VIII	$1\frac{1}{2}$	iss
3	III	9	IX	$7\frac{1}{2}$	viiss
4	IV	10	X		
5	V	15	XV		
6	VI	20	XX		

THE HOUSEHOLD SYSTEM

Liquid Volume in the Household System

Occasionally household measurements are used in prescribing liquid medication. Table 4.3 lists equivalent values, with their abbreviations, for units of liquid measurement in the household system.

▶ **TABLE 4.3**

Equivalent Measurements in the Household System

1 glass (usually)	=	ounces (℥ or oz) 8
1 measuring cup	=	ounces (℥ or oz) 8
1 teacup	=	ounces (℥ or oz) 6
1 ounce (℥)	=	2 tablespoons (T)
1 tablespoon (T)	=	3 teaspoons (t)
1 teaspoon (t)	=	60 drops (gtt)

Since these units are measured using household utensils, which are not necessarily accurate, the equivalents listed in Table 4.3 are only *approximate*. Unlike the metric system, which uses decimal numbers such as 0.5 and 3.75, the household system uses fractions such as $\frac{1}{2}$ and $3\frac{3}{4}$. Notice that the ounce is a unit of measurement in both the apothecary and household systems.

▶ **E X A M P L E 4.3**

The patient is to receive 15 drops of the gastrointestinal antispasmodic drug paregoric. How many teaspoons would the patient receive?

$$15 \text{ gtt} = ? \text{ t}$$

You want to cancel drops and obtain the equivalent amount in teaspoons.

$$15 \text{ gtt} \times \frac{? \text{ t}}{? \text{ gtt}} = ? \text{ t}$$

Because 60 gtt = 1 t, the fraction is $\frac{1 \text{ t}}{60 \text{ gtt}}$.

$$\overset{1}{\cancel{15 \text{ gtt}}} \times \frac{1 \text{ t}}{\underset{4}{\cancel{60 \text{ gtt}}}} = \frac{1}{4} \text{ t}$$

So, 15 drops is approximately the same as $\frac{1}{4}$ teaspoon, and the patient would receive $\frac{1}{4}$ teaspoon of paregoric.

▶ **E X A M P L E 4.4**

The prescriber directs the patient to take 2 ounces of a laxative agent, citrate of magnesia, at home whenever necessary. How many tablespoons would the patient take?

2 oz. = ? T

You want to cancel the ounces and obtain the equivalent amount in tablespoons.

$$2 \text{ oz} \times \frac{? \text{ T}}{? \text{ oz}} = ? \text{ T}$$

Because 2 T = 1 oz, the fraction is $\frac{2 \text{ T}}{1 \text{ oz}}$.

$$2 \text{ oz} \times \frac{2 \text{ T}}{1 \text{ oz}} = 4 \text{ T}$$

So, 2 ounces is approximately the same as 4 tablespoons, and the patient would take 4 tablespoons of citrate of magnesia whenever necessary.

Weight in the Household System

The only units of weight used in the household system are ounces (oz) and pounds (lb), as shown in Table 4.4.

▶ **TABLE 4.4**

Weight in the Household System
16 oz = 1 lb

▶ **EXAMPLE 4.5**

An infant weighs 8 pounds 11 ounces. What is the weight of the infant in ounces? First you change the 8 pounds to ounces.

8 lb = ? oz

You want to cancel the pounds and obtain the equivalent amount in ounces.

$$8 \text{ lb} = \frac{? \text{ oz}}{? \text{ lb}} = ? \text{ oz}$$

Because 16 oz = 1 lb, the fraction is $\frac{16 \text{ oz}}{1 \text{ lb}}$.

$$8 \text{ lb} \times \frac{16 \text{ oz}}{1 \text{ lb}} = 128 \text{ oz}$$

Now you add the extra 11 ounces.

128 oz + 11 oz = 139 oz

So, the 8-pound, 11-ounce infant weighs 139 ounces.

THE METRIC SYSTEM

Liquid Volume in the Metric System

The equivalents for the units of measurement for liquid volume in the metric system are shown in Table 4.5, along with their abbreviations.

▶ TABLE 4.5

Metric Equivalents of Liquid Volume

1 cubic centimeter (cc or cm³)	=	1 milliliter (mL or ml)
1000 milliliters (mL or ml)	=	1 liter (L)
1000 cubic centimeters (cc or cm³)	=	1 liter (L)

NOTES

The prefix "milli" means "$\frac{1}{1000}$". So a milliliter is $\frac{1}{1000}$ of a liter.

The milliliter (mL) and cubic centimeter (cc) are equivalent measurements. A 30 mL vial of meperidine hydrochloride (Demerol) is therefore the same as a 30 cc vial of meperidine hydrochloride.

Using dimensional analysis and the information in Table 4.5, you can convert a quantity written in one unit of metric volume to another. The next examples show how to do this.

▶ EXAMPLE 4.6

If the prescriber ordered 1.5 liters of 5% dextrose in water (D/W), how many cubic centimeters were ordered?

$$1.5 \text{ L} = ? \text{ cc}$$

You want to cancel the liters and obtain the equivalent amount in cubic centimeters.

$$1.5 \text{ L} \times \frac{? \text{ cc}}{? \text{ L}} = ? \text{ cc}$$

Since 1000 cc = 1 L (see Table 4.5), the fraction you want is $\frac{1000 \text{ cc}}{1 \text{ L}}$.

$$1.5 \text{ L} \times \frac{1000 \text{ cc}}{1 \text{ L}} = 1500 \text{ cc}$$

So the prescriber ordered 1500 cubic centimeters of 5% D/W.

NOTE

Write 1.5 liters instead of $1\frac{1}{2}$ liters because in the metric system quantities are written as decimal numbers instead of fractions.

▶ EXAMPLE 4.7

Your patient is to receive 1750 milliliters of 10% dextrose (D) in normal saline (NS). What is the same dose in liters?

1750 mL = ? L

You want to cancel the milliliters and obtain the equivalent amount in liters.

$$1750 \text{ mL} \times \frac{? \text{ L}}{? \text{ mL}} = ? \text{ L}$$

Because 1000 mL = 1 L, the fraction you want is $\frac{1 \text{ L}}{1000 \text{ mL}}$.

$$1750 \text{ mL} \times \frac{1 \text{ L}}{1000 \text{ mL}} = \frac{1750 \text{ L}}{1000} = 1.75 \text{ L}$$

So, 1750 milliliters of 10% D/NS is the same dose as 1.75 liters of 10% D/NS.

Weight in the Metric System

Drugs in dry form are measured by weight in the metric system. Metric equivalents for weight are shown in Table 4.6, along with their abbreviations.

▶ TABLE 4.6

Metric Equivalents of Weight

1 kilogram (kg)	=	1000 grams (g)
1 gram (g)	=	1000 milligrams (mg)
1 milligram (mg)	=	1000 micrograms (μg or mcg)

NOTE

"Kilo" means "thousand" (1000). So, a kilogram is 1000 grams.

"Milli" means "one thousandth" ($\frac{1}{1000}$). So, a milligram is $\frac{1}{1000}$ of a gram.

"Micro" means "one millionth" ($\frac{1}{1,000,000}$). So, a microgram is

$\frac{1}{1,000,000}$ of a gram.

Using dimensional analysis and the information in Table 4.6, you can convert a quantity written in one unit of metric weight to an equivalent quantity in another unit of metric weight. The following examples show you how to do this.

▶ EXAMPLE 4.8

The prescriber has ordered 500 micrograms of cyanocobalamin (vitamin B_{12}). How many milligrams in this dose?

500 μg = ? mg

You want to cancel the micrograms and obtain the equivalent amount in milligrams.

$$500 \; \mu g \times \frac{? \; mg}{? \; \mu g} = ? \; mg$$

Because 1000 μg = 1 mg, the fraction you want is $\frac{1 \; mg}{1000 \; \mu g}$.

$$\overset{1}{\cancel{500 \; \mu g}} \times \frac{1 \; mg}{\underset{2}{\cancel{1000 \; \mu g}}} = \frac{1 \; mg}{2} = 0.5 \; mg$$

So, 500 micrograms is the same as 0.5 milligram.

▶ EXAMPLE 4.9

The order reads 125 micrograms of digoxin (Lanoxin). How many milligrams of this anti-arrythmic medication would you administer to the patient?

$$125 \; mcg = ? \; mg$$

You want to cancel the micrograms and obtain the equivalent amount in milligrams.

$$125 \; mcg \times \frac{? \; mg}{? \; mcg} = ? \; mg$$

Because 1000 mcg = 1 mg, you have:

$$125 \; \cancel{mcg} \times \frac{1 \; mg}{1000 \; \cancel{mcg}} = 0.125 \; mg$$

So, 125 micrograms is the same as 0.125 milligram, and you would administer 0.125 milligram of digoxin.

▶ EXAMPLE 4.10

The order reads 0.016 gram of the analgesic medication morphine sulfate. How many milligrams would you administer?

$$0.016 \; g = ? \; mg$$

You want to cancel the grams and obtain the equivalent amount in milligrams.

$$0.016 \; g \times \frac{? \; mg}{? \; g} = ? \; mg$$

$$0.016 \; \cancel{g} \times \frac{1000 \; mg}{1 \; \cancel{g}} = 16 \; mg$$

So, 0.016 gram is the same as 16 milligrams, and you would administer 16 milligrams of morphine sulfate.

BY THE WAY

A dose is always expressed in the form of a number and a unit. Both are important. For example:

15 cc	2 capsules
2.5 mg	1.5 mL
3 tablets	0.5 L

When you write your answer, be sure to include the appropriate unit.

Prerequisite Equivalents

In order to do the exercises at the end of this chapter, you need to memorize the metric equivalents for volume and weight. To test yourself, fill in the missing numbers in the following chart and check your answers below before you start *Try These for Practice* and the exercises.

Volume

1. 1 mL = _____ cc = _____ cm^3

2. 1 L = _____ mL

3. 1 L = _____ cc

Weight

4. 1 kg = _____ g

5. 1 g = _____ mg

6. 1 mg = _____ μg

7. 1 mg = _____ mcg

8. 1 μg = _____ mcg

Answers: 1. 1 cc, 1 cm^3 2. 1000 mL   3. 1000 cc   4. 1000 g   5. 1000 mg   6. 1000 μg 7. 1000 mcg   8. 1 mcg

You will find the answers to *Try These for Practice* below. Answers to *Exercises* and *Cumulative Review* appear in Appendix A at the back of the book. Your instructor has the answers to the *Additional Exercises*.

Try These for Practice

Test your comprehension after reading the chapter.

1. You need to memorize all the apothecary, household, and metric equivalents. To test yourself, fill in the missing numbers in the following chart.

   Apothecary System

   a. qt 1   =   pt _____

   b. pt 1   =   ℥ _____

   c. ℥ 1   =   ʒ _____

   d. ʒ 1   =   ♏ _____

   Household System

   e. 1 glass   =   ℥ _____

   f. 1 measuring cup   =   ℥ _____

   g. 1 teacup   =   ℥ _____

   h. 1 oz   =   _____ T

   i. 1 T   =   _____ t

   j. 1 t   =   _____ gtt

   k. 1 lb   =   _____ oz

   Metric System

   l. 1 mL   =   _____ cc

   m. 1 g   =   _____ mg

n. 1 kg = _____ g

o. 1000 μg = _____ mg

2. According to the label in Figure 4.1, each capsule of Amoxil contains 250 mg. Convert 250 milligrams to grams.

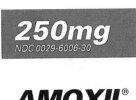

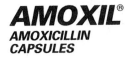

▶ **FIGURE 4.1 Drug label for Amoxil.**

3. A prescriber has ordered 1500 micrograms of cyanocobalamin (vitamin B₁₂). How many milligrams is this dose?

4. The prescriber ordered the following:

cranberry juice ℥ 12 q A.M. po convert 12 ounces to pints.

5. The prescriber has ordered 8 ounces of the food supplement Ensure. How many drams will you administer to the patient?

Answers: 1. a) pt 2 b) ℥ 16 c) ℨ 8 d) ℥ 8 e) ℥ 8 f) ℥ 8 g) ℥ 6 h) 2 T i) 3 t j) 60 gtt k) 16 oz l) 1 cc m) 1000 cc n) 1000 g o) 1 mg 2. 0.25 g 3. 1.5 mg 4. pt ¾ 5. ℥ 64

Exercises

Reinforce your understanding in class or at home.

1. 2500 g = _____ kg

2. 3.5 L = _____ cc

3. ℳ 120 = dr _____

4. ℥ 32 = ℨ _____

5. 0.006 g _____ mg

6. ℥ 24 = ℨ _____

7. 0.4 kg = _____ g   **8.** qt 4 = pt _____

9. ℥ 30 = ♏ _____   **10.** 3 t = _____ gtt

11. 25,000 mcg = _____ mg   **12.** 50 mL = _____ cc

13. The label in Figure 4.2 indicates the quantity of clonidine in 1 tablet. Indicate the number of grams of clonidine in 1 tablet. _____

NDC 0005-3182-23

Clonidine Hydrochloride Tablets, USP

 NEW PRODUCT APPEARANCE

CAUTION: Federal law prohibits dispensing without prescription.

100 TABLETS   STANDARD *Lederle* PRODUCTS

DOSAGE: See accompanying circular for complete directions for use.
Store at Controlled Room Temperature 15-30°C (59-86°F). Dispense in a tight, light-resistant container as defined in the USP.
This package not for household dispensing.

Control No.   Exp. Date

LEDERLE LABORATORIES DIVISION
American Cyanamid Company
Pearl River, NY 10965

21875
D1

▶ **FIGURE 4.2 Drug label for clonidine.**

14. How many milligrams would you administer to the patient if the order for the sedative drug triazolam (Halcion) was 0.075 gram? _____

15. According to the physician's order sheet in Figure 4.3, what is the dose of guaifenesin (Robitussin) in ounces? _____

✚ GENERAL HOSPITAL ✚

PRESS HARD WITH BALLPOINT PEN. WRITE DATE & TIME AND SIGN EACH ORDER

DATE	TIME	A.M. P.M.
3/8/01	11	

Robitussin dr. 4 po q6h

SIGNATURE
A. Giangrasso   M.D.

IMPRINT
273189   3/7/01
Abdul Danuish   2/1/75
2 Elm St.   Buddhist
Silver Springs, CO   Aetna
43612
Antony Giangrasso, M.D.

ORDERS NOTED   A.M. P.M.

DATE _3/8/01_ TIME _11:20_

❏ MEDEX ❏ KARDEX

NURSE'S SIG. _J. Olsen_

FILLED BY   DATE

PHYSICIAN'S ORDERS

▶ **FIGURE 4.3 Physician's order sheet.**

16. The prescriber ordered 5% D/W 0.7 L IV q8h. How many milliliters are contained in this amount of solution? _____

17. The prescriber ordered the following:

H$_2$O $\frac{1}{4}$ pt po q1h.

How many ounces should be given every hour? _____

18. The patient must receive 0.75 milligram of dexamethasone po stat ("immediately"). What is the equivalent dose in micrograms? _____

19. The prescriber ordered Navane 500 μg po stat (Figure 4.4). What is the equivalent dose in milligrams of this narcotic antipsychotic drug? _____

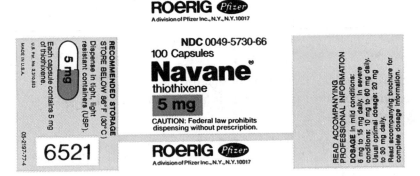

▶ FIGURE 4.4 Drug label for Navane.

20. The label in Figure 4.5 indicates that each capsule contains 100 milligrams of Vibramycin. Convert 100 milligrams to grams. _____

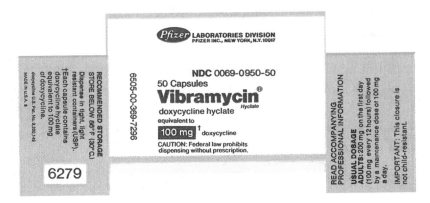

▶ FIGURE 4.5 Drug label for Vibramycin.

Additional Exercises

Now, on your own, test yourself! Ask your instructor to check your answers.

1. $\frac{1}{3}$ t = _____ gtt

2. 800 mcg = _____ mg

3. 18 oz = _____ teacups

4. 2.25 L = _____ mL

5. ℥ 12 = ℨ _____

6. 0.007 g = _____ mg

7. 0.3 mg = _____ g

8. 0.75 g = _____ mg

9. 0.002 L = _____ cc

10. $\frac{3}{4}$ qt = _____ pt

11. The prescriber ordered zalcitabine 375 μg po bid. How many milligrams of this antiviral drug would you administer to the patient? _____

12. How many ounces are contained in 5 tablespoons? _____

13. The prescriber ordered $\frac{1}{2}$ teaspoon of tincture of opium (paregoric) as an antidiarrheal agent. How many drops are contained in $\frac{1}{2}$ teaspoon? _____

14. How many drops are contained in 3 teaspoons of cimetidine (Tagamet), an antiulcer agent? _____

15. The prescriber ordered the following:

    caster oil dr 8 po 9 P.M.

    Convert this amount to ounces. _____

16. If an infant weighs 3.5 kilograms, what would be its weight in grams? _____

17. If the patient must receive ounces 4 of sodium phosphate (Phospho-Soda) po, how many drams of this laxative will you prepare? _____

18. How many milligrams are contained in the order written in Figure 4.6 for azithromycin? _____

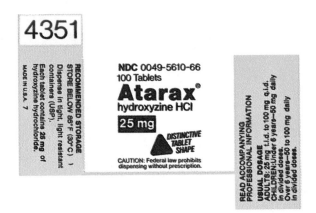

⊕ GENERAL HOSPITAL ⊕

PRESS HARD WITH BALLPOINT PEN. WRITE DATE & TIME AND SIGN EACH ORDER

DATE	TIME	A.M.
1/29/01	1	(P.M.)

azithromycin 0.5 g po bid

D/C ampicillin 500 mg po tid

sustagen po 600 ml per 12 h

soft diet

OOB

SIGNATURE   L. Ablon   M.D.

IMPRINT
129941   01/29/01
Kim Park   03/14/65
23 Jones Court   Prot
San Diego, CA 09774 Prud

Dr. Leon Ablon

ORDERS NOTED
DATE _1/29/01_ TIME _1:15_ A.M. (P.M.)

❑ MEDEX   ❑ KARDEX

NURSE'S SIG. ___C. Hill___

FILLED BY   DATE

PHYSICIAN'S ORDERS

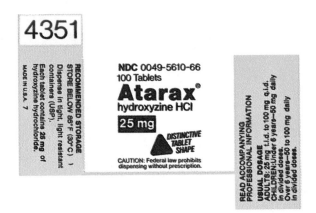

▶ **FIGURE 4.6 Physician's order sheet.**

19. Calculate the amount of fluid in milliliters a patient must receive each hour if the order is 0.1 liter per hour. _____

20. In Figure 4.7, each tablet of hydroxyzine HCl (Atarax) contains 25 milligrams. Convert this quantity to micrograms. _____

4351

RECOMMENDED STORAGE
STORE BELOW 86°F (30°C.)
Dispense in tight, light resistant
containers (USP).
Each tablet contains 25 mg. of
hydroxyzine hydrochloride.
MADE IN U.S.A. 7

NDC 0049-5610-66
100 Tablets

Atarax®
hydroxyzine HCl
25 mg

△ DISTINCTIVE TABLET SHAPE

CAUTION: Federal law prohibits
dispensing without prescription.

READ ACCOMPANYING
PROFESSIONAL INFORMATION

USUAL DOSAGE
ADULTS: 25 mg t.i.d. to 100 mg q.i.d.
CHILDREN: Under 6 years—50 mg daily
in divided doses.
Over 6 years—50 to 100 mg daily
in divided doses.

▶ **FIGURE 4.7 Drug label for Atarax.**

CUMULATIVE REVIEW EXERCISES

Review your mastery of earlier chapters.

1. 2.5 g = _____ mg   2. 200 mcg = _____ mg

3. ℥ 180 = ℈ _____

4. ℥ 4 = ℥ _____

5. 25 mg = _____ μg

6. 6 t = _____ T

7. 1200 cc = _____ L

8. 6000 mg = _____ g

9. 2.35 kg = _____ g

10. 2.5 g = _____ mg

11. How many teaspoons are contained in $\frac{1}{2}$ tablespoon? _____

12. How many milliliters are contained in 3.25 liters? _____

13. The prescriber ordered drams 6 of a preparation of magnesium hydroxide and aluminum hydroxide (Mylanta), an antacid. How many ounces would you administer to the patient? _____

14. If the prescriber ordered 30 drops of a drug, how many teaspoons would you administer to the patient? _____

15. The order reads as follows:

    orange juice 240 mL po qd

    Convert 240 milliliters to liters. _____

CHAPTER FIVE

Converting from One System of Measurement to Another

Converting from
One System of
Measurement to
Another

▶ **Objectives**

After completing this chapter, you will be able to

- State the equivalent units of weight for the metric, apothecary, and household systems.
- State the equivalent units of volume for the metric, apothecary, and household systems.
- State the equivalent units of length for the metric and household systems.
- Convert from one unit to its equivalent among the three systems.

When calculating drug dosages, you will sometimes need to convert a quantity expressed in one system of measurement to an equivalent quantity expressed in another. For example, you might need to convert a quantity measured in drams to the same quantity measured in milliliters. This chapter will show you how to use dimensional analysis to accomplish this conversion.

EQUIVALENTS OF COMMON UNITS OF MEASUREMENT

To get started, you will need to learn some basic equivalent values of the various units in the different systems. Tables 5.1 through 5.3 list some common equivalent values for weight, volume, and length in the metric, apothecary, and household systems of measurement. Although these equivalents are considered standards, many of them are approximations.

▶ **TABLE 5.1**

Equivalent Values for Units of Weight

Metric		Apothecary		Household
60 milligrams (mg)	=	grain (gr) 1		
1 gram (g)	=	grains (gr) 15		
1 kilogram (kg)			=	2.2 pounds (lb)
0.45 kilogram (kg)			=	1 pound (lb)

▶ **TABLE 5.2**

Equivalent Values for Units of Volume

Metric		Apothecary		Household
		minim (♏) 1	=	1 drop (gtt)
1 milliliter (mL)	=	minims (♏) 15 or 16	=	15 or 16 drops (gtt)
4 or 5 milliliters (mL)	=	dram (ʒ) 1	=	1 teaspoon (t)
		minims (♏) 60	=	1 teaspoon (t)
		minims (♏) 60	=	60 drops (gtt)
15 milliliters (mL)	=	ounce (ʒ) ½	=	1 T
30 milliliters (mL)	=	ounce (ʒ) 1	=	1 ounce (ʒ) or 2 T
500 milliliters (mL)	=	ounces (ʒ) 16	=	1 pint (pt)
1000 milliliters (mL)	=	ounces (ʒ) 32	=	1 quart (qt)

NOTE

Here are some useful equivalents:

1 t = 60 gtt = ♏ 60 = ʒ 1 = 4 or 5 mL

2 T = ʒ 1 = ʒ 8 = 30 or 32 mL

▶ **TABLE 5.3**

Equivalent Values for Units of Length

Metric		Household
1 centimeter (cm)	=	0.4 inch (in)
2.5 centimeters (cm)	=	1 inch (in)

You can use dimensional analysis to convert from one system to another in exactly the same way you converted from one unit to another within the same system. Multiply the original measurement by a fraction that is equal to 1. This fraction will have the original units on the bottom and the new units on the top. Figure 5.1 depicts some useful equivalents of volume measurements among the three systems.

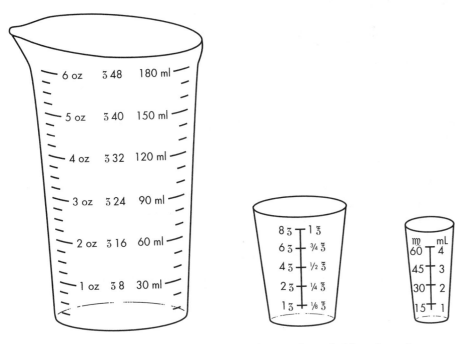

▶ **FIGURE 5.1 Units of measure in the apothecary, household, and metric systems.**

METRIC-TO-APOTHECARY CONVERSIONS

▶ **EXAMPLE 5.1**

Convert 600 milligrams to grains.

600 mg = gr ?

You want to cancel the milligrams and obtain the equivalent amount in grains.

$$600 \text{ mg} \times \frac{\text{gr ?}}{\text{? mg}} = \text{gr ?}$$

Because 60 mg = gr 1, the fraction is $\frac{\text{gr 1}}{60 \text{ mg}}$.

$$600 \text{ mg} \times \frac{\text{gr } 1}{60 \text{ mg}} = \frac{\text{gr } 600}{60} = \text{gr } 10$$

So, 600 milligrams are equivalent to grains 10.

▶ **EXAMPLE 5.2**

Convert 20 milligrams to grains.

$$20 \text{ mg} = \text{gr ?}$$

You want to cancel the milligrams and obtain the equivalent amount in grains.

$$20 \text{ mg} \times \frac{\text{gr ?}}{\text{? mg}} = \text{gr ?}$$

Because 60 mg = gr 1, the fraction is $\frac{\text{gr } 1}{60 \text{ mg}}$.

$$\overset{1}{\cancel{20 \text{ mg}}} \times \frac{\text{gr } 1}{\underset{3}{\cancel{60 \text{ mg}}}} = \text{gr } \frac{1}{3}$$

So, 20 milligrams are equivalent to grain $\frac{1}{3}$.

▶ **EXAMPLE 5.3**

The label for clonidine hydrochloride is shown in Figure 5.2. Convert the milligrams in 1 tablet to grains.

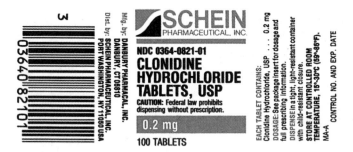

▶ **FIGURE 5.2 Drug label for clonidine hydrochloride.**

$$0.2 \text{ mg} = \text{gr ?}$$

You want to cancel the milligrams and get the answer in grains.

$$0.2 \text{ mg} \times \frac{\text{gr ?}}{\text{? mg}} = \text{gr ?}$$

Because gr 1 = 60 mg, the fraction is $\frac{\text{gr } 1}{60 \text{ mg}}$.

$$0.2 \ \text{mg} \times \frac{\text{gr } 1}{60 \ \text{mg}} = \frac{\text{gr } 0.2}{60} \times \frac{10}{10} = \text{gr} \frac{2}{600} = \text{gr} \frac{1}{300}$$

So, 0.2 mg is equivalent to grains $\frac{1}{300}$.

In Example 5.3, we multiplied both the numerator and the denominator of the fraction $\frac{\text{gr } 0.2}{60}$ by 10 to eliminate the decimal number.

▶ **EXAMPLE 5.4**

Convert 2 grams to grains.

$$2 \ \text{g} = \text{gr ?}$$

You want to cancel the grams and obtain the equivalent amount in grains.

$$2 \ \text{g} \times \frac{\text{gr ?}}{? \ \text{g}} = \text{gr ?}$$

Because 1 g = gr 15, the fraction is $\frac{\text{gr } 15}{1 \ \text{g}}$.

$$2 \ \text{g} \times \frac{\text{gr } 15}{1 \ \text{g}} = \text{gr } 30$$

So, 2 grams are equivalent to grains 30.

▶ **EXAMPLE 5.5**

Convert 0.25 gram to grains.

$$0.25 \ \text{g} = \text{gr ?}$$

You want to cancel the gram and obtain the equivalent amount in grains.

$$0.25 \ \text{g} \times \frac{\text{gr ?}}{? \ \text{g}} = \text{gr ?}$$

Because 1 g = gr 15, the fraction is $\frac{\text{gr } 15}{1 \ \text{g}}$.

$$0.25 \ \text{g} \times \frac{\text{gr } 15}{1 \ \text{g}} = \text{gr } 3.75 = \text{gr } 3\frac{3}{4}$$

So, 0.25 gram is equivalent to grains $3\frac{3}{4}$.

NOTE

Grains are expressed in fractions and whole numbers. Therefore, grains 3.75 should be expressed as grains $3\frac{3}{4}$.

APOTHECARY-TO-METRIC CONVERSIONS

▶ **EXAMPLE 5.6**

Convert grain $\frac{2}{3}$ to milligrams.

$$\text{gr } \frac{2}{3} = ? \text{ mg}$$

You want to cancel the grain and obtain the equivalent amount in milligrams.

$$\text{gr } \frac{2}{3} \times \frac{? \text{ mg}}{\text{gr }?} = ? \text{ mg}$$

Because 60 mg = gr 1, the fraction is $\frac{60 \text{ mg}}{\text{gr } 1}$.

$$\cancel{\text{gr}} \frac{2}{\cancel{3}_{1}} \times \frac{\overset{20}{\cancel{60} \text{ mg}}}{\cancel{\text{gr}} 1} = 40 \text{ mg}$$

So, grain $\frac{2}{3}$ is equivalent to 40 milligrams.

▶ **EXAMPLE 5.7**

Convert grains 5 to milligrams.

$$\text{gr } 5 = ? \text{ mg}$$

You want to cancel the grains and obtain the equivalent amount in milligrams.

$$\text{gr } 5 \times \frac{? \text{ mg}}{\text{gr }?} = ? \text{ mg}$$

Because 60 mg = gr 1, the fraction is $\frac{60 \text{ mg}}{\text{gr } 1}$.

$$\cancel{\text{gr}} 5 \times \frac{60 \text{ mg}}{\cancel{\text{gr}} 1} = 300 \text{ mg}$$

So, grains 5 are equivalent to 300 milligrams.

▶ **EXAMPLE 5.8**

Convert grains $7\frac{1}{2}$ to grams.

$$\text{gr } 7\frac{1}{2} = ? \text{ g}$$

You want to cancel the grains and obtain the equivalent amount in grams.

$$\text{gr } \frac{15}{2} \times \frac{? \text{ g}}{\text{gr }?} = ? \text{ g}$$

Since 1 g = gr 15, the fraction is $\frac{1\,g}{gr\,15}$.

$$\cancel{gr}\,\frac{\overset{1}{\cancel{15}}}{2}\times\frac{1\,g}{\underset{1}{\cancel{gr\,15}}}=\frac{1}{2}\,g=0.5\,g$$

So, grains $7\frac{1}{2}$ are equivalent to 0.5 gram.

> ### NOTE
>
> Grams are expressed in decimals or whole numbers. Therefore, $\frac{1}{2}$ gram is expressed as 0.5 gram.

▶ **EXAMPLE 5.9**

Convert grains $\frac{3}{4}$ to grams.

$$gr\,\frac{3}{4}=?\,g$$

You want to cancel the grains and obtain the equivalent amount in grams.

$$gr\,\frac{3}{4}\times\frac{?\,g}{gr\,?}=?\,g$$

Because 1 g = gr 15, the fraction is $\frac{1\,g}{gr\,15}$.

$$\cancel{gr}\,\frac{\overset{1}{\cancel{3}}}{4}\times\frac{1\,g}{\underset{5}{\cancel{gr\,15}}}=\frac{1}{20}\,g=0.05\,g$$

So, grains $\frac{3}{4}$ is equivalent to 0.05 gram.

HOUSEHOLD-TO-APOTHECARY OR HOUSEHOLD-TO-METRIC CONVERSIONS

▶ **EXAMPLE 5.10**

Convert 6 teaspoons to milliliters.

$$6\,t=?\,mL$$

You want to cancel the teaspoons and obtain the equivalent in milliliters.

$$6\,t\times\frac{?\,mL}{?\,t}=?\,mL$$

You can either use 4 mL = 1 t or 5 mL = 1 t. For this calculation, use 5 mL = 1 t; the fraction is therefore $\frac{5 \text{ mL}}{1 \text{ t}}$.

$$6 \text{ t} \times \frac{5 \text{ mL}}{1 \text{ t}} = 30 \text{ mL}$$

So, 6 teaspoons are equivalent to 30 milliliters.

BY THE WAY

If you used the equivalent 4 mL = 1 t in this example, the answer would be 24 milliliters instead of 30 milliliters. This illustrates the approximate nature of the equivalents among systems.

> **EXAMPLE 5.11**

Change $\frac{1}{3}$ teaspoon to drops.

$$\frac{1}{3} \text{ t} = ? \text{ gtt}$$

You want to cancel the teaspoon and obtain the equivalent amount in drops.

$$\frac{1}{3} \text{ t} \times \frac{? \text{ gtt}}{? \text{ t}} = ? \text{ gtt}$$

Since 60 gtt = 1 t, the fraction is $\frac{60 \text{ gtt}}{1 \text{ t}}$.

$$\frac{1}{3} \text{ t} \times \frac{\overset{20}{\cancel{60} \text{ gtt}}}{\cancel{\text{t}}} = 20 \text{ gtt}$$

So, $\frac{1}{3}$ teaspoon is equivalent to 20 drops.

> **EXAMPLE 5.12**

Dixie is 5 feet 9 inches tall. What is her height in centimeters?

5 ft 9 in   means   5 ft + 9 in

First determine Dixie's height in inches. To do this, convert 5 feet to inches.

5 ft = ? in

You want to cancel feet and obtain the equivalent height in inches.

$$5 \text{ ft} \times \frac{? \text{ in}}{? \text{ ft}} = ? \text{ in}$$

Because 1 ft = 12 in, the fraction is $\frac{12 \text{ in}}{1 \text{ ft}}$.

$$5 \text{ ft} \times \frac{12 \text{ in}}{1 \text{ ft}} = 60 \text{ in}$$

Second, add the extra 9 inches.

$$60 \text{ in} + 9 \text{ in} = 69 \text{ in}$$

Now convert 69 inches to centimeters.

$$69 \text{ in} = ? \text{ cm}$$

You want to cancel inches and obtain the equivalent length in centimeters.

$$69 \text{ in} \times \frac{? \text{ cm}}{? \text{ in}} = ? \text{ cm}$$

Because 1 in = 2.5 cm, the fraction is $\frac{2.5 \text{ cm}}{1 \text{ in}}$.

$$69 \text{ in} \times \frac{2.5 \text{ cm}}{1 \text{ in}} = 172.5 \text{ cm}$$

So, Dixie is 172.5 centimeters tall.

▶ **EXAMPLE 5.13**

Jennifer weighs 103 pounds 8 ounces. What is her weight in kilograms?

$$103 \text{ lb } 8 \text{ oz} \quad \text{means} \quad 103 \text{ lb} + 8 \text{ oz}$$

First determine Jennifer's weight in pounds. To do this, convert 8 ounces to pounds.

$$8 \text{ oz} = ? \text{ lb}$$

You want to cancel ounces and obtain the equivalent amount in pounds.

$$8 \text{ oz} \times \frac{? \text{ lb}}{? \text{ oz}} = ? \text{ lb}$$

Because 1 lb = 16 oz, the fraction is $\frac{1 \text{ lb}}{16 \text{ oz}}$.

$$\overset{1}{8 \text{ oz}} \times \frac{1 \text{ lb}}{\underset{2}{16 \text{ oz}}} = \frac{1}{2} \text{ lb}$$

So, Jennifer weighs 103 lb + $\frac{1}{2}$ lb or 103.5 pounds.

Second, convert 103.5 pounds to kilograms.

$$103.5 \text{ lb} = ? \text{ kg}$$

You want to cancel pounds and obtain the equivalent amount in kilograms.

$$103.5 \text{ lb} \times \frac{? \text{ kg}}{? \text{ lb}} = ? \text{ kg}$$

Because 1 kg = 2.2 lb, the fraction is $\frac{1 \text{ kg}}{2.2 \text{ lb}}$.

$$103.5 \text{ lb} \times \frac{1 \text{ kg}}{2.2 \text{ lb}} = 47.0 \text{ kg}$$

So, Jennifer weighs 47 kilograms.

If we use the equivalent 1 lb = 0.45 kg instead of 2.2 lb = 1 kg, then our calculations would be

$$103.5 \text{ lb} \times \frac{0.45 \text{ kg}}{1 \text{ lb}} = 46.575 \text{ kg}$$

This answer is different from the previous result because of the approximate nature of the equivalents among systems.

PREREQUISITE EQUIVALENTS

In order to do the exercises at the end of this chapter, you need to memorize all the equivalents presented so far. To test yourself, fill in the missing numbers in the following chart. Check your answers on the next page before you start *Try These for Practice* and the exercises.

Metric System

1. 1 mL   =   1 cc   =   _____ cm^3
2. 1 L   =   _____ mL
3. 1 kg   =   _____ g
4. 1000 mg   =   _____ g
5. 1000 μg =   _____ mg
6. 1μg   =   _____ mcg

Household System

7. 1 glass   =   ʒ _____
8. 1 teacup   =   ʒ _____
9. ʒ 1   =   _____ T
10. 1 T   =   _____ t
11. 1 t   =   _____ gtt
12. 1 lb   =   _____ oz
13. 1 ft   =   _____ in

Apothecary System

14. 1 qt   =   _____ pt
15. 1 pt   =   ʒ _____

16. ℥ 1 = ʒ _____
17. ℥ 1 = ♏ _____

Mixed Systems

18. ʒ 1 = _____ t = ♏ _____ = _____ gtt = _____ mL
19. ℥ 1 = _____ T = ʒ _____ = _____ mL
20. 1 measuring cup = _____ glass = ℥ _____ = _____ pt
21. gr 1 = _____ mg
22. 1 g = gr _____
23. 1 mL = _____ gtt
24. 1 kg = _____ lb
25. 1 lb = _____ kg
26. 1 in = _____ cm

Answers 1. 1 mL = 1 cm³   2. 1 L = 1000 mL   3. 1 kg = 1000 g   4. 1000 mg = 1 g
5. 1000 µg = 1 mg   6. 1 µg = 1 mcg   7. ʒ 8   8. ℥ 6   9. 2 T   10. 3 t   11. 60 gtt
12. 16 oz   13. 12 in   14. 2 pt   15. ʒ 16   16. ℥ 8   17. ♏ 60   18. ʒ 1 = 1 t = ♏ 60 = 60 gtt = 4 or 5 mL   19. ℥ 1 = 2 T = ʒ 8 = 30 or 32 mL   20. 1 measuring cup = 1 glass = ℥ 8 = ½ pt
21. gr 1 = 60 mg   22. 1 g = gr 15   23. 1 mL = 15 gtt   24. 1 kg = 2.2 lb   25. 1 lb = 0.45 kg
26. 1 in = 2.5 cm

PRACTICE SETS

You will find the answers to *Try These for Practice* below. Answers to *Exercises* and *Cumulative Review* appear in Appendix A at the back of the book. Your instructor has the answers to the Additional Exercises.

Try These for Practice

Test your comprehension after reading the chapter.

1. The prescriber has ordered grains 30 of acetylsalicylic acid (Aspirin). Convert this quantity to milligrams. _____

2. If a patient has an order for 0.5 milligram of cosyntropin (Cortrosyn) IM, how many grains will you administer to the patient? _____

3. The prescriber ordered atropine sulfate gr $\frac{1}{500}$ sc stat. Convert this quantity to milligrams. _____

4. A child weighs 54 pounds. Convert this weight to kilograms. _____

5. The patient is to receive 4 milliliters of diphenhydramine (Benadryl). How many minims will you administer to the patient? _____

Answers 1. 1800 mg   2. gr $\frac{1}{120}$ 3. 0.12 mg   4. 24.3 or 24.5 kg   5. ℥ 60

Exercises

Reinforce your understanding in class or at home.

1. Convert 75 micrograms to milligrams. _____

2. How many grams does 2.25 kilograms equal? _____

3. 0.003 g = _____ mg

4. 0.005 mg = _____ mcg

5. 6.25 L = _____ mL

6. 0.6 mg = gr _____

7. 0.4 mg = _____ g

8. 0.2 mg = _____ mcg

9. 2400 mL = _____ L

10. gr $3\frac{3}{4}$ = _____ mg

11. $2\frac{1}{2}$ t = _____ gtt

12. gr $\frac{1}{600}$ = _____ mg

13. The prescriber ordered atropine sulfate 0.2 mg sc q6h prn. What is the equivalent dose in micrograms? _____

14. The order reads grains 4 of a drug. Change this order to grams. _____

15. A prescriber has ordered 25 milligrams of captopril (Capoten). What is the equivalent quantity in micrograms? _____

16. According to the medication administration record in Figure 5.3, how many milligrams of glipizide will you give the patient each day? _____

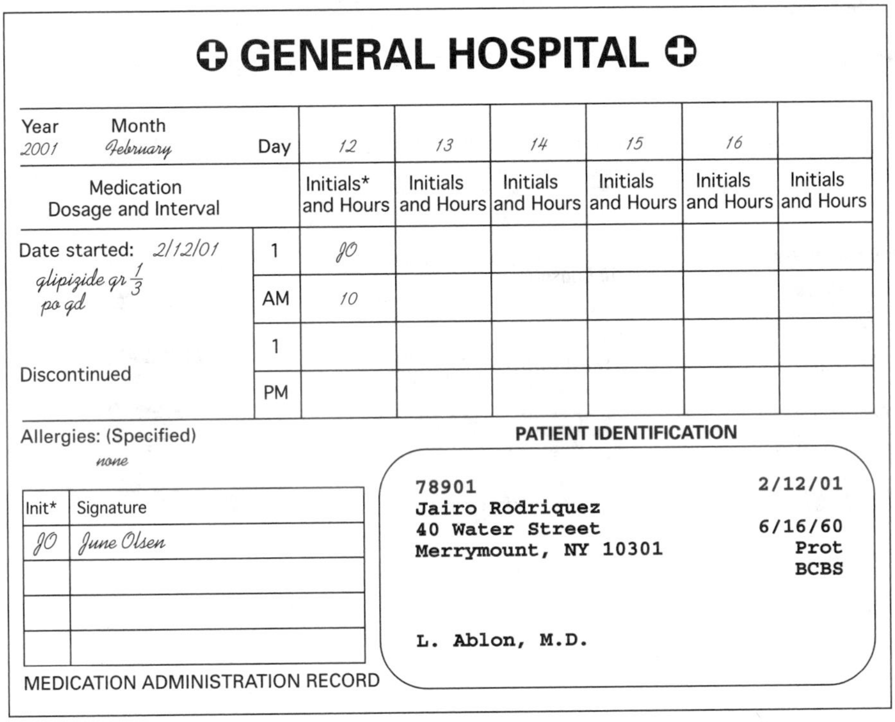

✚ GENERAL HOSPITAL ✚

Year 2001 Month February		Day	12	13	14	15	16	
Medication Dosage and Interval			Initials* and Hours	Initials and Hours	Initials and Hours	Initials and Hours	Initials and Hours	Initials and Hours
Date started: 2/12/01 glipizide gr $\frac{1}{3}$ po qd	1		JO					
	AM		10					
Discontinued	1							
	PM							

Allergies: (Specified)
none

Init*	Signature
JO	June Olsen

PATIENT IDENTIFICATION

```
78901                           2/12/01
Jairo Rodriquez
40 Water Street                 6/16/60
Merrymount, NY 10301              Prot
                                  BCBS


    L. Ablon, M.D.
```

MEDICATION ADMINISTRATION RECORD

▶ **FIGURE 5.3 Medication administration record.**

17. Using the information in Figure 5.4, calculate the number of grams in each tablet. _____

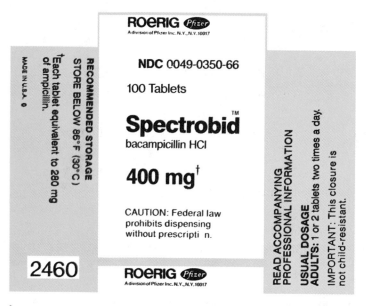

▶ FIGURE 5.4 Drug label for Spectrobid.

18. Read the information on the label in Figure 5.5 and change the milligrams to grains. _____

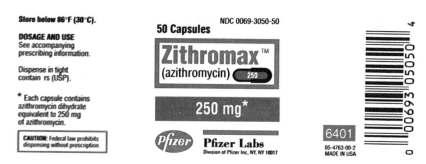

▶ FIGURE 5.5 Drug label for Zithromax.

19. Using the information in Figure 5.6, calculate the number of grams in 1 capsule. _____

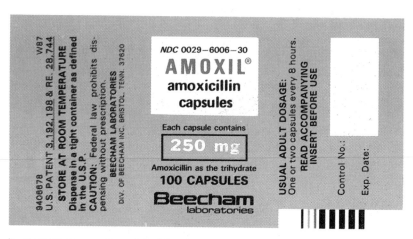

▶ FIGURE 5.6 Drug label for Amoxil.

20. The prescriber ordered K-Lyte/Cl 50. Calculate the number of grams in 1 tablet from the label in Figure 5.7. _____

NDC 0087-0757-42
100 EFFERVESCENT TABLETS
FRUIT PUNCH FLAVOR
K-Lyte/Cl® 50

EACH TABLET IN SOLUTION PROVIDES THE EQUIVALENT OF 50 mEq (3730 mg) POTASSIUM CHLORIDE (SUPPLIED BY 2.24 g POTASSIUM CHLORIDE, 2.0 g POTASSIUM BICARBONATE AND 3.65 g L-LYSINE MONOHYDROCHLORIDE) AND 1.0 g CITRIC ACID.

50 mEq POTASSIUM CHLORIDE (3730 mg)

CAUTION: Federal Law Prohibits Dispensing Without Prescription

BRISTOL LABORATORIES
A Bristol-Myers Company
Evansville, IN 47721

Made in U.S.A.

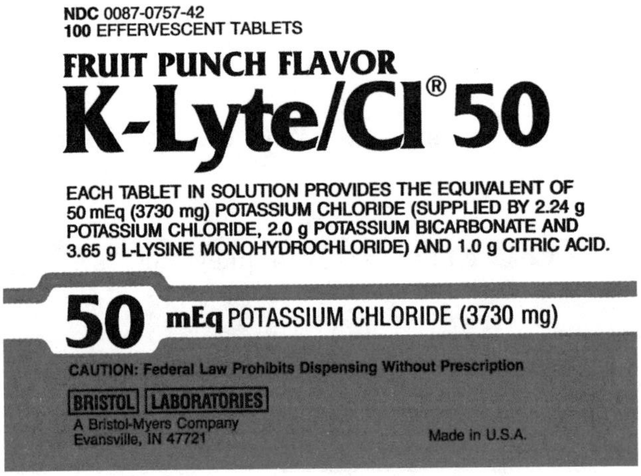

▶ **FIGURE 5.7 Drug label for K-Lyte/Cl 50.**

Additional Exercises

Now, on your own, test yourself! Ask your instructor to check your answers.

1. From the medication administration record in Figure 5.8, calculate the number of grains of digoxin you would prepare. _____

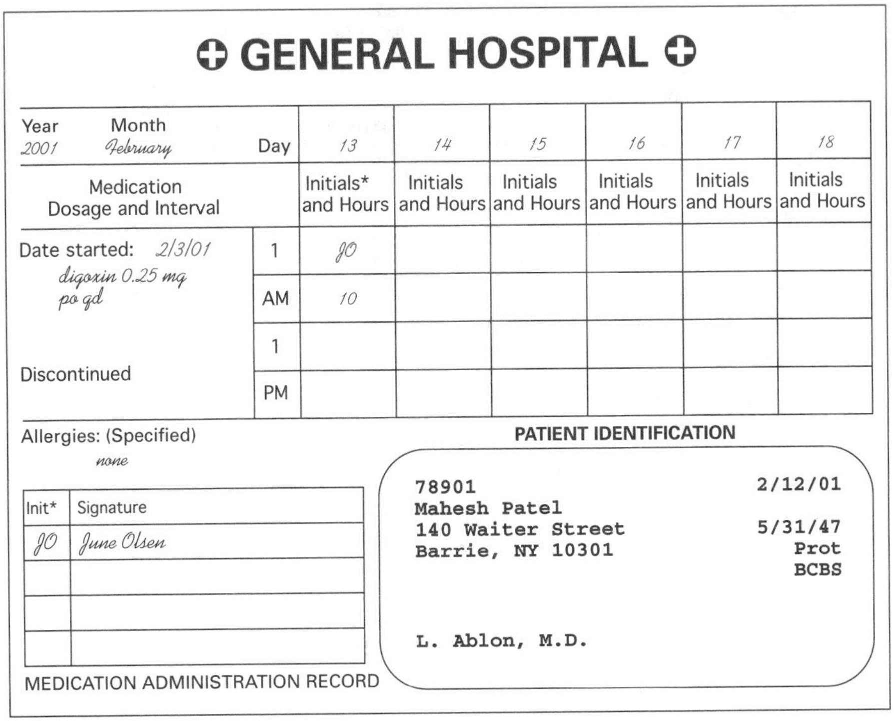

✛ GENERAL HOSPITAL ✛

Year 2001 Month February	Day	13	14	15	16	17	18
Medication Dosage and Interval		Initials* and Hours	Initials and Hours	Initials and Hours	Initials and Hours	Initials and Hours	Initials and Hours
Date started: 2/3/01 digoxin 0.25 mg po qd	1	JO					
	AM	10					
Discontinued	1						
	PM						

Allergies: (Specified)
none

Init*	Signature
JO	June Olsen

PATIENT IDENTIFICATION

78901   2/12/01
Mahesh Patel
140 Waiter Street   5/31/47
Barrie, NY 10301   Prot
                                         BCBS

L. Ablon, M.D.

MEDICATION ADMINISTRATION RECORD

▶ **FIGURE 5.8 Medication administration record.**

2. If a physician orders grain $\frac{1}{150}$ of atropine sulfate, how many milligrams would you administer of this anti-arrhythmic drug? _____

3. The order is 0.5 milligram of digoxin (Lanoxin). Change this quantity to grains. _____

4. The prescriber ordered isoniazid 350 mg po tid. What is the dose of this antitubercular drug in grams? _____

5. An order reads 0.004 gram. Change this quantity to milligrams. _____

6. gr 15 = _____ mg

7. A capsule of acetaminophen (Tylenol), an antipyretic drug, contains 0.5 gram. How much is this in milligrams? _____

8. Using the information in Figure 5.9, calculate the number of grams that are contained in 1 capsule. _____

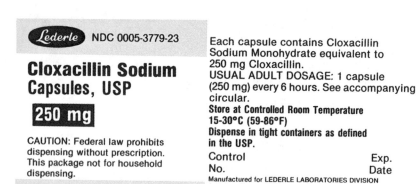

Lederle NDC 0005-3779-23

Cloxacillin Sodium Capsules, USP

250 mg

CAUTION: Federal law prohibits dispensing without prescription. This package not for household dispensing.

100 CAPSULES D1

Each capsule contains Cloxacillin Sodium Monohydrate equivalent to 250 mg Cloxacillin.
USUAL ADULT DOSAGE: 1 capsule (250 mg) every 6 hours. See accompanying circular.
Store at Controlled Room Temperature 15-30°C (59-86°F)
Dispense in tight containers as defined in the USP.

Control   Exp.
No.   Date
Manufactured for LEDERLE LABORATORIES DIVISION American Cyanamid Company, Pearl River, N.Y. 10965 by BIOCRAFT LABORATORIES, INC. Elmwood Park, New Jersey 07407

▶ FIGURE 5.9 Drug label for cloxacillin sodium.

9. 5000 μg = _____ mg

10. Convert 2500 grams to kilograms. _____

11. Change 10,000 micrograms to milligrams. _____

12. 0.005 mg = _____ g

13. 5.5 g = _____ mg

14. 0.012 g = _____ mg

15. 3.75 L = _____ mL

16. The order reads quinidine gluconate 200 mg po q12h. How many grains of this anti-arrhythmic drug are contained in 200 milligrams? _____

17. The order reads 0.02 gram of loratadine (Claritin). How many milligrams equals 0.02 gram? _____

18. Read the information on the label in Figure 5.10. Each tablet contains 100 mg of Darvon-N. Change the milligrams to grains. _____

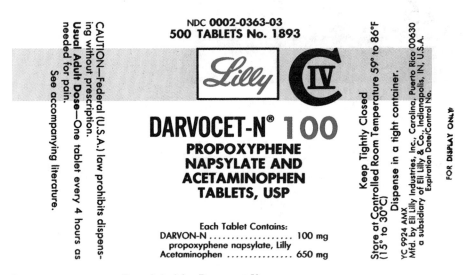

▶ **FIGURE 5.10** Drug label for Darvocet-N.

19. The label in Figure 5.11 is for Cephradine. How many milligrams are contained in 100 capsules? _____

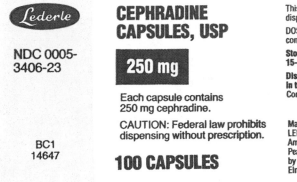

▶ **FIGURE 5.11** Drug label for cephradine.

20. The drug in Figure 5.12 is K-Lyte/Cl. Convert the milligrams to grams. _____

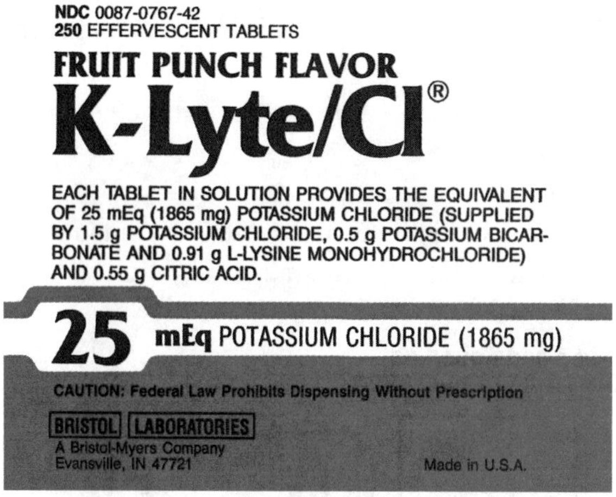

NDC 0087-0767-42
250 EFFERVESCENT TABLETS
FRUIT PUNCH FLAVOR
K-Lyte/Cl®

EACH TABLET IN SOLUTION PROVIDES THE EQUIVALENT OF 25 mEq (1865 mg) POTASSIUM CHLORIDE (SUPPLIED BY 1.5 g POTASSIUM CHLORIDE, 0.5 g POTASSIUM BICARBONATE AND 0.91 g L-LYSINE MONOHYDROCHLORIDE) AND 0.55 g CITRIC ACID.

25 mEq POTASSIUM CHLORIDE (1865 mg)

CAUTION: Federal Law Prohibits Dispensing Without Prescription

BRISTOL LABORATORIES
A Bristol-Myers Company
Evansville, IN 47721   Made in U.S.A.

▶ FIGURE 5.12 Drug label for K-Lyte/Cl.

CUMULATIVE REVIEW EXERCISES

Review your mastery of earlier chapters.

1. 9 mg = _____ mcg

2. 3 t = ℥ _____

3. 0.25 g = gr _____

4. 3 teacups = _____ oz

5. 0.06 g = _____ mg

6. 40 gtt = drams _____

7. 30 mg = gr _____

8. minims 120 = _____ t

9. ℨ 16 = ℥ _____

10. 4 T = _____ mL

11. The order reads 2.25 mg of reserpine (Serpasil), an antihypertensive drug. What would be the equivalent amount in grams? _____

12. The prescriber ordered 2.75 liters of 5% D/W. Convert this quantity to milliliters. _____

13. Read the information on the label in Figure 5.13. Calculate the number of grains in each tablet. _____

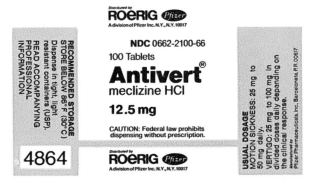

▶ **FIGURE 5.13 Drug label for Antivert.**

14. How many grams are equal to the number of milligrams contained in 1 capsule of the drug cefaclor (Ceclor) shown in Figure 5.14? _____

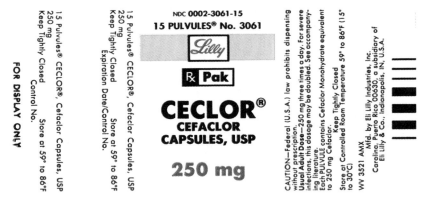

▶ **FIGURE 5.14 Drug label for Ceclor.**

15. The label for Vibramycin is shown in Figure 5.15. Convert the milligrams to grams. _____

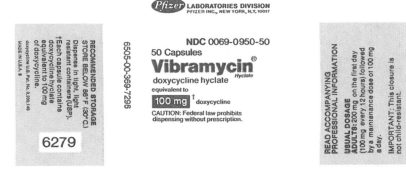

▶ **FIGURE 5.15 Drug label for Vibramycin.**

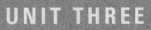

Common Medical Preparations

CHAPTER SIX

Calculating Oral Medication Doses

> ### ▷ Objectives
>
> *After completing this chapter, you will be able to*
>
> - Calculate doses by body weight.
> - Calculate doses by body surface area.
> - Do multistep conversion problems.
> - Calculate doses for oral medications in liquid form.
> - Calculate doses for oral medications in tablet, capsule, and caplet form.
> - Calculate doses for oral medications from the information given on drug labels.

In this chapter you will learn the computations necessary to calculate doses of oral medication in liquid, tablet (tab), capsule (cap), or caplet (cap) form.

ONE-STEP CONVERSIONS

In the calculations you have done in previous chapters, all the equivalents have come from standard tables. For example, 60 mg = gr 1. In this section, the equivalent used will depend on the strength of the drug that is available. In the following examples, the equivalent used is found on the label of the drug container.

▶ **EXAMPLE 6.1**

The order reads 50 milligrams po of Antivert, an antivertigo drug. Read the drug label in Figure 6.1 and determine how many tablets you would administer to the patient.

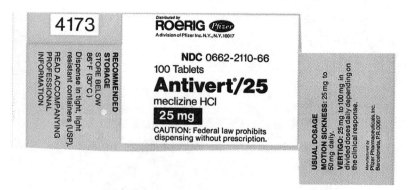

▶ **FIGURE 6.1 Drug label for Antivert.**

You want to convert the order, 50 milligrams, to tablets.

50 mg = ? tab

You want to cancel the milligrams and obtain the equivalent amount in tablets.

$$50 \text{ mg} \times \frac{? \text{ tab}}{? \text{ mg}} = ? \text{ tab}$$

Because the label states that 1 tab = 25 mg, the fraction is $\frac{1 \text{ tab}}{25 \text{ mg}}$.

$$50 \text{ mg} \times \frac{1 \text{ tab}}{25 \text{ mg}} = 2 \text{ tab}$$

So, 50 milligrams is equivalent to 2 tablets, and you would give 2 tablets of Antivert to the patient.

▶ **EXAMPLE 6.2**

The order reads as follows:

Navane 40 mg po qd

The label is shown in Figure 6.2. How many capsules will you administer to the patient?

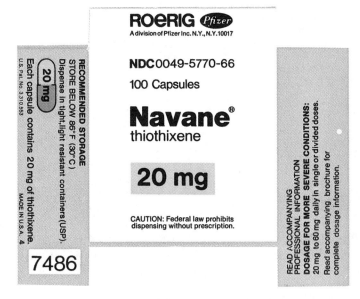

▶ **FIGURE 6.2 Drug label for Navane.**

You want to convert 40 milligrams to capsules.

40 mg = ? cap

You want to cancel the milligrams and calculate the equivalent amount in capsules.

$$40 \text{ mg} \times \frac{? \text{ cap}}{? \text{ mg}} = ? \text{ cap}$$

Because the label indicates that each capsule contains 20 milligrams, you use the equivalent $\frac{1 \text{ cap}}{20 \text{ mg}}$.

$$\overset{2}{\cancel{40 \text{ mg}}} \times \frac{1 \text{ cap}}{\underset{1}{\cancel{20 \text{ mg}}}} = 2 \text{ cap}$$

So, you would administer 2 capsules of Navane to the patient.

___

EXAMPLE 6.3

How many tablets should you give a patient if the order is for grain $\frac{1}{2}$ of codeine sulfate and each tablet contains grain $\frac{1}{4}$?

In this problem you want to convert the order grain $\frac{1}{2}$ to tablets.

$$\text{gr } \frac{1}{2} = ? \text{ tab}$$

You want to cancel the grain and determine the equivalent amount in tablets.

$$\text{gr } \frac{1}{2} \times \frac{? \text{ tab}}{? \text{ gr}} = ? \text{ tab}$$

Because 1 tab = gr $\frac{1}{4}$, the fraction is $\frac{1 \text{ tab}}{\text{gr} \frac{1}{4}}$.

$$\cancel{\text{gr}} \frac{1}{2} \times \frac{1 \text{ tab}}{\cancel{\text{gr}} \frac{1}{4}} = \frac{1 \text{ tab}}{\frac{2}{4}} = 1 \text{ tab} \div \frac{2}{4} = 1 \text{ tab} \times \frac{4}{2} = 2 \text{ tab}$$

So, grain $\frac{1}{2}$ is equivalent to 2 tablets, and you should give the patient 2 tablets of codeine sulfate.

▶ EXAMPLE 6.4

The order reads 6 milligrams of the antihypertensive drug Cardura. The label indicates that each scored tablet contains 4 milligrams of Cardura. How many scored tablets should be given to the patient po?

You want to convert the order, 6 milligrams, to tablets.

$\quad$ 6 mg = ? tab

You want to cancel the milligrams and obtain the equivalent amount in tablets.

$$6 \text{ mg} \times \frac{? \text{ tab}}{? \text{ mg}} = ? \text{ tab}$$

Since each tablet contains 4 milligrams, the equivalent fraction is $\frac{1 \text{ tab}}{4 \text{ mg}}$.

$$6 \cancel{\text{ mg}} \times \frac{1 \text{ tab}}{4 \cancel{\text{ mg}}} = 1\frac{1}{2} \text{ tab}$$

So, 6 milligrams is equivalent to $1\frac{1}{2}$ tablets, and the patient should be given $1\frac{1}{2}$ tablets of Cardura.

▶ EXAMPLE 6.5

The prescriber orders 0.3 milligram of the antiadrenergic drug clonidine. Examine the drug label shown in Figure 6.3 and determine how many of these tablets you would give the patient.

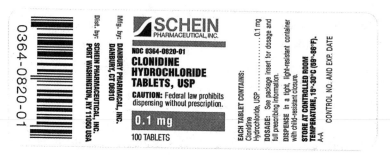

▶ FIGURE 6.3 Drug label for clonidine.

You want to convert 0.3 milligram to tablets.

0.3 mg = ? tab

You want to cancel the milligrams and obtain the equivalent amount in tablets.

$$0.3 \text{ mg} \times \frac{? \text{ tab}}{? \text{ mg}} = ? \text{ tab}$$

Because 1 tab = 0.1 mg, the equivalent fraction is $\frac{1 \text{ tab}}{0.1 \text{ mg}}$.

$$0.3 \text{ mg} \times \frac{1 \text{ tab}}{0.1 \text{ mg}} = \frac{0.3}{0.1} \text{ tab} = 3 \text{ tab}$$

So, 0.3 milligram is equivalent to 3 tablets, and you would give 3 tablets of clonidine to the patient.

DOSAGE BY BODY WEIGHT

Sometimes the amount of medication prescribed depends on the patient's body weight. A patient who weighs more will receive more of the drug, and a patient who weighs less will receive less of the drug.

▶ **E X A M P L E   6 . 6**

The prescriber orders 15 milligrams per kilogram of methsuximide (Celontin) for a patient who weighs 80 kilograms. How much of this anticonvulsant drug should the patient receive?

N O T E

The expression 15 mg/kg means that the patient is to receive 15 milligrams of the drug for each kilogram of body weight. So you will use the equivalent 15 mg (of drug) = 1 kg (of body weight).

You want to convert body weight to dosage.

80 kg (of body weight) = ? mg (of drug)

$$80 \text{ kg (of body weight)} \times \frac{? \text{ mg (of drug)}}{? \text{ kg (of body weight)}} = \text{mg (of drug)}$$

So, you use the fraction $\frac{15 \text{ mg}}{1 \text{ kg}}$, which relates dosage to body weight.

$$80 \text{ kg} \times \frac{15 \text{ mg}}{1 \text{ kg}} = 1200 \text{ mg}$$

So, the patient should receive 1200 milligrams of methsuximide.

▶ **EXAMPLE 6.7**

The order is 6 milligrams per kilogram of the antitubercular drug, rifampin (Rifadin). How many milligrams would you administer to a patient who weighs 75 kilograms?

You want to convert body weight to dosage.

$$75 \text{ kg} = ? \text{ mg}$$

$$75 \text{ kg} \times \frac{? \text{ mg}}{? \text{ kg}} = ? \text{ mg}$$

You use the equivalent 6 mg = 1 kg. So, the fraction you use is $\frac{6 \text{ mg}}{1 \text{ kg}}$.

$$75 \text{ kg} \times \frac{6 \text{ mg}}{1 \text{ kg}} = 450 \text{ mg}$$

So, the patient should receive 450 milligrams of rifampin.

CALCULATING DOSAGE BY BODY SURFACE AREA

In many cases, body surface area (BSA) is a more important factor than weight in determining appropriate drug dosages. This is particularly true of pediatric drugs and drugs that are used for cancer therapy.

A patient's BSA, which is measured in square meters (m^2), can be determined by using either of the mathematical formulas below or by using a nomogram.

Formula for metric units

$$BSA = \sqrt{\frac{\text{weight in kg} \times \text{height in centimeters}}{3600}}$$

Formula for household units

$$BSA = \sqrt{\frac{\text{weight in lb} \times \text{height in inches}}{3131}}$$

▶ **EXAMPLE 6.8**

Find the BSA of an adult who is 183 cm tall and weighs 92 kg.

Because we are using metric units (kg and cm), we use the formula

$$BSA = \sqrt{\frac{\text{weight in kg} \times \text{height in centimeters}}{3600}}$$

$$= \sqrt{\frac{92 \times 183}{3600}}$$

At this point we need a calculator with a square root key.

$$= \sqrt{4.6767}$$

$$= 2.16 \text{ m}^2$$

NOTE

In this book, we will round off BSA to two decimal places.

▶ **EXAMPLE 6.9**

What is the BSA of a man who is 4 feet 10 inches tall and weighs 142 pounds? First you convert 4 feet 10 inches to 58 inches.

Because we are using household units (lb and in), we use the formula

$$\text{BSA} = \sqrt{\frac{\text{weight in lb} \times \text{height in inches}}{3131}}$$

$$= \sqrt{\frac{142 \times 58}{3131}}$$

$$= \sqrt{2.6305}$$

$$= 1.62 \text{ m}^2$$

NOMOGRAM

BSA can also be approximated by using nomograms. As Figure 6.4 shows, if a straight line is drawn on the nomogram from the patient's height (left column) to the patient's weight (right column), the line will cross the center column at the approximate BSA of this patient.

In Example 6.8, we used the formula to calculate the BSA of a 183 cm, 92 kg patient to be 2.16 m². Now let's use the adult nomogram to do the same problem. In Figure 6.5, you can see that the line from 183 cm to 92 kg intersects the BSA column at about 2.20 m².

NOTE

Whether formulas or nomograms are used to obtain body surface area, the results are only approximations. This explains why we obtained both 2.16 m² (using the formula) and 2.20 m² (using the nomogram) as BSA for the same patient.

In Example 6.9, using the formula we calculated the BSA of a 4 ft 10 in, 142 lb patient to be 1.62 m². If we use the adult nomogram to determine the BSA (see Figure 6.6), we get 1.59 m².

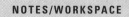
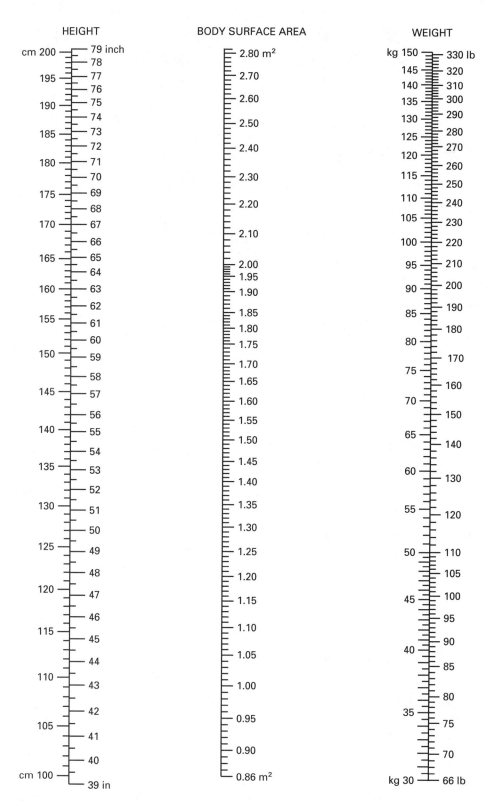

▶ FIGURE 6.4 Adult nomogram. *Source:* From *Davis's Drug Guide for Nurses,*
5th ed. (p. 1276) by J. H. Deglin and A. H. Vallerand, 1997,
Philadelphia: Davis.

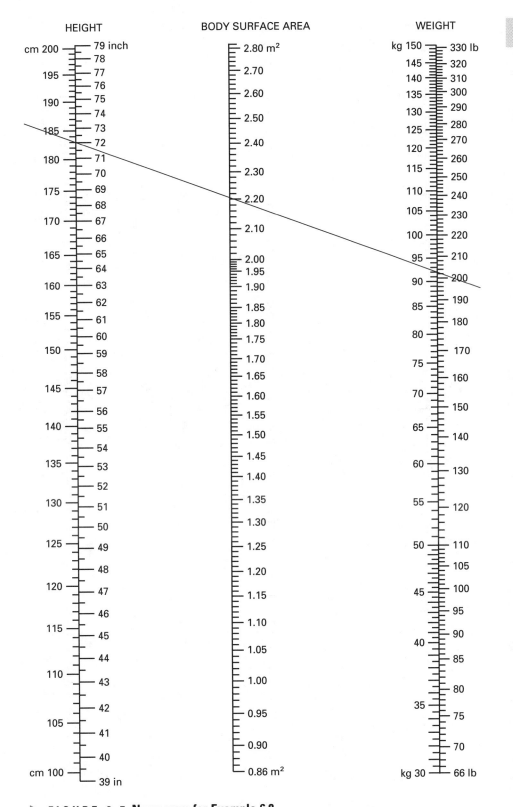

FIGURE 6.5 Nomogram for Example 6.8.

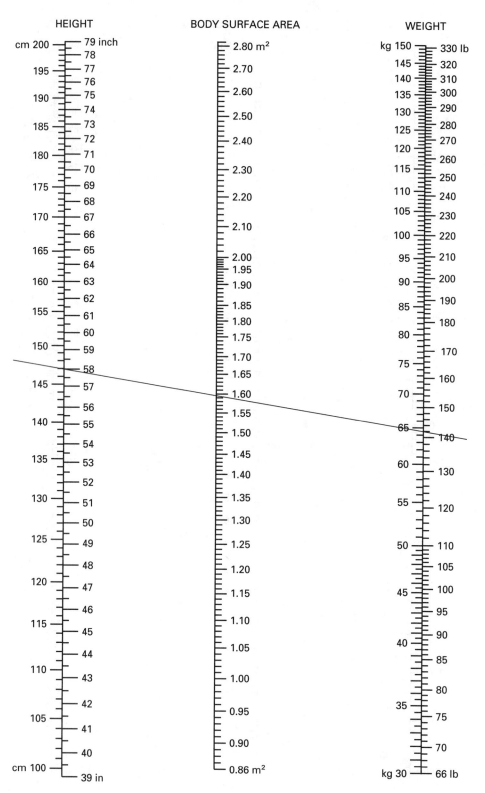

HEIGHT

BODY SURFACE AREA

WEIGHT

▶ F I G U R E 6.6 Nomogram for Example 6.9.

▶ **E X A M P L E   6 . 1 0**

The order is 40 mg/m^2 of the corticosteroid prednisone (Deltasone). How many milligrams of this adrenocorticoid drug would you administer to an adult patient weighing 88 kg with a height of 150 cm?

The first step is to determine the BSA of the patient. This can be done by formula or nomogram.

Using the formula, you get

$$\text{BSA} = \sqrt{\frac{88 \times 150}{3600}}$$

$$= \sqrt{3.6667}$$

$$= 1.91 \text{ m}^2$$

With the adult nomogram, you get 1.81 m^2. So, you can use either 1.91 m^2 or 1.81 m^2 as the BSA. If you chose to use 1.81 m^2, you want to convert BSA to dosage in mg.

$$1.81 \text{ m}^2 = ? \text{ mg}$$

$$1.81 \text{ m}^2 \times \frac{? \text{ mg}}{\text{m}^2} = ? \text{ mg}$$

You use the equivalent 40 mg/m^2, so the fraction you use is $\frac{40 \text{ mg}}{\text{m}^2}$.

$$1.81 \text{ m}^2 \times \frac{40 \text{ mg}}{\text{m}^2} = 72.4 \text{ mg}$$

However, if you use the BSA of 1.91 m^2, the calculations would be similar and the last step would be

$$1.91 \text{ m}^2 \times \frac{40 \text{ mg}}{\text{m}^2} = 76.4 \text{ mg}$$

So, you would administer between 72.4 mg and 76.4 mg of prednisone to the patient.

▶ **E X A M P L E   6 . 1 1**

The prescriber ordered 0.15 mg/m^2 of digoxin for a patient who has a BSA of 1.65 m^2. How many milligrams of this anti-arrhythmic drug would you administer to your patient?

In this case, you know the BSA. You want to convert the BSA 1.65 m^2 to dosage.

$$1.65 \text{ m}^2 = ? \text{ mg (of drug)}$$

$$1.65 \text{ m}^2 \times \frac{? \text{ mg}}{\text{m}^2} = ? \text{ mg (of drug)}$$

So, you use the fraction $\frac{0.15 \text{ mg}}{\text{m}^2}$, which relates dosage to BSA.

$$1.65 \text{ m}^2 \times \frac{0.15 \text{ mg}}{\text{m}^2} = 0.25 \text{ mg}$$

So, the patient should receive 0.25 mg of digoxin.

MULTISTEP CONVERSIONS

Sometimes drug dosage calculations involve more than one step. For example, suppose you want to find out how many seconds are in 2 hours. You can do this conversion in two steps.

Step 1   Change hours to minutes. Because 60 minutes is 1 hour, the fraction to change hours to minutes is $\frac{60 \text{ min}}{1 \text{ hr}}$.

$$2 \text{ hr} \times \frac{60 \text{ min}}{1 \text{ hr}}$$

Step 2   Change minutes to seconds. Because 60 seconds is 1 minute, the fraction to change minutes to seconds is $\frac{60 \text{ sec}}{1 \text{ min}}$.

$$2 \text{ hr} \times \frac{60 \text{ min}}{1 \text{ hr}} \times \frac{60 \text{ sec}}{1 \text{ min}}$$

Cancel hours and minutes.

$$2 \text{ hr} \times \frac{60 \text{ min}}{1 \text{ hr}} \times \frac{60 \text{ sec}}{1 \text{ min}} = \frac{2 \times 60 \times 60}{1} \text{ sec} = 7200 \text{ sec}$$

This is the general method you will use in the following examples. When you do this kind of calculation, you must make sure that each equivalent fraction you use is equal to 1 and that it gives the units needed.

▶ EXAMPLE 6.12

The order is 600 milligrams of acetylsalicylic acid (aspirin); grains 5 caplets are available. How many caplets of this antipyretic should be given to the patient?

In this problem, you need to convert 600 milligrams to grains and then convert grains to caplets.

$$600 \text{ mg} \longrightarrow \text{gr ?} \longrightarrow \text{? cap}$$

This is done in two steps as follows:

Step 1   Change milligrams to grains.

$$600 \text{ mg} \times \frac{\text{gr ?}}{\text{? mg}}$$

Step 2   Change grains to caplets.

$$600 \text{ mg} \times \frac{\text{gr ?}}{\text{? mg}} \times \frac{\text{? cap}}{\text{gr ?}} = \text{? cap}$$

Because gr 1 = 60 mg, the first fraction is $\frac{\text{gr } 1}{60 \text{ mg}}$. Since 1 cap = gr 5, the second fraction is $\frac{1 \text{ cap}}{\text{gr } 5}$.

$$\overset{10}{\cancel{600}} \text{ mg} \times \frac{\cancel{\text{gr }} 1}{\cancel{60} \text{ mg}} \times \frac{1 \text{ cap}}{\cancel{\text{gr }} 5} = 2 \text{ cap}$$

So, 600 milligrams are equivalent to 2 caplets, and 2 caplets of aspirin should be given to the patient.

NOTE

Equivalent values for units of weight are given in Table 5.1. By this point, however, you should have all the equivalent values memorized.

▶ **EXAMPLE 6.13**

The order is 0.4 milligram per kilogram tid of piroxicam (Feldene) for a patient who weighs 50 kilograms. Read the drug label in Figure 6.7 and determine the number of capsules of this anti-inflammatory drug you would give to the patient.

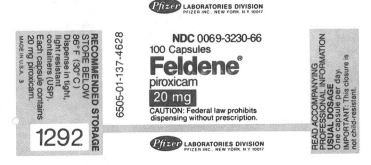

▶ **FIGURE 6.7 Drug label for Feldene.**

In this problem you want to convert 50 kilograms to milligrams and then convert milligrams to capsules.

$$50 \text{ kg} \longrightarrow ? \text{ mg} \longrightarrow ? \text{ cap}$$

This is done in two steps.

Step 1   Change body weight in kilograms to dosage in milligrams.

$$50 \text{ kg} \times \frac{? \text{ mg}}{? \text{ kg}}$$

Step 2   Change milligrams to capsules.

$$50 \text{ kg} \times \frac{? \text{ mg}}{? \text{ kg}} \times \frac{? \text{ cap}}{? \text{ mg}} = ? \text{ cap}$$

Because the patient is to receive 0.4 milligram of piroxicam per kilogram of body weight, the first equivalent fraction is $\frac{0.4\ mg}{1\ kg}$. Because the label indicates that 1 cap = 20 mg, the second equivalent fraction is $\frac{1\ cap}{20\ mg}$.

$$50\ \cancel{kg} \times \frac{0.4\ \cancel{mg}}{1\ \cancel{kg}} \times \frac{1\ cap}{20\ \cancel{mg}} = \frac{20}{20}\ cap = 1\ cap$$

So, the patient should receive 1 capsule of piroxicam.

▶ E X A M P L E   6.14

The order is 0.5 gram of the antibiotic cefaclor (Ceclor). Read the label shown in Figure 6.8 and calculate how many capsules should be given.

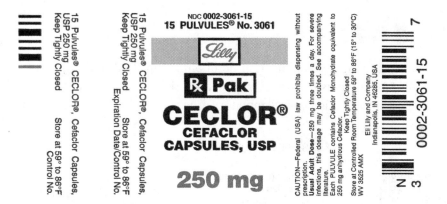

▶ F I G U R E   6.8 Drug label for Ceclor.

In this problem you want to convert 0.5 gram to milligrams and then convert milligrams to capsules.

$$0.5\ g \longrightarrow ?\ mg \longrightarrow ?\ cap$$

Do the two steps on one line as follows:

$$0.5\ g \times \frac{?\ mg}{?\ g} \times \frac{?\ cap}{?\ mg} = ?\ cap$$

Because 1000 mg = 1 g, the first equivalent fraction is $\frac{1000\ mg}{1\ g}$. Because 250 mg = 1 cap, the second equivalent fraction is $\frac{1\ cap}{250\ mg}$.

$$0.5\ \cancel{g} \times \frac{1000\ \cancel{mg}}{1\ \cancel{g}} \times \frac{1\ cap}{250\ \cancel{mg}} = \frac{500}{250}\ cap = 2\ cap$$

So, 0.5 gram is equivalent to 2 capsules, and 2 capsules of Ceclor should be given to the patient.

NOTE

Sometimes prescribed oral medications are in liquid form. The calculations for these drugs follow the same format you have been using. The label will always state how much drug is contained in a certain amount of liquid.

EXAMPLE 6.15

The prescriber orders 0.5 gram of the antibiotic erythromycin (EryPed 200). Study the label shown in Figure 6.9 and calculate how many milliliters you will administer.

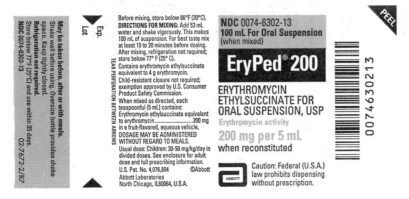

▶ **FIGURE 6.9 Drug label for EryPed.**

In this problem you want to convert 0.5 gram to milligrams and then convert milligrams to milliliters.

$$0.5 \text{ g} \longrightarrow \text{? mg} \longrightarrow \text{? mL}$$

You do the two steps on one line as follows:

$$0.5 \text{ g} \times \frac{\text{? mg}}{\text{? g}} \times \frac{1 \text{ mL}}{\text{? mg}} = \text{? mL}$$

Because 1000 mg = 1 g, the first equivalent fraction is $\frac{1000 \text{ mg}}{1 \text{ g}}$. The label on the bottle indicates that 5 mL contains 200 milligrams of erythromycin. So, the second equivalent fraction is $\frac{5 \text{ mL}}{200 \text{ mg}}$.

$$0.5 \text{ g} \times \frac{\overset{5}{\cancel{1000} \text{ mg}}}{1 \text{ g}} \times \frac{5 \text{ mL}}{\underset{1}{\cancel{200} \text{ mg}}} = 12.5 \text{ mL}$$

So, you would administer 12.5 mL of erythromycin.

▶ **E X A M P L E   6 . 1 6**

The patient is to receive 0.374 gram of the antibiotic cefaclor (Ceclor). Read the information on the drug label in Figure 6.10 and determine how many milliliters you would administer.

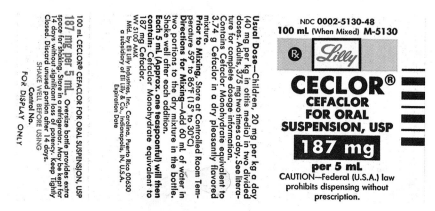

▶ **F I G U R E   6 . 1 0 Drug label for Ceclor.**

The label on the bottle reads 187 milligrams per 5 milliliters. This means that each 5 milliliters of liquid contains 187 milligrams of cefaclor. In this problem you want to convert 0.374 gram to milligrams and then get its equivalent in milliliters.

$$0.374 \text{ g} \longrightarrow ? \text{ mg} \longrightarrow ? \text{ mL}$$

Do this on one line as follows:

$$0.374 \text{ g} \times \frac{? \text{ mg}}{? \text{ g}} \times \frac{? \text{ mL}}{? \text{ mg}} = ? \text{ mL}$$

Because 1000 mg = 1 g, the first equivalent fraction is $\frac{1000 \text{ mg}}{1 \text{ g}}$. Because 5 mL = 187 mg, the second equivalent fraction is $\frac{5 \text{ mL}}{187 \text{ mg}}$.

$$0.374 \text{ g} \times \frac{1000 \text{ mg}}{1 \text{ g}} \times \frac{5 \text{ mL}}{187 \text{ mg}} = 10 \text{ mL}$$

So, you would administer 10 milliliters of cefaclor.

▶ **E X A M P L E   6 . 1 7**

The prescriber orders 0.0075 gram po of clorazepate (Tranxene), an antianxiety drug. Study the information on the label shown in Figure 6.11 and calculate the number of tablets of this drug you would administer.

The label on the bottle reads 7.5 milligrams per tablet. In this problem you want to convert 0.0075 gram to milligrams and then get its equivalent in tablets.

$$0.0075 \text{ g} \longrightarrow ? \text{ mg} \longrightarrow ? \text{ tab}$$

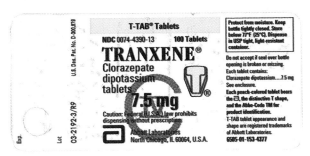

Do this on one line as follows:

$$0.0075 \text{ g} \times \frac{? \text{ mg}}{? \text{ g}} \times \frac{? \text{ tab}}{? \text{ mg}} = ? \text{ tab}$$

Because 1000 mg = 1 g, the first equivalent fraction is $\frac{1000 \text{ mg}}{1 \text{ g}}$. Because 1 tab = 7.5 mg, the second equivalent fraction is $\frac{1 \text{ tab}}{7.5 \text{ mg}}$.

$$0.0075 \cancel{\text{g}} \times \frac{1000 \cancel{\text{mg}}}{1 \cancel{\text{g}}} \times \frac{1 \text{ tab}}{7.5 \cancel{\text{mg}}} = 1 \text{ tab}$$

So, you would administer 1 tablet of Tranxene.

NOTE

In Example 6.18, the unit value is milliequivalents. Electrolytes are usually measured in milliequivalents, which is abbreviated mEq. Recently, pharmaceutical companies have begun to label their electrolytes in milligrams as well as milliequivalents. For example, oral potassium chloride might be labeled

10 mEq = 750 mg (see label 6.12)

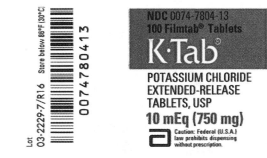

▶ **FIGURE 6.12 Drug label for K-Tab**

EXAMPLE 6.18

The order for Mr. Jones is 15 milliequivalents of potassium chloride (K-Lor, Kay Ciel). The label on the bottle reads 10 milliequivalents in 5 cubic centimeters. How many drams of this electrolyte would you administer?

In this problem you want to change 15 milliequivalents to drams. You must first convert 15 milliequivalents to cubic centimeters and then convert cubic centimeters to drams.

$$15 \text{ mEq} \longrightarrow ? \text{ cc} \longrightarrow \text{Ʒ } ?$$

Do this on one line as follows:

$$15 \text{ mEq} \times \frac{? \text{ cc}}{? \text{ mEq}} \times \frac{\text{Ʒ } ?}{? \text{ cc}} = \text{Ʒ } ?$$

The label on the bottle indicates that every 5 cubic centimeters of liquid contains 10 milliequivalents of potassium chloride. So, the first fraction is $\frac{5 \text{ cc}}{10 \text{ mEq}}$. Because Ʒ 1 = 5 cc, the second fraction is $\frac{\text{Ʒ } 1}{5 \text{ cc}}$.

$$15 \text{ mEq} \times \frac{5 \text{ cc}}{10 \text{ mEq}} \times \frac{\text{Ʒ } 1}{5 \text{ cc}} = \text{Ʒ}\frac{15}{10} \text{ or } \text{Ʒ } 1\frac{1}{2}$$

So, you would administer drams $1\frac{1}{2}$ of potassium chloride to the patient.

PRACTICE READING LABELS

Calculate the following doses using the labels shown. (You will find the answers to *Practice Reading Labels* in Appendix A at the back of the book.)

1. Cephalexin 1 g = _____ cap

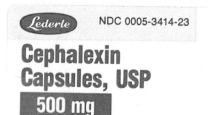

Lederle NDC 0005-3414-23

Cephalexin Capsules, USP

500 mg

CAUTION: Federal law prohibits dispensing without prescription. This package not for household dispensing.

100 CAPSULES BC1 18121

Each capsule contains cephalexin monohydrate equivalent to 500 mg cephalexin. Usual Adult Dose: 250 mg every 6 hours. For more severe infections, dose may be increased, not to exceed 4 g a day. See accompanying literature. **Store at Controlled Room Temperature 15-30°C (59-86°F). Keep Tightly Closed.** Dispense in tight containers as defined in the USP.

Control No.   Exp. Date

Manufactured for LEDERLE LABORATORIES DIVISION American Cyanamid Company Pearl River, NY 10965 by BIOCRAFT LABORATORIES, INC., Elmwood Park, NJ 07407

2. Voltaren 0.15 g = _____ tab

Exp
Lot
Dispense in tight container (USP).
Do not store above 86°F.
Protect from moisture.
Dosage: See package insert.
PHARMACIST: Container closure is not child-resistant.
GEIGY Pharmaceuticals Division of CIBA–GEIGY Corporation Ardsley, NY 10502

NDC **0028-0164-01** FSC **8830**
6505-01-290-4661

Voltaren® **75**mg
diclofenac sodium

100 enteric-coated tablets

Caution: Federal law prohibits dispensing without prescription.

Geigy

3 0028-0164-01 1

644253

3. Declomycin 0.3 g = _____ tab

Declomycin®
Lederle

Demeclocycline Hydrochloride
Tablets 300 mg (Film Coated)

CAUTION: Federal law prohibits
dispensing without prescription.
This package not for household
dispensing.
48 TABLETS   94439   D7

Exp. Date

Control No.

NDC 0005-9270-29

Average Adult Dosage:
600 mg daily divided into two
doses. See Accompanying Literature.
Store at Controlled Room Temperature
15-30ºC (59-86ºF)
Dispense in tight containers
as defined in the USP.   Made in U.S.A.

LEDERLE LABORATORIES DIVISION
American Cyanamid Company
Pearl River, N.Y. 10965

4. Vibramycin 200 mg = _____ cap

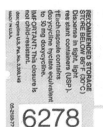

RECOMMENDED STORAGE
STORE BELOW 86°F (30°C)
Dispense in tight, light
resistant containers (USP).
†Each capsule contains
doxycycline hyclate equivalent
to 50 mg doxycycline.
IMPORTANT: This closure is
not child-resistant.
MADE IN U.S.A.
doxycycline U.S. Pat. No. 3,200,149
05-2169-77-5

6505-00-812-254

NDC 0069-0940-50
50 Capsules

Vibramycin®
Hyclate

equivalent to
50 mg† doxycycline

CAUTION: Federal law prohibits
dispensing without prescription.

6278

READ ACCOMPANYING
PROFESSIONAL INFORMATION

USUAL DOSAGE
Adults: 200 mg on the first day (100 mg
every 12 hours) followed by a maintenance
dose of 100 mg a day.
Children above eight years of age: Under
100 lb —2 mg/lb on the first day followed
by 1 mg/lb on subsequent days.
Over 100 lb —See adult dosage.

5. DynaCirc CR 0.01 g = _____ tab

Store and dispense: Below 86°F (30°C) in
a tight container, protected from moisture
and humidity.
See package insert for dosage information.
20522103
2212-41
LOT
EXP.

⚠ **SANDOZ**   NDC 0078-0236-05

DynaCirc CR®
(isradipine)
Controlled Release Tablets
10 mg GITS

100 Tablets

CAUTION: Federal law prohibits
dispensing without prescription.

3 0078-0236-05 8

Sandoz Pharmaceuticals Corporation
East Hanover, New Jersey 07936

6. Vistaril 200 mg = _____ cap

RECOMMENDED STORAGE
STORE BELOW 86° F (30°C)
Dispense in tight, light
resistant containers (USP).
Each capsule contains
hydroxyzine pamoate
equivalent to **100mg**
hydroxyzine hydrochloride.
MADE IN U.S.A. 5

Pfizer **LABORATORIES DIVISION**
PFIZER INC., NEW YORK, N.Y. 10017

NDC 0069-5430-66
100 Capsules

Vistaril®
hydroxyzine pamoate
equivalent to
100mg of hydroxyzine HCl

TARTRAZINE
DYE FREE

CAUTION: Federal law prohibits
dispensing without prescription.

4377

READ ACCOMPANYING
PROFESSIONAL INFORMATION

DOSAGE
ADULTS: 25 mg t.i.d. to 100 mg q.i.d.
CHILDREN: Under 6 years—50 mg
daily in divided doses.
Over 6 years—50 to 100 mg
daily in divided doses.

7. Ceclor 112 mg = _____ mL

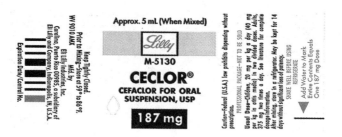

8. Atarax 50 mg = _____ tab

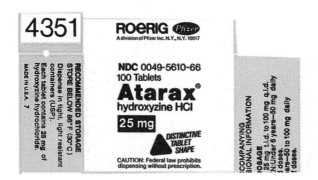

9. Clonidine hydrochloride gr $\dfrac{1}{600}$ = _____ tab

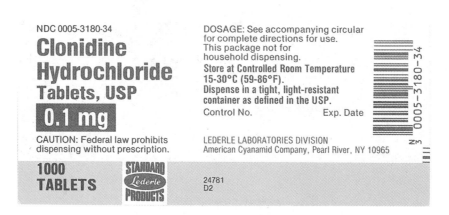

10. DynaCirc CR 5000 μg = _____ tab

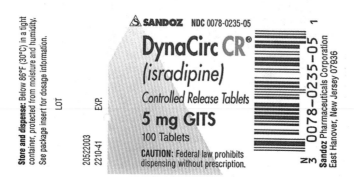

11. Ceclor 0.5 g = _____ cap

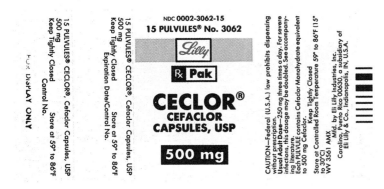

12. Cataflam 0.1 g = _____ tab

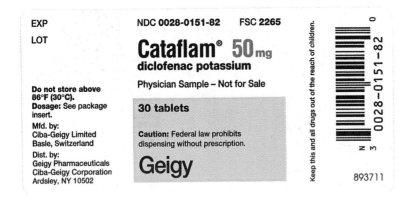

13. Parlodel 1.25 mg = _____ tab

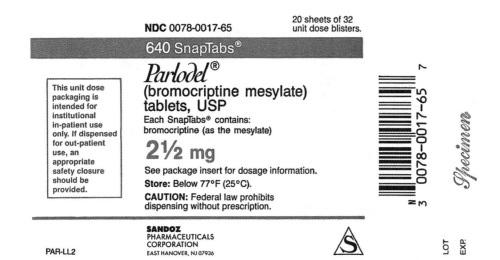

14. Tegretol 0.4 g = _____ tab

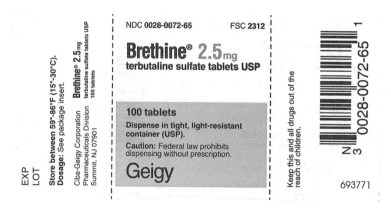

15. Terbutaline 7.5 mg = _____ tab

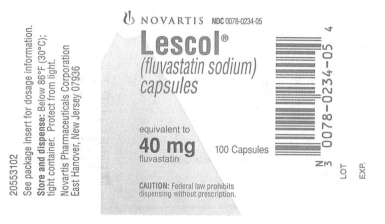

16. Fluvastatin sodium 0.08 g = _____ cap

17. Restoril 0.03 g = _____ cap

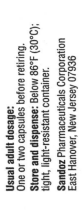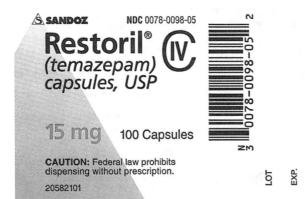

Usual adult dosage:
One or two capsules before retiring.
Store and dispense: Below 86°F (30°C);
tight, light-resistant container.
Sandoz Pharmaceuticals Corporation
East Hanover, New Jersey 07936

△ SANDOZ   NDC 0078-0098-05

Restoril® (IV)
(temazepam)
capsules, USP

15 mg   100 Capsules

CAUTION: Federal law prohibits
dispensing without prescription.

20582101

LOT   EXP.

18. Nortriptyline HCl 0.1 g = _____ cap

Store and dispense:
Below 86°F (30°C); tight container.
See package insert for dosage
information.
Novartis Pharmaceuticals Corporation
East Hanover, New Jersey 07936

NOVARTIS   NDC 0078-0078-05

Pamelor®
(nortriptyline HCl)
capsules, USP

equivalent to
50 mg   100 Capsules
base

CAUTION: Federal law prohibits
dispensing without prescription.

20575202

LOT   EXP.

19. Augmentin 400 mg = _____ mL

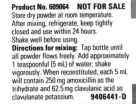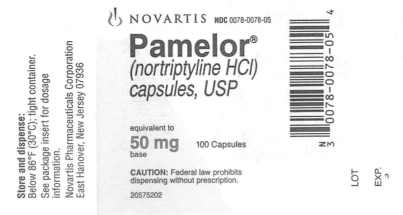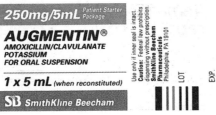

Product No. 609064   **NOT FOR SALE**
Store dry powder at room temperature.
After mixing, refrigerate, keep tightly
closed and use within 24 hours.
Shake well before using.
Directions for mixing: Tap bottle until
all powder flows freely. Add approximately
1 teaspoonful (5 mL) of water; shake
vigorously. When reconstituted, each 5 mL
will contain 250 mg amoxicillin as the
trihydrate and 62.5 mg clavulanic acid as
clavulanate potassium.   **9406441-D**

250mg/5mL Patient Starter
Package

AUGMENTIN®
**AMOXICILLIN/CLAVULANATE
POTASSIUM
FOR ORAL SUSPENSION**

1 x 5 mL *(when reconstituted)*

SB **SmithKline Beecham**

Use only if inner seal is intact.
Caution: Federal law prohibits
dispensing without prescription.
**SmithKline Beecham
Pharmaceuticals**
Philadelphia, PA 19101

LOT   EXP.

20. Cloxacillin sodium 1000 mg = _____ cap

Lederle   NDC 0005-3780-23

Cloxacillin Sodium Capsules, USP

500 mg

CAUTION: Federal law prohibits dispensing without prescription. This package not for household dispensing.

100 CAPSULES   D1

Each capsule contains Cloxacillin Sodium Monohydrate equivalent to 500 mg Cloxacillin.
USUAL ADULT DOSAGE: 1 capsule (500 mg) every 6 hours. See accompanying circular.
Store at Controlled Room Temperature 15-30°C (59-86°F)
Dispense in tight containers as defined in the USP.

Control No.   Exp. Date

Manufactured for LEDERLE LABORATORIES DIVISION American Cyanamid Company, Pearl River, N.Y. 10965 by BIOCRAFT LABORATORIES, INC. Elmwood Park, New Jersey 07407

21. Imipramine parnoate 0.075 g = _____ cap

NDC 0028-0020-26   FSC 2002

Tofranil-PM® 75 mg*
imipramine pamoate

*Each capsule contains imipramine pamoate equivalent to 75 mg of imipramine hydrochloride

30 capsules

Do not store above 86°F.

Geigy

Dispense in tight container (USP).

Caution: Federal law prohibits dispensing without prescription.

Tofranil-PM® 75 mg* imipramine pamoate *Each capsule contains imipramine pamoate equiv. to 75 mg of imipramine HCl. 30 capsules

Exp Lot

642606

6505-00-502-9595 Dosage: See package insert. GEIGY Pharmaceuticals Division of CIBA–GEIGY Corp. Ardsley, NY 10502

22. Temazepam 0.03 g = _____ cap

SANDOZ   NDC 0078-0099-05

Restoril® (IV)
(temazepam)
capsules, USP

30 mg   100 Capsules

CAUTION: Federal law prohibits dispensing without prescription.
20582201

Usual adult dosage:
One capsule before retiring.
Store and dispense: Below 86°F (30°C); tight, light-resistant container.

Sandoz Pharmaceuticals Corporation East Hanover, New Jersey 07936

LOT   EXP.

23. Haloperidol gr $\dfrac{1}{120}$ = _____ tab

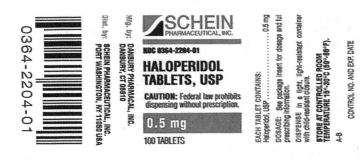

24. Parlodel 0.005 g = _____ cap

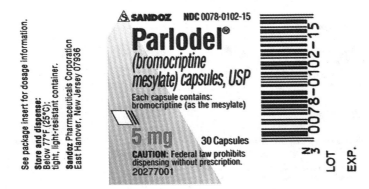

25. Clomipramine 100 mg = _____ cap

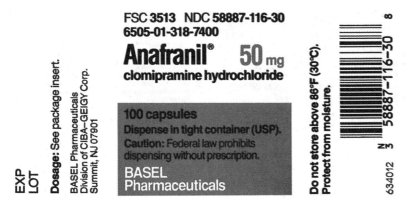

26. Femara 0.01 g = _____ tab

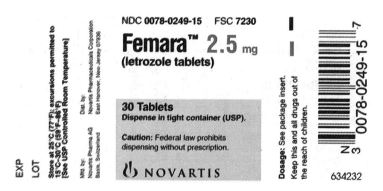

27. Ritalin HCl 0.04 g = _____ tab

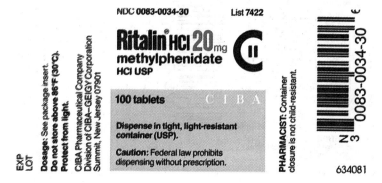

28. Biaxin 0.5 g = _____ tab

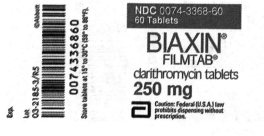

29. Restoril 15 mg = _____ cap

SANDOZ   NDC 0078-0140-05

Restoril® CIV
(temazepam)
capsules, USP

7.5 mg   100 Capsules

CAUTION: Federal law prohibits
dispensing without prescription.

20582001

See package insert for dosage information.
Store and dispense: Below 86°F (30°C);
tight, light-resistant container.

Sandoz Pharmaceuticals Corporation
East Hanover, New Jersey 07936

0078-0140-05

LOT   EXP.

30. Depacon 0.125 g = _____ mL

CONTAINS NO PRESERVATIVES:
Discard any unused solution.
Store at controlled room
temperature 15° - 30°C (59° -
86°F).

Exp.

Lot

Each mL contains: valproate
sodium equivalent to 100 mg
valproic acid, edetate disodium
0.4 mg, and water for injection. pH
adjusted with sodium hydroxide
and/or hydrochloric acid.
See enclosure.
TM - Trademark
Abbott Laboratories
North Chicago, IL 60064, U.S.A.

06-8192-2/R1

List No. 1564
Sterile 5 mL Single Dose Vial

DEPACON™
VALPROATE SODIUM INJECTION
500 mg/5 mL Vial
Valproic Acid Activity
For Intravenous Infusion Only

A female patient was admitted to the hospital with the following diagnoses: Rt. side congestive heart failure (CHF) chronic hypertension, ventricular arrhythmia. Her orders include the following:

- Digoxin 0.5 mg 12 noon, 6 PM, 12 midnight po 7/8/01
- Digoxin 0.25 mg po daily beginning at 10 AM 7/9/01
- Cardura 4 mg at hs
- Inderal 20 mg po tid
- Multivitamin 1 qd
- Lasix 20 mg qd
- Low-fat, low-sodium ADA diet, 1500 calories
- K-lor 20 mEq per day
- Isordil 10 mg sl qd
- Fluids 240 mL q4h × 6 per day

1. How many milligrams of digoxin did the patient receive on 7/8/01?

2. How many milligrams of digoxin are contained in a tablet labeled 250 μg?

3. Cardura tablets are available in 1, 2, 4, and 8 mg tablets. If 2 mg tablets were available, how many tablets would you administer to the patient?

4. Digoxin is available in 125 μg tablets. How many tablets would you administer to the patient at 10 A.M. on 7/9/01?

5. Inderal is available in 0.02 g tablets. How many tablets will you administer to the patient in a 24-hour period?

6. How many milliliters of fluid will the patient receive per day? How many liters of fluid will she receive in 7 days?

7. Isordil sl indicates that the medication will be administered

_____ .

8. If each 10 mEq of K-lor contains 750 mg, how many grams of K-lor will Mrs. Lindor receive in one day?

9. If the drug Inderal is to be administered TID, q8h, and her Cardura will be given at 10 PM, at what other times would you administer the Inderal so she receives both her Inderal and Cardura at 10 PM?

Answers to Case Study 6 appear in back of book.

You will find the answers to *Try These for Practice* below. Answers to *Exercises* and *Cumulative Review* appear in Appendix A at the back of the book. Your instructor has the answers to the *Additional Problems*.

Try These for Practice

Test your comprehension after reading the chapter.

1. The prescriber has ordered 0.2 mg of the gastric acid inhibitor medication misoprostol (Cytotec). How many tablets will you administer to the patient if each tablet contains 200 micrograms? _____

2. The patient is to receive grain $\frac{1}{50}$ of the antigout medication colchicine (Colsalide). Each tablet contains 0.6 milligram. How many tablets will you administer? _____

3. The order reads as follows:

    zidovudine 100 mg po qid

    Tablets are grain $1\frac{1}{2}$ each. How many tablets will you administer to the patient? _____

4. The prescriber ordered 40 mg/m^2 of the anti-ulcer drug famotidine (Pepcid). The patient's BSA is 1.5 m^2. If the drug is dispensed 5 mL/40 mg, how many mL would you prepare? _____

5. The drug meclizine has been prescribed for a patient. The dose ordered is 0.625 milligram per kilogram, and the patient weighs 80 kilograms. Read the label in Figure 6.13 and calculate the number of tablets you will administer to the patient. _____

Answers: 1. 1 tab   2. 2 tab   3. 1 tab   4. 7.5 mL   5. 2 tab

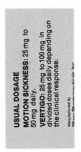

▶ **FIGURE 6.13 Drug label for Antivert.**

Exercises

Reinforce your understanding in class or at home.

1. Amantadine hydrochloride (Symmetrel) is an antiviral drug, and 0.2 gram has been ordered for a patient. Each capsule contains 100 milligrams. How many capsules will you administer to the patient? _____

2. If a patient is unable to swallow Symmetrel capsules, the patient must receive the oral suspension labeled 50 milligrams per 5 milliliters. How many milliliters equal 200 milligrams? _____

3. The order reads 0.4 gram of cyclosporine (Sandimmune) po. If each capsule contains 100 milligrams, how many capsules of this immunosuppressant drug equals the prescribed dose? _____

4. The patient has been prescribed 0.01 gram po of the antihistamine drug loratadine (Claritin). Each tablet contains 10 milligrams. How many tablets will you administer? _____

5. The order reads as follows:

    Estradiol 0.004 g transdermal

    See Figure 6.14. How many patches would you apply? _____

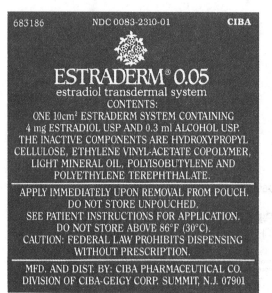

▶ **FIGURE 6.14 Drug label for Estraderm.**

6. Ten milligrams of the antihypertensive drug amlodipine (Norvasc) is ordered for your patient. If each tablet contains 0.005 grams, how many tablets will you give your patient? _____

7. The order in Problem 6 has been reduced to 5 milligrams po. How many tablets equal this dose? _____

8. Read the first order on the medication administration record in Figure 6.15. Name the drug and the number of tablets you will administer to the patient if the label reads 100 milligrams per tablet. _____

⊕ GENERAL HOSPITAL ⊕

Year 20*01* Month *December* Day		17	18	19	20	21	22
Medication Dosage and Interval		Initials* and Hours	Initials and Hours	Initials and Hours	Initials and Hours	Initials and Hours	Initials and Hours
Date started: *12/17/01*	I	*LA*	*LA*				
Zoloft 0.2 g *po qd*	AM	*10*	*10*				
	I						
Discontinued:	PM						
Date started: *12/18/01*	I						
Dalmane 15 mg *po hs*	AM						
	I		*JO*				
Discontinued:	PM		*10*				

Allergies: (Specify)	PATIENT IDENTIFICATION
penicillin, codeine	

Init*	Signature
LA	*Leon Ablon*
JO	*June Olsen*

```
226310                          12/17/01
Susan Jackson                    1/30/63
80 Martin Ave.                     Epis
Little Rock, AR                     HIP
76412

Dr. Anthony Giangrasso
```

MEDICATION ADMINISTRATION RECORD

▶ **FIGURE 6.15 Medication administration record.**

9. Read the second order from the MAR in Figure 6.15. Name the drug and the number of capsules you will administer if each capsule contains 0.015 g of this sedative drug? _____

10. Your patient is to receive 0.125 milligram of the cardiac glycoside digoxin (Lanoxin) po. Each scored tablet contains 0.25 milligram. How many tablets will you administer to the patient? _____

11. The order reads Tenormin 50 mg qd. Each tablet contains 25 milligrams. How many tablets equal 50 mg? _____

12. A patient with tuberculosis has an order for the antitubercular drug ethambutol hydrochloride (Myambutol). Each tablet contains 400 milligrams. If the order is 1.6 grams po, how many tablets will you administer to the patient? _____

13. The prescriber has ordered 20 milligrams of piroxicam (Feldene), and each capsule contains 0.01 gram. How many capsules of this nonsteroidal anti-inflammatory drug (NSAID) will you give the patient? _____

14. If the order in Problem 13 was changed to 0.375 gram po of the NSAID naproxen (Naprosyn) and each scored tablet contained 250 milligrams, how many tablets would you administer to the patient? _____

15. The order reads trimethadione 13 mg/kg po qd. The patient weighs 46 kilograms. Each capsule contains 300 milligrams. How many capsules of this anticonvulsant drug will equal the prescribed dose? _____

16. The prescriber has ordered 0.01 gram tid sublingual (under the tongue) of the anti-anginal medication erythrityl tetranitrate (Cardilate) for a patient. If each tablet contains 5 milligrams, how many tablets equal this dosage? _____

17. A patient is 5 feet 3 inches tall and weighs 150 pounds. Use the adult nomogram to estimate her BSA. The order is 60 mg/m^2 of the antibiotic doxycycline (Vibramycin), and the oral suspension is labeled 25 milligrams per 5 milliliters. How many milliliters would you give to the patient? _____

18. The patient has been prescribed 0.45 mg of clonidine hydrochloride (Catapres), an antihypertensive drug. The drug is available in 0.3 mg scored tablets. How many tablets equals the prescribed dose? _____

19. A patient is 183 centimeters tall and weighs 80 kilograms. The prescriber has written the order for clozapine (Clozaril) 50 mg/m^2. Each tablet contains 100 mg of clozapine. How many tablets would you administer to this patient? (Use the formula to estimate the BSA.) _____

20. The order reads: azithromycin 7.2 mg/kg po qd. Each capsule contains 250 milligrams. How many capsules will you prepare of this antiviral drug for a patient weighing 154 pounds? _____

Now, on your own, test yourself! Ask your instructor to check your answers.

1. The order is 2.5 milligrams per kilogram of a drug for a patient weighing 68 kilograms. Each capsule contains 50 milligrams. How many capsules would you administer to the patient? _3.4 Capsules_

2. Calculate the number of tablets a patient would be given if the order is 0.5 milligram and each tablet contains grain $\frac{1}{120}$. _____

3. The order reads as follows:

    delavirdine 220 mg/m^2

    How many tablets of this antiviral drug will you administer if each tablet contains 400 mg? The patient is 6 feet 3 inches tall and weighs 150 lb? (Use the formula to approximate the BSA.) _____

4. A patient has been prescribed 0.01 gram bid of a central nervous system (CNS) stimulant, methylphenidate hydrochloride (Ritalin). If each tablet contains 10 milligrams, how many tablets equal 0.01 gram? _____

5. Aminophylline (Phyllocontin) is frequently ordered for patients with chronic obstructive disease—specifically, bronchial asthma. The usual dosage is 600 milligrams po qid. Your patient's order is 0.6 gram po qid. Is this an appropriate dosage for this patient? _____

6. The prescriber has ordered 0.5 gram po q8h of the antibiotic erythromycin (E-Mycin) for the treatment of Lyme disease. Is this an appropriate dosage for a patient weighing 74 kilograms when the usual dosage is 6.75 milligrams per kilogram? _____

7. The prescriber ordered the following:

    elixir of digoxin 250 mcg po qd

    The label reads 0.5 milligram per milliliter. How many milliliters would you administer to the patient? _____

8. A patient has been prescribed 2.5 milligrams sl of isosorbide dinitrate (Isordil). Each tablet contains grain $\frac{1}{24}$. How many tablets will you administer to this patient of this anti-anginal drug? _____

9. The order reads thyroid 16.25 mg/m^2. If each tablet contains 32.5 mg, how many tablets would you administer to a patient who is 164 cm tall and weighs 94 kg? (Use the nomogram to approximate the BSA.) _____

10. The BSA of the patient is 2.13 m². The physician ordered indinavir (Crixivan) 375 mg/m². How many capsules would you administer if the label reads 0.25 g per capsule? _____

11. Your patient must receive 1.4 milligrams per kilogram of the antihypertensive drug metoprolol tartrate (Lopressor). The drug is available in the form of 50 mg tablets. If your patient weighs 72 kilograms, how many tablets will you administer? _____

12. Read the first order on the medication administration record (MAR) in Figure 6.16. How many milliliters will you prepare of the anticonvulsant drug if the label reads 100 milligrams per 4 milliliters? _____

✚ GENERAL HOSPITAL ✚

Year 20*01* Month *June* Day		3	4	5	6	7	8
Medication Dosage and Interval		Initials* and Hours	Initials and Hours	Initials and Hours	Initials and Hours	Initials and Hours	Initials and Hours
Date started: 06/3/01 *Dilantin 0.2 g po tid*	I	AG	LA	LA			
	AM	10	10	10			
	I	AG AG	LA LR	LA LR			
Discontinued: 06/5/01	PM	2 6	2 6	2 6			
Date started: 6/3/01 *ciprofloxacin 0.25 g bid*	I	AG	LA	LA			
	AM	10	10	10			
	I	AG	LR	LR			
Discontinued: 6/5/01 6:30 P.M.	PM	6	6	6			
Date started: 6/3/01 *propranolol 0.12 g po daily*	I	AG	LA	LA			
	AM	6	6	6			
	I						
Discontinued: 6/5/01	PM						

Allergies: (Specify)
  none

Init*	Signature
AG	*Anthony Giangrasso*
LA	*Leon Ablon*
LR	*Laura Reese*

MEDICATION ADMINISTRATION RECORD

PATIENT IDENTIFICATION

705432   6/3/01

David Vyas   12/1/32
10-01 4th Ave.   Muslim
Brooklyn, NY   11209   GHI-CBP

June Olsen, M.D.

▶ **FIGURE 6.16 Medication administration record.**

13. Read the second order on the MAR in Figure 6.16. The ciprofloxacin label reads 100 milligrams per milliliter. How many milliliters of this antibiotic will you prepare for Mr. Vyas? _____

14. Read the third order on the MAR in Figure 6.16. If the drug propanolol (Inderal) is available in 120 mg capsules, how many capsules will you administer? _____

15. Your patient must receive grains $\frac{5}{6}$ of Anafranil, an antidepressant medication. Consult the label in Figure 6.17 and calculate how many capsules you will administer to your patient. _____

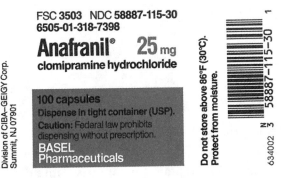

▶ FIGURE 6.17 Drug label for Anafranil.

16. The prescriber ordered 200 milligrams po bid of indomethacin (Indocin), an anti-inflammatory drug used in the treatment of rheumatoid arthritis. The capsules are labeled 0.05 gram. How many capsules equal the prescribed dosage? _____

17. The order for Indocin in Problem 16 has been changed to 3 milligrams per kilogram per day. The patient weighs 50 kilograms. How many milligrams equal this dosage? _____

18. The order reads as follows:

    tolazamide 0.25 g po qd

    Each tablet contains 250 milligrams. How many tablets of this antidiabetic agent will you administer to the patient? _____

19. A patient has been prescribed 1.5 grams po of diflunisal (Dolobid). How many tablets of this anti-inflammatory drug will you administer if each tablet is labeled 500 milligrams? _____

20. The order reads as follows:

    Lotensin 0.01 g po

Read the label in Figure 6.18 and calculate the number of tablets you would administer. _____

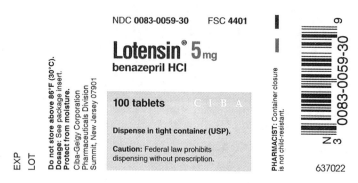

FIGURE 6.18 Drug label for Lotensin.

CUMULATIVE REVIEW EXERCISES

Review your mastery of earlier chapters.

1. The order for Margaret Jones is grain $\frac{1}{4}$ po of the sedative quazepam (Doral). What is the equivalent in milligrams? _____

2. The patient must receive 0.005 gram po of terbutaline sulfate (Brethine). How many tablets will you administer to this patient of this bronchodilating drug if each tablet contains 5 milligrams? _____

3. ℥ 10 = ℈ _____

4. 0.2 g = gr _____

5. 40 mg = _____ g

6. 2500 mg = gr _____

7. gr $\overline{\text{VIISS}}$ = _____ mg

8. The order is 250 milligrams of trimethobenzamide hydrochloride (Tigan). Give the equivalent in grains of this antiemetic drug. _____

9. The order reads didanosine (Videx) 1.1 mg/lb. The patient weighs 110 lb. If each tablet contains 125 mg, how many tablets will the patient receive? _____

10. The order reads cefpodoxime 267 mg/m^2. The patient weighs 130 lb and has a height of 56 inches. The label reads 100 mg/5 mL. How many mL would you administer to the patient? Use the nomogram to estimate the BSA. _____

11. The order is Biaxin 315 mg/m². The patient is 67 in tall and weighs 116 lb. Each scored tablet contains 500 mg. How many tablets of this antibiotic drug would you administer to the patient? _____

12. The prescriber ordered 0.015 gram po of glipizide (Glucotrol), and the tablets contain 5 milligrams of the drug. How many tablets will you administer of this oral antidiabetic drug? _____

13. The patient must receive 1000 milligrams po of the antibiotic sulfisoxazole (Gantrisin). The drug label reads 500 milligrams per 5 milliliters. How many milliliters will you give the patient? _____

14. A prescriber orders 0.2 gram of the sedative drug ethchlorvynol (Placidyl) for a patient with insomnia. Read the label in Figure 6.19 and determine how many capsules you will administer to the patient. _____

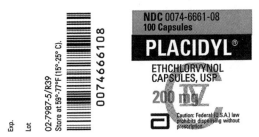

▶ FIGURE 6.19 Drug label for Placidyl.

15. The patient has been prescribed 0.0625 milligram po of digoxin (Lanoxin), an anti-arrhythmic inotropic drug. The elixir is labeled 0.05 milligram per milliliter. How many milliliters will you administer to the patient? _____

CHAPTER SEVEN

Syringes

▷ Objectives

After completing this chapter, you will be able to

- Identify the various types of syringes.
- Identify the parts of a syringe.
- Determine the amount of solution in a syringe.
- Understand prepackaged cartridges.
- Read and use USP units.

A *hypodermic syringe* (inserted beneath the skin) is an instrument used in parenteral therapy to administer sterile liquid medications by injection. The medication is introduced into a body space, such as a vein, a muscle, subcutaneous tissue, cardiac muscle, subarachnoid space, or bone tissue. Figure 7.1 illustrates the parts of a syringe: the plunger, barrel, and hollow needle, which must all be connected separately. The plunger, needle, and the inside of the barrel must always be sterile.

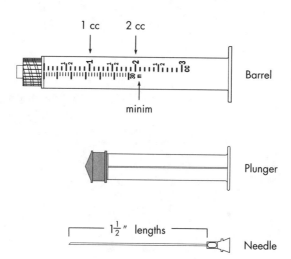

1 cc   2 cc

Barrel

minim

Plunger

$1\frac{1}{2}''$ lengths

Needle

▶ **FIGURE 7.1 A needle, plunger, and barrel**

COMMON TYPES OF SYRINGES

There are many types of syringes in common use. They include syringes with such capacities as

1 cc	10 cc	30 cc	100 cc
3 cc	12 cc	35 cc	
5 cc	20 cc	50 cc	
6 cc	25 cc	60 cc	

The circumference and length of a syringe increase with its capacity. Many syringes are calibrated in minims and in tenths of a cubic centimeter. These two scales of measurement frequently appear together on the same syringe, particularly the 3 cc syringe.

> **NOTE**
>
> All syringes in this text are drawn at 75% of actual size.

The syringe shown in Figure 7.2 has a capacity of 3 cubic centimeters or minims 30. The minims scale is on one side of the barrel, where each marking represents minim 1 and the longer lines represent minims 5. On the other side is the milliliter or cubic centimeter scale. Each line represents 0.1 milliliter or 0.1 cubic centimeter, and the longer lines represent 0.5 milliliter or $\frac{1}{2}$ cubic centimeter (more commonly written as 0.5 cc). The 3 cc syringe is the most commonly used syringe for subcutaneous (sc) and intramuscular (IM) injections.

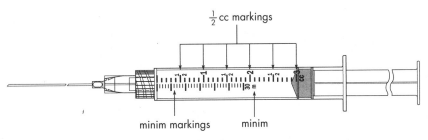

▶ **FIGURE 7.2** A 3 cc syringe

BY THE WAY

A cubic centimeter is the same as a milliliter:

1 cc = 1 mL

Figure 7.3 shows a 10 cc syringe. Notice that this syringe has neither incremental markings of 0.5 cubic centimeter nor a minims scale. Each line represents 0.2 cubic centimeter, and the longer lines represent 1 cubic centimeter. This syringe can be used to draw venous or arterial blood as well as to add sterile diluent to a vial or ampule of powdered medication.

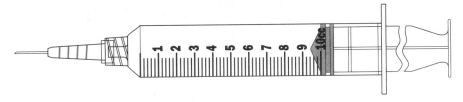

▶ **FIGURE 7.3** A 10 cc syringe

A 20 cc syringe is shown in Figure 7.4. Each line on the scale represents 1 cubic centimeter, and the longer line indicates 5 cubic centimeters. The 20 cc syringe can be used to inject large volumes of sterile liquids.

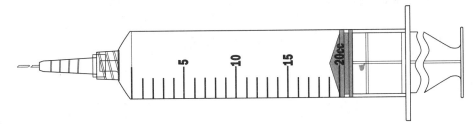

▶ **FIGURE 7.4** A 20 cc syringe

Figure 7.5 shows a 20 cc syringe filled with liquid up to the 12 cc mark.

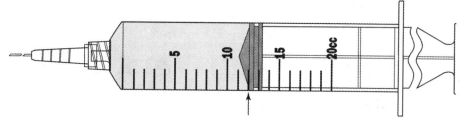

▶ **FIGURE 7.5 A partially filled 20 cc syringe**

The liquid volume in a syringe is read from the *top ring*, **not** the bottom ring or the raised section in the middle of the plunger tip.

▶ **EXAMPLE 7.1**

How much liquid is in the 10 cc syringe in Figure 7.6?

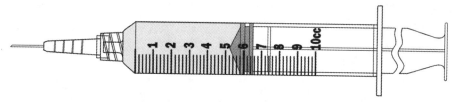

▶ **FIGURE 7.6 A partially filled 10 cc syringe**

The top ring of the plunger is at the fourth line above 5 cubic centimeters. Because each line measures 0.2 cubic centimeter, the fourth line measures 0.8 cubic centimeter. So, the amount of fluid in the syringe is 5.8 cubic centimeters.

▶ **EXAMPLE 7.2**

How much liquid is in the 3 cc syringe in Figure 7.7?

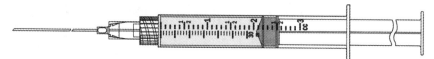

▶ **FIGURE 7.7 A partially filled 3 cc syringe**

The top ring of the plunger is at the second line above 2 cubic centimeters. Because each line measures 0.1 cubic centimeter, the two lines measure 0.2 cubic centimeter. So, the amount of liquid in the syringe is 2.2 cubic centimeters.

►EXAMPLE 7.3

How much liquid is in the 3 cc syringe in Figure 7.8?

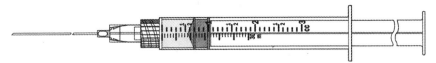

► FIGURE 7.8 A partially filled 3 cc syringe

The top ring of the plunger is at the second line above $\frac{1}{2}$ cubic centimeter. Because each short line measures 0.1 cubic centimeter, the two lines measure 0.2 cubic centimeter. So, the amount of liquid in the syringe is 0.7 cubic centimeter.

OTHER TYPES OF SYRINGES

Other types of syringes that are available for administering medications include the prepackaged cartridge, the tuberculin syringe, and the insulin syringe.

A *prepackaged cartridge* is a syringe that is prefilled with medication. If the medication order is for the exact amount of drug in the prepackaged cartridge, the possibility of measurement error by the medication administrator is eliminated. The prepackaged cartridge syringe shown in Figure 7.9 is calibrated so that each line measures 0.1 milliliter and the thicker lines measure 0.5 milliliter. Note that the prepackaged cartridges are measured in millimeters rather than cubic centimeters.

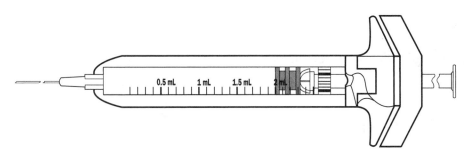

► FIGURE 7.9 A prepackaged cartridge

►EXAMPLE 7.4

How much medication is in the prepackaged cartridge shown in Figure 7.10?

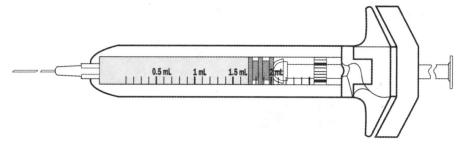

▶ **FIGURE 7.10 A partially filled prepackaged 2 mL syringe**

The top of the plunger is at two lines above 1.5 milliliters. Because each line measures 0.1 milliliter, the two lines measure 0.2 milliliter. So the prepackaged cartridge contains 1.7 milliliters.

The *tuberculin syringe* shown in Figure 7.11 is a small, slender syringe used to inject small quantities of liquids. It has a capacity of 1 cubic centimeter. Each line on the syringe represents 0.01 cubic centimeter, and the longer lines represent 0.05 cubic centimeter. This syringe is used for intradermal injection (injection directly beneath the skin) as well as for injection of small quantities of medication that might be prescribed for pediatric or adult patients.

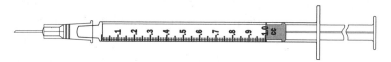

▶ **FIGURE 7.11 A tuberculin syringe**

▶ **EXAMPLE 7.5**

How much liquid is in the tuberculin syringe shown in Figure 7.12?

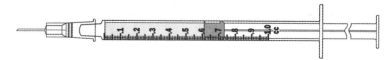

▶ **FIGURE 7.12 A partially filled tuberculin syringe**

The top ring of the plunger is at one line above 0.60 milliliter. Because each line represents 0.01 milliliter, the amount of liquid in the syringe is 0.61 milliliter.

The *insulin syringe* is used to measure insulin. Insulin is a hormone used to treat patients with insulin-dependent diabetes mellitus (IDDM). It is available in both short-acting and long-acting preparations. Insulin can also be prescribed for patients who are hyperglycemic as a result of certain medical therapies. Insulin is supplied in standardized units of potency rather than by weight or volume. These standardized units are called *USP units*, which is often shortened to *units* and abbreviated u.

The insulin syringe is calibrated in units. Figure 7.13 shows an insulin syringe with a capacity of 50 units ($\frac{1}{2}$ cubic centimeter), where each line on the scale measures 1 unit (0.01 cubic centimeter).

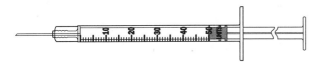

▶ **FIGURE 7.13 A 50 u insulin syringe**

A 100 u insulin syringe is shown in Figure 7.14. Each line on its scale measures 2 units (0.02 cubic centimeter).

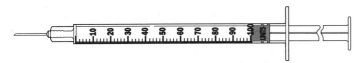

▶ **FIGURE 7.14 A 100 u insulin syringe**

NOTE

The top ring of an insulin syringe plunger is flat. As mentioned earlier, other types of syringes have a peak in the center of the top ring. With both types of syringes, the liquid volume is measured from the *top ring*.

▶ **EXAMPLE 7.6**

How much liquid is in the 50 u insulin syringe shown in Figure 7.15?

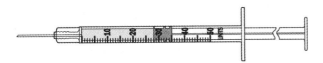

▶ **FIGURE 7.15 A partially filled 50 u insulin syringe**

The top ring of the plunger is at three lines above 25. Because each line represents 1 unit, the amount of liquid in the syringe is 28 units.

▶ **E X A M P L E   7 . 7**

How much liquid is in the 100 u insulin syringe shown in Figure 7.16?

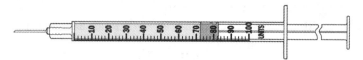

▶ **F I G U R E   7 . 1 6   A partially filled 100 u insulin syringe**

The top ring of the plunger is at one line above 70. Because each line represents 2 units, the amount of liquid in the syringe is 72 units.

▶ **E X A M P L E   7 . 8**

Explain what you would do to fill a medication order for 55 units of NPH insulin.

There are no calculations necessary. You would simply draw 55 units into an insulin syringe as shown in Figure 7.17.

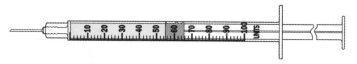

▶ **F I G U R E   7 . 1 7   The correctly filled insulin syringe**

▶ **E X A M P L E   7 . 9**

Explain what you would do to fill a medication order for 26 units of Humulin R insulin.

There are no calculations necessary. You would draw 26 units of Humulin R insulin into the insulin syringe as shown in Figure 7.18.

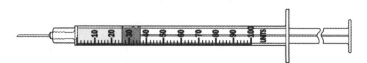

▶ **F I G U R E   7 . 1 8   The correctly filled insulin syringe**

▶ **EXAMPLE 7.10**

The prescriber ordered 15 units of Humulin R insulin and 45 units of NPH insulin in the same syringe for a total of 60 units sc. Explain how you would fill this order.

You would first draw 15 units of Humulin R insulin into a 100 u insulin syringe and then draw 45 units of NPH insulin into the same syringe, as shown in the four steps of Figure 7.19a and 7.19b.

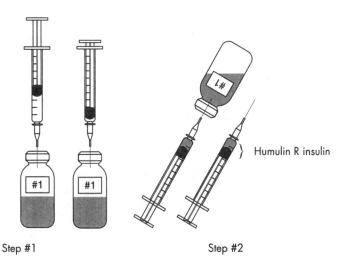

Step #1   Step #2

▶ **F I G U R E   7 . 1 9 A   Filling the insulin syringe: Humulin R insulin from vial #1.**

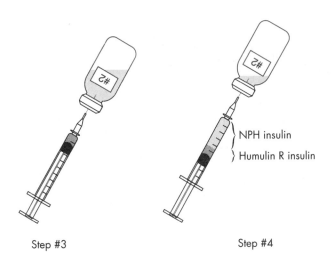

Step #3   Step #4

▶ **F I G U R E   7 . 1 9 B   The correctly filled insulin syringe: Adding NPH insulin from vial #2.**

BY THE WAY

It is recommended that Humulin R insulin be drawn into the syringe first.

You will find the answers to *Try These for Practice*, *Exercises*, and *Cumulative Review Exercises* in Appendix A at the back of the book. Your instructor has the answers to the *Additional Exercises*.

Try These for Practice

Test your comprehension after reading the chapter.

In problems 1 through 4, identify the type of syringe shown in the figure. Then, for each quantity, place an arrow at the appropriate level of measurement on the syringe.

1. _____ syringe; 0.3 cc

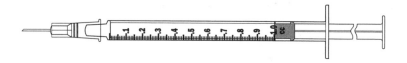

2. _____ syringe; 5.2 cc

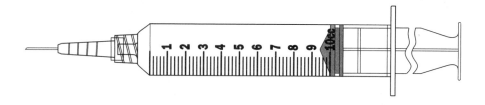

3. _____ syringe; 12 u

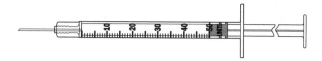

4. _____ syringe; 22 u

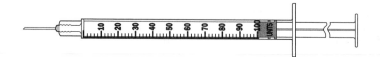

5. The prescriber ordered 0.2 mg of Corvert. Read the label in Figure 7.20, do the calculation, and place an arrow at the appropriate level of measurement on the syringe below.

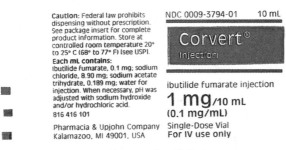

Caution: Federal law prohibits dispensing without prescription. See package insert for complete product information. Store at controlled room temperature 20° to 25° C (68° to 77° F) [see USP].
Each mL contains:
Ibutilide fumarate, 0.1 mg; sodium chloride, 8.90 mg; sodium acetate trihydrate, 0.189 mg; water for injection. When necessary, pH was adjusted with sodium hydroxide and/or hydrochloric acid.
816 416 101
Pharmacia & Upjohn Company
Kalamazoo, MI 49001, USA

NDC 0009-3794-01   10 mL

Corvert®
Injection

ibutilide fumarate injection
1 mg/10 mL
(0.1 mg/mL)
Single-Dose Vial
For IV use only

▶ **FIGURE 7.20 Corvert drug label**

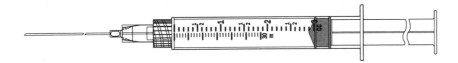

Exercises

Reinforce your understanding in class or at home.

In problems 1 through 16, identify the type of syringe shown in the figure. Then, for each quantity, place an arrow at the appropriate level of measurement on the syringe.

1. _____ syringe; 9.8 cc

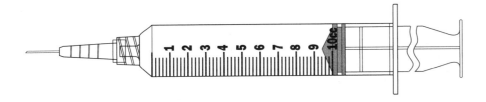

2. _____ syringe; 1.1 cc

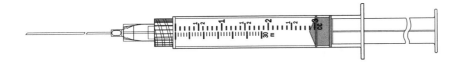

3. _____ syringe; 0.8 mL

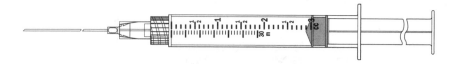

4. _____ syringe; 40 u

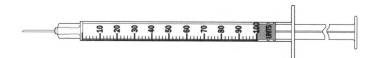

5. _____ syringe; 35 u

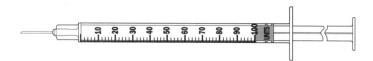

6. _____ syringe; ℥ 8

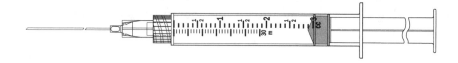

7. _____ syringe; 3 cc

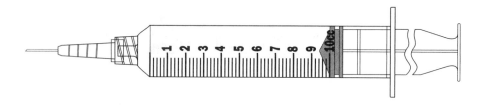

8. _____ syringe; 90 u

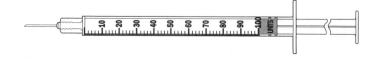

9. _____ syringe; 2.7 cc

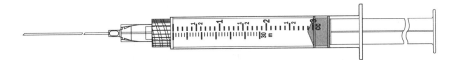

10. _____ syringe; 0.6 cc

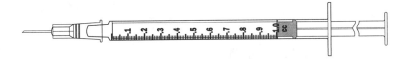

11. _____ syringe; 8 u

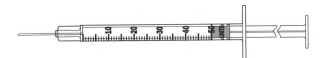

12. _____ syringe; 6.6 cc

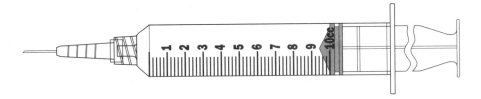

13. _____ syringe; 78 u

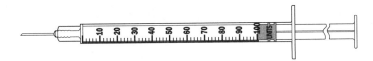

14. _____ syringe; 36 u

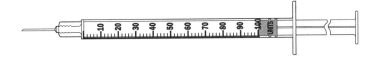

15. _____ syringe; 3.4 cc

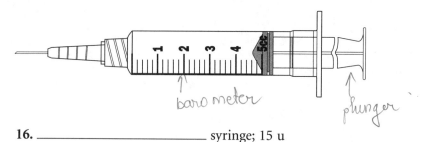

baro meter   plunger

16. _____ syringe; 15 u

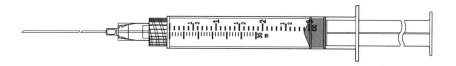

In problems 17 through 20, read the order and use the appropriate label (found at the end of the *Exercises*); calculate the dosage if necessary, and place an arrow at the appropriate level of measurement on the syringe.

17. order: Fragmin 7500 u sc _____ cc

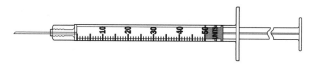

18. order: Humulin BR insulin 42 units sc _____ units

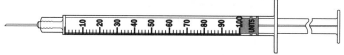

19. order: lymphocyte immune globulin 75 mg IV _____ cc

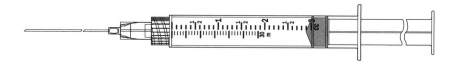

20. order: irinotecan hydrochloride 50 mg IV _____ cc

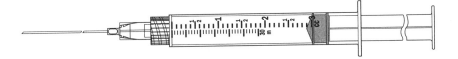

NDC 0009-7529-02
2 mL

CAMPTOSAR™
Injection
irinotecan hydrochloride
injection
40 mg/2 mL
(20 mg/mL)
—on basis of trihydrate

**INTRAVENOUS
USE ONLY**
See package insert
for complete
product information.

Store at controlled
room temperature
15° to 30° C
(59° to 86° F).

Protect from freezing.

817 060 000

Pharmacia & Upjohn
Company
Kalamazoo, MI 49001

NDC 0009-7224-01   5 mL

Lymphocyte Immune
Globulin, Anti-Thymocyte
Globulin (Equine)
Atgam®
Sterile Solution

250 mg protein
(50 mg per mL)

Caution: Federal (USA) law prohibits
dispensing without prescription.
For I.V. use only. For suggested dose,
refer to package insert.
U.S. License No. 1216.
ATTENTION—May contain particles; this is
normal. Use 0.2μ to 1.0μ in-line filter.
See insert.   816 661 000
Pharmacia & Upjohn Company
Kalamazoo, MI 49001, USA

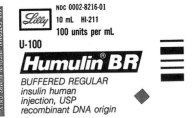

NDC 0002-8216-01
10 mL   HI-211
100 units per mL
U-100
Humulin® BR
BUFFERED REGULAR
insulin human
injection, USP
recombinant DNA origin

FOR DISPLAY ONLY

FOR EXTERNAL INSULIN PUMPS ONLY—
DO NOT MIX WITH OTHER INSULIN PRODUCTS

Important:
See enclosed circular.
If pregnant or nursing, see carton.
Keep in a cold place. Avoid freezing.
Eli Lilly & Co., Indianapolis, IN 46285, U.S.A.
WV 4190 AMX   Neutral
Exp. Date/Control No.

NDC 0013-2436-06

Fragmin®

dalteparin sodium injection
10,000 IU (anti-Xa) per mL
For subcutaneous injection
9.5 mL multiple-dose vial

Contains benzyl alcohol as a preservative.
Usual dosage: See package insert for complete
product information.
Store at controlled room temperature
20° to 25°C (68° to 77°F) (See USP).
Manufactured for: Pharmacia & Upjohn Company,
Kalamazoo, MI 49001, USA

EXP
LOT

Additional Exercises

Now, on your own, test yourself! Ask your instructor to check your answers.

In problems 1 through 16, identify the type of syringe shown in the figure. Then, for each quantity, place an arrow at the appropriate level of measurement on the syringe.

1. _____ syringe; 42 u

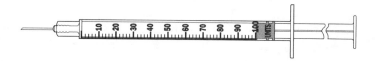

2. _____ syringe; 30 u

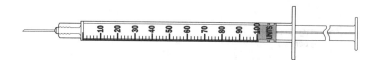

3. _____ syringe; 3.4 cc

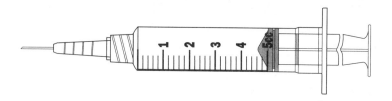

4. _____ syringe; 1.6 cc

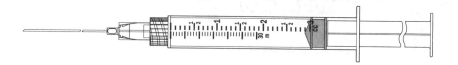

5. _____ syringe; 11 cc

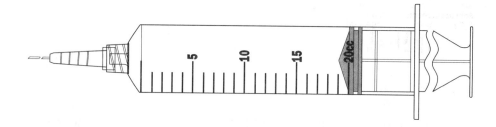

6. _____ syringe; 18 cc

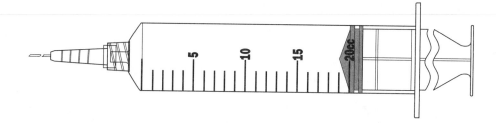

7. _____ syringe; 22 u

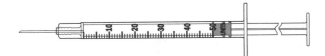

8. _____ syringe; 48 u

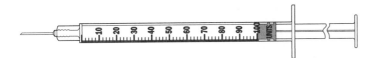

9. _____ syringe; 0.4 cc

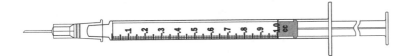

10. _____ syringe; 12 u

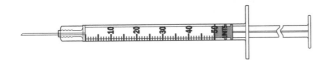

11. _____ syringe; 6.8 cc

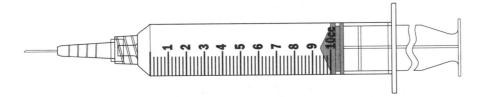

12. _____ syringe; 18 u

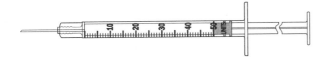

13. _____ syringe; 7.8 cc

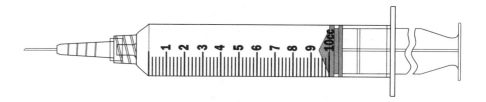

14. _____ syringe; 20 cc

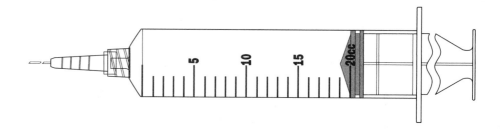

15. _____ syringe; 88 u

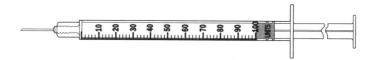

16. _____ syringe; 1.7 cc

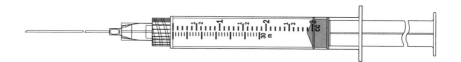

In problems 17 through 20, read the order and use the appropriate label (found at the end of the *Additional Exercises*), calculate the dosage if necessary, and place an arrow at the appropriate level of measurement on the syringe.

17. order: Depacon 0.6 g IV _____ cc

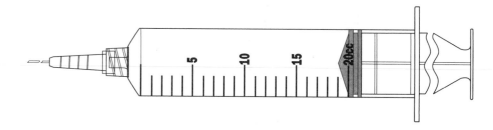

18. order: Nubain 56 mg IV _____ cc

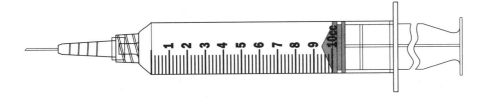

19. order: verapamil 7.5 mg IV _____ cc

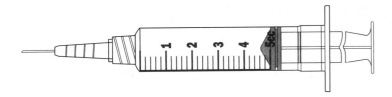

20. order: Methadone 8 mg _____ cc

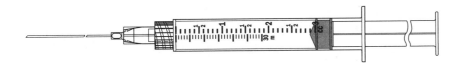

CONTAINS NO PRESERVATIVES:
Discard any unused solution.
Store at controlled room
temperature 15° - 30°C (59° -
86°F).

Exp.

Lot

Each mL contains: valproate
sodium equivalent to 100 mg
valproic acid, edetate disodium
0.4 mg, and water for injection. pH
adjusted with sodium hydroxide
and/or hydrochloric acid.
See enclosure.
TM - Trademark

Abbott Laboratories
North Chicago, IL 60064, U.S.A.

06-8192-2/R1

List No. 1564
Sterile 5 mL Single Dose Vial

DEPACON™
VALPROATE SODIUM INJECTION
500 mg/5 mL Vial
Valproic Acid Activity
For Intravenous Infusion Only

NDC 0044-181

ISOPTIN®
verapamil HCl

INTRAVENOUS

10 mg/4 mL

Knoll Pharmaceuticals
Whippany, NJ 07981

1 mL POISON
No. 456 **C Ⅱ**
DOLOPHINE®
HCl
METHADONE
HCl **10** mg

Sub. Q. or I.M.
YU 6001 AMU
LILLY, INDPLS.

FOR DISPLAY ONLY

NUBAIN®
(nalbuphine HCl)

10 mg/ml injection

10 ml VIAL

Each ml contains: 10 mg nalbuphine HCl,
0.1% sodium chloride, 0.94% sodium
citrate hydrous, 1.26% citric acid anhy-
drous, 0.1% sodium metabisulfite and
0.2% of a 9:1 mixture of methyl and
propylparaben, as preservatives. pH is
adjusted with hydrochloric acid.

FOR IM, SC OR IV USE
DOSAGE: Read accompanying product
information.
CAUTION: Federal law prohibits dispens-
ing without prescription.
Store at controlled room temperature
(59°-86°F, 15°-30°C).
PROTECT FROM EXCESSIVE LIGHT
Du Pont Pharmaceuticals, Inc.
Subsidiary of
E. I. du Pont de Nemours & Co. (Inc.)
Manati, Puerto Rico 00701 XC

LOT:

EXP:

CUMULATIVE REVIEW EXERCISES

Review your mastery of earlier chapters.

1. gr 10 = _____ mg

2. 1200 mL = _____ L

3. The prescriber ordered Prilosec 0.020 g po qd. Each capsule contains 20 milligrams. How many capsules will you administer to the patient?

   _____

4. The order reads: morphine sulfate gr $\frac{1}{6}$ IM q4h prn. Change grain $\frac{1}{6}$ to milligrams. _____

5. The prescriber ordered Ceclor 250 mg po q 12h. The label reads 375 milligrams per 5 milliliters. How many milliliters will you administer to the patient? _____

6. Change grain $\frac{1}{240}$ to milligrams. _____

7. The prescriber ordered 120 mL H_2O po q2h for 12h. How many ounces should the patient receive? _____

8. ℥ 16 = ʒ _____

9. 0.6 mg = gr _____

10. 0.004 g = gr _____

11. The prescriber ordered Feldene 20 mg po qd. Each capsule contains 0.02 gram. How many capsules will you administer to the patient?

    _____

12. The prescriber ordered 0.3 milligram of clonidine hydrochloride. If each tablet contains 0.1 milligram, how many tablets will you administer to the patient? _____

13. Read the information on the label in Figure 7.21, and calculate the number of tablets equal to 0.6 gram. _____

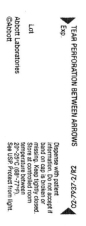
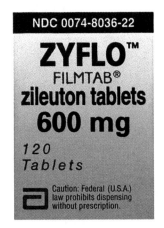

▶ **FIGURE 7.21 Drug label for Zyflo**

14. Read Figure 7.22. Calculate the number of tablets required to make 1.5 g. _____

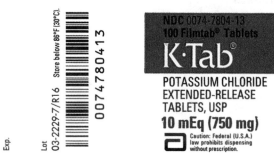

▶ **FIGURE 7.22 Drug label for K-Tab**

15. The prescriber ordered Norvir 160 mg q6h po. Read the label in Figure 7.23. How many milliliters equal 160 mg? _____

NDC 0074-1940-63
240 mL

NORVIR®

(RITONAVIR ORAL SOLUTION)

80 mg per mL

Shake well before each use.

DO NOT REFRIGERATE

Use within 30 days from dispensing.

Ⴈ R͟x only 02-8141-2/R2

▶ F I G U R E 7.23 Drug label for Norvir

CHAPTER EIGHT

Preparation of Solutions

▶ **Objectives**

After completing this chapter, you will be able to

- Use the strength of a solution, given in ratio form or percentage form, to calculate drug doses.
- Understand the relationships among the amount of solution, the strength of the solution, and the amount of pure drug that the solution contains.
- Do the calculations necessary to prepare solutions from pure drugs.
- Do the calculations necessary to prepare solutions by diluting stock solutions.

In this chapter you will learn about solutions. Although most solutions are prepared in the pharmacy by the pharmacist, nurses must understand the concepts involved and be able to prepare solutions, especially in home care situations.

Drugs are manufactured in both pure and diluted form. A pure drug contains only the drug and nothing else. A drug is frequently diluted by dissolving a quantity of pure drug in a liquid to form a solution. This solution is called a ***stock solution.*** The pure drug (either dry or liquid) is called the ***solute.*** The liquid added to the pure drug to form the solution is called the ***solvent*** or ***diluent.*** The solvents most commonly used are sterile water and normal saline solution.

STRENGTH OF SOLUTIONS

The strength of a solution can be stated as a ***ratio*** or a ***percentage.***

- The ratio 1:2 (read "1 to 2") means that there is 1 part of the drug in 2 parts of solution. This solution is also referred to as a $\frac{1}{2}$ strength solution or a 50% solution.

- The ratio 1:10 (read "1 to 10") means that there is 1 part of the drug in 10 parts of solution. This solution is also referred to as a 10% solution.

- A 5% solution means that there are 5 parts of the drug in 100 parts of solution.

- A $2\frac{1}{2}$% solution means that there are $2\frac{1}{2}$ parts of the drug in 100 parts of solution.

PURE DRUGS IN LIQUID FORM

For a pure drug that is in liquid form, the ratio 1:40 means there is 1 milliliter of pure drug in every 40 milliliters of solution. So 40 milliliters of a 1:40 acetic acid solution means that 1 milliliter of pure acetic acid is diluted with water to make a total of 40 milliliters of solution. You would prepare this solution by placing 1 milliliter of pure acetic acid in a graduated cylinder and adding water until the level in the graduated cylinder reaches 40 milliliters. See Figure 8.1.

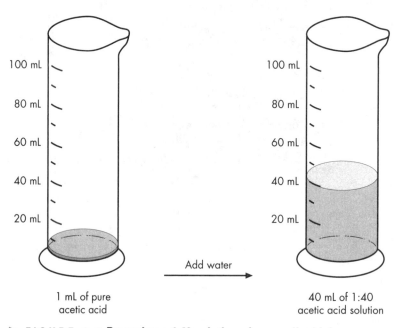

▶ **FIGURE 8.1 Preparing a 1:40 solution of a pure liquid drug**

A 1% solution means that there is 1 part of the drug in 100 parts of solution. So you would prepare 100 milliliters of a 1% creosol solution by placing

1 milliliter of pure creosol in a graduated cylinder and adding water until the level in the graduated cylinder reaches 100 milliliters. See Figure 8.2.

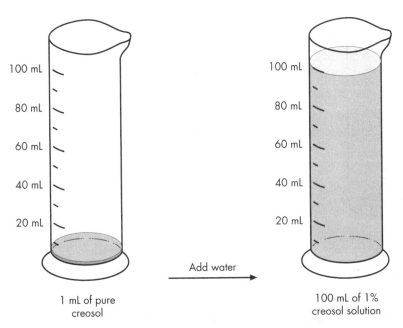

100 mL

80 mL

60 mL

40 mL

20 mL

1 mL of pure creosol

Add water

100 mL

80 mL

60 mL

40 mL

20 mL

100 mL of 1% creosol solution

▶ **FIGURE 8.2 Preparing a 1% solution of a pure liquid drug**

PURE DRUGS IN DRY FORM

The ratio 1:20 means 1 part of the pure drug in 20 parts of solution, or 2 parts of the pure drug in 40 parts of solution, or 3 parts in 60, or 4 parts in 80, and so on. When a pure drug is in *dry* form, the ratio 1:20 means 1 *gram* of pure drug in every 20 *milliliters* of solution. So 100 milliliters of a 1:20 potassium permanganate solution means *5 grams* of pure potassium permanganate dissolved in water to make a total of *100 milliliters* of the solution. If each tablet is 5 grams, then you would prepare this solution by placing 1 tablet of the pure potassium permanganate in a graduated cylinder and adding water until the level in the graduated cylinder reaches 100 milliliters.

BY THE WAY

A 1:20 solution is the same as a 5% solution.

A 5% potassium permanganate solution means 5 grams of pure potassium permanganate in 100 milliliters of solution. So, a 5% potassium permanganate solution is written as $\frac{5g}{100 \text{ mL}}$ or $\frac{1g}{20 \text{ mL}}$. See Figure 8.3.

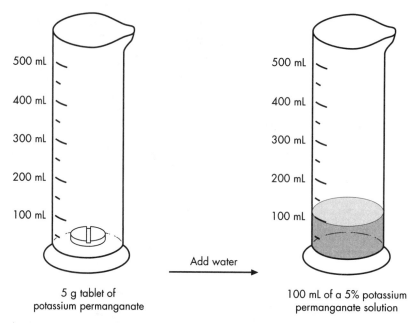

5 g tablet of
potassium permanganate

Add water

100 mL of a 5% potassium
permanganate solution

▶ FIGURE 8.3 Preparing a 5% solution of a pure dry drug

PREPARING SOLUTIONS FROM PURE DRUGS

The formula below shows the relationships among the amount of solution, the strength of the solution, and the amount of pure drug that the solution contains. You can use this formula to prepare a prescribed solution of a certain strength from a pure drug.

> **NOTE**
>
> Amount of solution $\times$ Strength = Amount of pure drug

Amount of solution: Use *milliliters* (or *cubic centimeters*).
Strength: Always write as a fraction for calculations.

> For liquids:
> 1:40 acetic acid solution is written as $\frac{1 \text{ mL}}{40 \text{ mL}}$.
> 5% acetic acid solution is written as $\frac{5 \text{ mL}}{100 \text{ mL}}$.

> For tablets or powder:
> 1:20 potassium permanganate solution is written as $\frac{1 g}{20 \text{ mL}}$.
> 12% potassium permanganate solution is written as $\frac{12 g}{100 \text{ mL}}$.

Amount of pure drug:
Use *milliliters* or *cubic centimeters* for liquids.
Use *grams* for tablets or powders.

EXAMPLE 8.1

How many grams of magnesium sulfate (Epsom salts) would you need to prepare 100 milliliters of a 20% solution?

Because magnesium sulfate is in dry form, it is measured in grams. So, a 20% solution contains 20 grams of magnesium sulfate in 100 milliliters of solute.

Amount of solution is 100 milliliters.
Strength is 20% or $\frac{20}{100}$, so you use $\frac{20\,g}{100\,mL}$.

$$100\,mL \times \frac{20\,g}{100\,mL} = \text{Amount of pure drug}$$

$$\overset{1}{\cancel{100\,mL}} \times \frac{20\,g}{\underset{1}{\cancel{100\,mL}}} = 20\,g$$

So, you need 20 grams of magnesium sulfate to prepare 100 milliliters of a 20% solution.

EXAMPLE 8.2

How many grams of dextrose would you need to prepare 1000 milliliters of a 5% solution?

Amount of solution is 1000 milliliters.
Strength is 5% or $\frac{5}{100}$, so you use $\frac{5\,g}{100\,mL}$.

$$1000\,mL \times \frac{5\,g}{100\,mL} = \text{Amount of pure drug}$$

$$\overset{10}{\cancel{1000\,mL}} \times \frac{5\,g}{\underset{1}{\cancel{100\,mL}}} = 50\,g$$

So, you need 50 grams of dextrose to prepare 1000 milliliters of a 5% solution.

EXAMPLE 8.3

How would you prepare 2000 milliliters of a 1:10 Clorox solution?

Because Clorox is a liquid, it is measured in milliliters. So, a 1:10 solution means 1 milliliter of Clorox in 10 milliliters of solution.

Amount of solution is 2000 milliliters.
Strength is 1:10 or $\frac{1}{10}$. You use $\frac{1\,mL}{10\,mL}$.

$$\overset{200}{\cancel{2000\,mL}} \times \frac{1\,mL}{\underset{1}{\cancel{10\,mL}}} = 200\,mL$$

So, you need 200 milliliters of Clorox to prepare 2000 milliliters of a 1:10 solution. This means that 200 milliliters of Clorox is diluted with water to 2000 milliliters of solution.

> ### EXAMPLE 8.4

How would you prepare 250 milliliters of a $\frac{1}{2}$% creosol solution? Creosol comes in liquid form, so a $\frac{1}{2}$% solution means 0.5 milliliter of creosol in 100 milliliters of solution. (*Remember:* $\frac{1}{2} = 0.5$.)

Amount of solution is 250 milliliters.
Strength is $\frac{1}{2}$% or $\frac{0.5}{100}$, so you use $\frac{0.5 \text{ mL}}{100 \text{ mL}}$.

$$\overset{5}{\cancel{250 \text{ mL}}} \times \frac{0.5 \text{ mL}}{\underset{2}{\cancel{100 \text{ mL}}}} = 1.25 \text{ mL}$$

So, you need 1.25 milliliters of creosol to prepare 250 milliliters of a $\frac{1}{2}$% creosol solution. This means that 1.25 milliliters of creosol is diluted with water to 250 milliliters of solution.

> ### EXAMPLE 8.5

How would you prepare 3 liters of a 1% urinary antiseptic solution using 5 g tablets of Neosporin?

Because the pure Neosporin is in dry form, it is measured in grams. So, a 1% solution means 1 gram of Neosporin in 100 milliliters of solution.

You must find the amount of pure drug necessary and convert to tablets.

Amount of solution is 3 liters.
Strength is 1% or $\frac{1}{100}$, so you use $\frac{1 \text{ g}}{100 \text{ mL}}$.

Because you are working in milliliters, change 3 liters to 3000 milliliters.

Because each tablet contains 5 grams, you use the fraction $\frac{1 \text{ tab}}{5 \text{ g}}$.

$$\overset{30}{\cancel{3000 \text{ mL}}} \times \frac{1 \cancel{\text{ g}}}{\underset{1}{\cancel{100 \text{ mL}}}} \times \frac{1 \text{ tab}}{5 \cancel{\text{ g}}} = 6 \text{ tab}$$

So, you dissolve 6 tablets of Neosporin in water and dilute to 3000 milliliters.

DILUTING STOCK SOLUTIONS

A stock solution is one in which a pure drug is already dissolved in a liquid. The strength of each stock solution is written on the label. If the order is for a stronger solution, you will need to prepare a new solution. However, if the order is for a weaker solution, you can dilute the stock solution to the prescribed strength. To find out how much stock solution to mix, use the following formula.

$$\frac{\text{Amount prescribed} \times \text{Strength prescribed}}{\text{Strength of stock}} = \text{Amount of stock}$$

▶ **E X A M P L E 8.6**

How would you prepare 1 liter of a 10% glucose solution from a 50% stock solution of glucose?

Amount prescribed is 1 liter, so you use 1000 milliliters.
Strength prescribed is 10%, so you use $\frac{10\ mL}{100\ mL}$.
Strength of stock is 50%, so you use $\frac{50\ mL}{100\ mL}$.

$$\frac{1000\ mL \times \dfrac{10\ \cancel{mL}}{100\ \cancel{mL}}}{\dfrac{50\ \cancel{mL}}{100\ \cancel{mL}}} = \text{Amount of stock}$$

$$1000\ mL \times \frac{10}{100} \div \frac{50}{100} =$$

$$1000\ mL \times \frac{\overset{1}{\cancel{10}}}{\underset{1}{\cancel{100}}} \times \frac{\overset{1}{\cancel{100}}}{\underset{5}{\cancel{50}}} = 200\ mL$$

So, you would take 200 milliliters of the 50% stock solution of glucose and dilute it with water to 1000 milliliters.

▶ **E X A M P L E 8.7**

How would you prepare 2500 milliliters of a 1:10 boric acid solution from a 40% stock solution of this antiseptic?

Amount prescribed is 2500 milliliters.
Strength prescribed is 1:10, so you use $\frac{1\ mL}{10\ mL}$.
Strength of stock is 40%, so you use $\frac{40\ mL}{100\ mL}$.

$$\frac{2500\ mL \times \dfrac{1\ \cancel{mL}}{10\ \cancel{mL}}}{\dfrac{40\ \cancel{mL}}{100\ \cancel{mL}}} = \text{Amount of stock}$$

Diluting Stock Solutions   167

$$2500 \text{ mL} \times \frac{1}{10} \div \frac{40}{100} =$$

$$\overset{250}{\cancel{2500}} \text{ mL} \times \frac{1}{\underset{1}{\cancel{10}}} \times \frac{100}{40} = 625 \text{ mL}$$

So, you would take 625 milliliters of the 40% stock solution of boric acid and dilute with water to 2500 milliliters.

▶ **E X A M P L E 8.8**

How would you prepare 500 milliliters of a 1:25 solution from a 1:4 stock solution of the antiseptic Argyrol?

Amount prescribed is 500 milliliters.

Strength prescribed is 1:25, so you use $\frac{1 \text{ mL}}{25 \text{ mL}}$.

Strength of stock is 1:4, so you use $\frac{1 \text{ mL}}{4 \text{ mL}}$.

$$\frac{500 \text{ mL} \times \dfrac{1 \cancel{\text{mL}}}{25 \cancel{\text{mL}}}}{\dfrac{1 \cancel{\text{mL}}}{4 \cancel{\text{mL}}}} = \text{Amount of stock}$$

$$500 \text{ mL} \times \frac{1}{25} \div \frac{1}{4} =$$

$$\overset{20}{\cancel{500}} \text{ mL} \times \frac{1}{\underset{1}{\cancel{25}}} \times \frac{4}{1} = 80 \text{ mL}$$

So, you would take 80 milliliters of a 1:4 stock solution of Argyrol and dilute it with water to 500 milliliters.

You have now learned how to prepare solutions by using formulas. In the following problems, you will use dimensional analysis to determine the amount of solution that contains a given amount of pure drug.

▶ **E X A M P L E 8.9**

How many milliliters of a 20% magnesium sulfate solution will contain 40 grams of the pure drug, magnesium sulfate?

You want to convert the 40 grams of pure drug to milliliters of solution.

$$40 \text{ g} = ? \text{ mL}$$

You want to cancel the grams and obtain the equivalent amount in milliliters.

$$40 \text{ g} \times \frac{? \text{ mL}}{? \text{ g}} = ? \text{ mL}$$

In a 20% solution there are 20 grams of pure drug per 100 mL of solution. So, the fraction is

$$\frac{100 \text{ mL}}{20 \text{ g}}$$

$$\overset{2}{\cancel{40 \text{ g}}} \times \frac{100 \text{ mL}}{\underset{1}{\cancel{20 \text{ g}}}} = 200 \text{ mL}$$

So, 200 milliliters of a 20% magnesium sulfate solution contains 40 grams of the pure drug, magnesium sulfate.

► **EXAMPLE 8.10**

How many milliliters of a 1:40 acetic acid solution will contain 25 milliliters of acetic acid?

You want to convert the 25 milliliters of pure acetic acid to milliliters of solution.

25 mL (of pure drug) = ? mL (of solution)

There may be some confusion in the meaning of the previous line because there are milliliters on both sides of the equal sign. To aid your understanding, the parentheses are included to indicate whether "mL" refers to the amount of pure drug or to the amount of solution.

You want to cancel the milliliters of pure drug and obtain the equivalent amount in milliliters of solution.

$$25 \text{ mL (of pure drug)} \times \frac{? \text{ mL (of solution)}}{? \text{ mL (of pure drug)}} = ? \text{ mL (of solution)}$$

In a 1:40 acetic acid solution there is 1 milliliter of pure acetic acid in 40 milliliters of solution. So, the fraction is

$$\frac{40 \text{ mL (of solution)}}{1 \text{ mL (of pure drug)}}$$

$$25 \cancel{\text{ mL}} \times \frac{40 \text{ mL}}{1 \cancel{\text{ mL}}} = 1000 \text{ mL}$$

So, 1000 milliliters of a 1:40 acetic acid solution contains 25 milliliters of pure acetic acid.

A 94-year-old female patient has a medical history of long-standing hypertension and diabetes mellitus type II. She is 5 feet tall and weighs 115 pounds. She makes an appointment with her primary physician. Her current medications are Inderal 20 mg tid, Isordil 20 mg tid, and one multivitamin per day.

Her physician examines her and finds the following symptoms: BP, 220/132; P, 110 irregular; R, 32; T, 100F. She complains of urinary burning, has pedal edema + 3, and has gained 6 pounds. The physician orders 60 mg furosemide stat IV, a chest x-ray, electrocardiogram, CBC, and SMA 18. Within 30 minutes she begins to diurese, and in 1 hour she is sent home with the following orders:

- Inderal 40 mg po tid
- Lasix 20 mg q12h
- K-Lor 20 mEq q12h
- Isordil 20 mg qid
- multivitamin 1 qd
- Zithromax 600 mg qd × 5 days
- Glucotrol 0.01 g qd ac breakfast
- hydroxyzine 0.05 g hs prn
- trovafloxacin 0.1 g qd × 7 days

1. How many tablets of Inderal will you administer to the patient if each tablet contains 0.04 g? _____

2. Calculate the number of grams of Lasix the patient will receive per day and per week. _____

3. Each packet of K-Lor contains 40 mEq. The directions state: Add packet to 4 oz of juice. How many milliliters equal the dose of potassium? _____

Read the labels found at the end of this case study to answer questions 4 through 6.

4. How many tablets of azithromycin will you administer to this client? _____

5. How many tablets of trovafloxacin will you administer to the patient? _____

6. Determine how many tablets of glipizide you will administer ac breakfast. _____

7. Change the hydroxyzine order to milligrams, and determine the number of tablets you will administer. _____

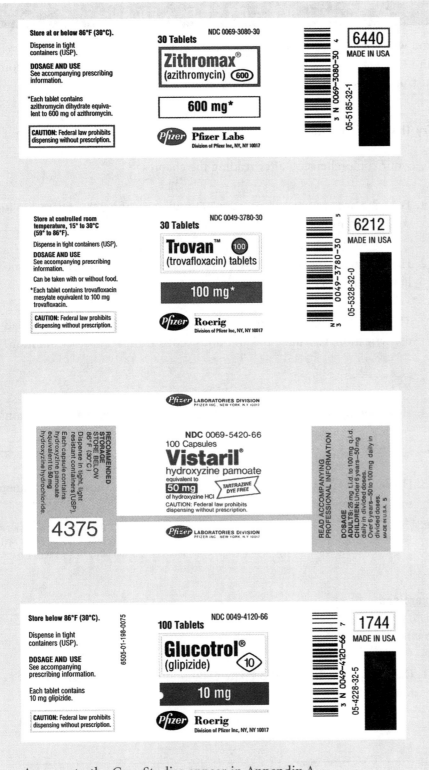

Answers to the Case Studies appear in Appendix A.

You will find the answers to *Try These for Practice* below. Answers to *Exercises* and *Cumulative Review* appear in Appendix A at the back of the book. Your instructor has the answers to the *Additional Exercises*.

Try These for Practice

Test your comprehension after reading the chapter.

1. Describe how you would prepare 500 milliliters of a 0.9% normal saline solution from the pure drug (sodium chloride). _____

2. How many grams of Epsom salt crystals are required to make 200 milliliters of a $2\frac{1}{2}$% solution? _____

3. The prescriber has ordered 4 liters of a 1% neomycin solution for bladder irrigation. Calculate the amount needed from a 2% stock solution.

   _____

4. How would you prepare 300 mL of a 1:25 solution from a 1:5 solution?

   _____

5. How would you prepare 4000 milliliters of 5% potassium permanganate solution from 5 g tablets? _____

Answers: 1. Take 4.5 g of sodium chloride, and dilute with water to 500 mL.   2. 5 g   3. 2 L   4. Take 60 mL of the 1:5 solution, and dilute with water to 300 mL.   5. Take 40 tablets, dissolve and dilute with water to 4000 mL.

Exercises

Reinforce your understanding in class or at home.

1. Describe how you would prepare 2000 milliliters of a 2% solution of formaldehyde, a disinfectant, from a 100% solution.

   _____

   _____

2. Explain how to prepare 500 milliliters of a 3% solution of Betadine from a 15% stock solution.

NOTES/WORKSPACE

_____

_____

_____

3. How would you prepare 1000 milliliters of a 10% Weskodyne solution, a disinfectant, from pure drug?

_____

_____

_____

4. How would you prepare 250 milliliters of a 0.45% solution from sodium chloride crystals?

_____

_____

_____

5. Describe how you would prepare 2500 milliliters of a 1:1000 aluminum acetate (Burow's) solution, an antiseptic, from 0.5 g tablets.

_____

_____

_____

6. You must prepare 200 milliliters of a 2% boric acid solution, a mild antiseptic. How would you prepare this from boric acid crystals?

_____

_____

_____

7. Explain how to prepare a 1% ammonium chloride solution (1 liter) from 1 g tablets.

_____

_____

_____

8. Use the information found on the label in Figure 8.4 to determine the number of grams of calcium chloride contained in 5 milliliters of this solution.

_____

_____

_____

10%   NDC 0186-1166-04

Calcium Chloride Injection, USP

1 gram (100 mg/mL) 27.3 mg (1.4 mEq) Ca+ +/mL

2.04 mOsm/mL (calc.)

For IV Use Only   Caution: Federal law prohibits dispensing without prescription.

ASTRA®

Astra Pharmaceutical Products, Inc.
Westborough, MA 01581

10mL Single Dose Vial
Not for multiple uses.
Discard unused portion.
CAUTION: Must not be injected IM, SC or into body tissues.
Each mL contains 100 mg calcium chloride dihydrate and hydrochloric acid to adjust pH to between 5.5-7.5.
See insert for dosage.
Store at 15°-30° C.

070701R01

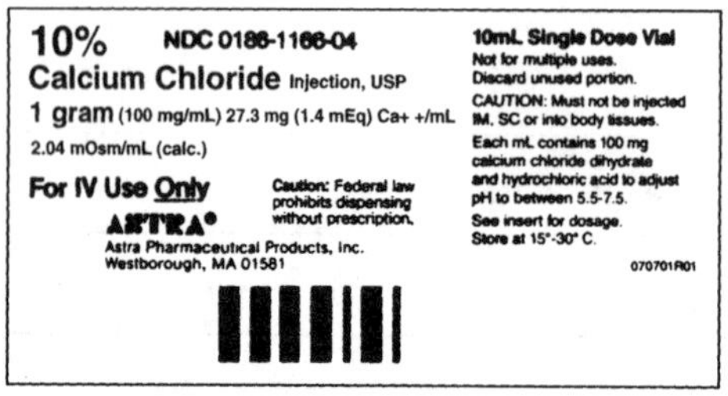

▶ **FIGURE 8.4 Drug label for 10% calcium chloride**

9. Describe how to prepare 600 milliliters of a 2.5% solution from a 3% solution of the antiseptic hydrogen peroxide.

_____

_____

_____

10. Read the label in Figure 8.5 and determine how many milliliters of this solution will contain 0.005 g epinephrine.

_____

_____

_____

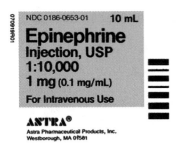

▶ FIGURE 8.5 Drug label for 1:10,000 epinephrine

11. Describe how to prepare 4000 milliliters of a 1:50 solution of the antiseptic potassium permanganate from 0.5 g tablets.

_____

_____

_____

12. How would you prepare 1000 milliliters of a 10% Lysol solution, a disinfectant, from a 25% stock solution?

_____

_____

_____

13. Using the information on the label in Figure 8.6, determine the number of grams of mannitol contained in 40 milliliters of this solution.

_____

_____

_____

50 mL

25%

MANNITOL

**Injection USP
for IV use only**

▶ FIGURE 8.6 Drug label for mannitol

14. How would you prepare 4000 milliliters of a 1:40 solution from a 1:20 solution?

_____

_____

_____

15. How many milliliters of a 20% serum albumin solution will contain 60 grams of serum albumin?

_____

_____

_____

16. Describe how to prepare 500 milliliters of a 0.025% solution from a 1% solution.

_____

_____

_____

17. If 3 grams of pure drug are added to a container of sterile water and the total amount is now 1000 milliliters, what would be the strength of this solution?

_____

_____

_____

18. How would you prepare 1.25 liters of 10% aluminum acetate (Burow's) solution from 1 g tablets?

_____

_____

_____

19. The information found in the second order on the physician's order sheet in Figure 8.7 is, "Cleanse abdominal wound with 1:1000 Zephiran chloride q shift" (*q shift* means "every shift"). Describe how you would pre-pare 500 milliliters of this solution from a 2% solution.

_____

_____

_____

✚ GENERAL HOSPITAL ✚

PRESS HARD WITH BALLPOINT PEN. WRITE DATE & TIME AND SIGN EACH ORDER

DATE	TIME	A.M.
7/8/01	3	(P.M.)

1. Apply flourocinonide 0.05% to affected skin qid

2. Cleanse abdominal wound with 1:1000 Zephiran

   chloride q shift

3. Tube feeding: 1/3 strength Meritine 240 mL q4h via

   Gastrostomy tube

IMPRINT
873667   7/8/01
Gene Martin   3/3/30
330Ocean Pkwy   Jewish
Huntington, NY   Aetna
41001
Dr. Leon Ablon

ORDERS NOTED
DATE _7/8/01_   TIME _3:10_ A.M. (P.M.)
❏ MEDEX   ❏ KARDEX
NURSE'S SIG. _A. Giangrasso_

FILLED BY   DATE

SIGNATURE
                L. Ablon   M.D.

PHYSICIAN'S ORDERS

▶ **FIGURE 8.7 Physician's order sheet**

20. Read the information in the first order from the physician's order sheet in Figure 8.7. How would you prepare 250 milliliters of 0.05% fluocinonide (Lidex) solution from a 1% solution?

_____

_____

_____

Additional Exercises

Now, on your own, test yourself! Ask your instructor to check your answers.

1. Read the physician's third order in Figure 8.7. How would you prepare the tube feeding from $\frac{1}{2}$ strength Meritine? _____

_____

_____

2. A 25% solution of serum albumin has been ordered for a patient. If the prescriber wants the patient to have 75 grams of serum albumin, how many milliliters will the patient receive? _____

3. If the serum albumin was a 25% solution and the order was 150 milliliters, how many grams of serum albumin would the patient receive?

_____

4. The prescriber has requested that 500 milligrams of lidocaine be added to 500 milliliters of 5% D/W. How many milliliters of 2% lidocaine must be added to the 5% D/W? _____

5. A dentist is to inject a 1% solution of lidocaine as a nerve block for a patient. He will give the patient a total of 5 milliliters. How many grams of lidocaine will the patient receive? _____

6. The prescriber has ordered 500 mL of 0.9% sodium chloride solution as a cleansing agent. How many 1 g tablets of sodium chloride are necessary to make this solution? _____

7. How would you prepare 250 milliliters of a 10% magnesium sulfate solution from pure drug? _____

_____

_____

8. Describe how a 2.5% solution of hexachlorophene would be prepared from a 3% solution (200 milliliters).

_____

_____

_____

9. Your patient is to have a tube feeding of 240 mL of $\frac{1}{2}$ strength Isocal, a nutritional supplement. Each can contains 240 milliliters. How many milliliters of water should be added to the Isocal for a $\frac{1}{2}$ strength solution? (*Hint:* $\frac{1}{2}$ strength means 50% solution.) _____

10. The prescriber has ordered a norepinephrine (Levophed) lavage for a patient having a gastric bleed. Each ampule contains 4 milligrams per 4 milliliters of Levophed, and the prescriber has ordered 1000 milliliters of normal saline with 0.04 gram of Levophed, how many milliliters of Levophed will be added to the normal saline? _____

11. Explain how to prepare 1000 milliliters of a 1:50,000 silver nitrate solution from a 1:1000 stock solution of silver nitrate.

_____

_____

_____

12. You have a 100% Clorox solution available. How would you prepare 1 gallon of a 10% solution?

_____

_____

_____

13. Describe how you would prepare 100 mL of a 1:100 solution of creosol from 500 mg tablets.

_____

_____

_____

14. Read the information on the label in Figure 8.8 and calculate the amount of dextrose in 20 milliliters of the solution. _____

_____

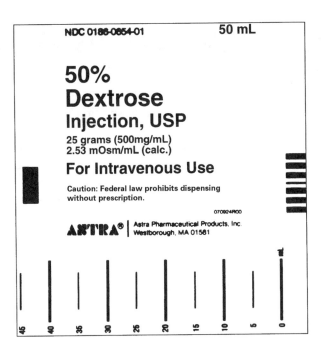

NDC 0186-0654-01   **50 mL**

50%
Dextrose
Injection, USP

25 grams (500mg/mL)
2.53 mOsm/mL (calc.)

For Intravenous Use

Caution: Federal law prohibits dispensing without prescription.

070924R00

ASTRA® | Astra Pharmaceutical Products, Inc.
Westborough, MA 01581

► **FIGURE 8.8 Drug label for 50% dextrose**

15. A physician has prescribed a $\frac{1}{2}$% acetic acid solution to treat an external ear canal infection. How would you prepare 25 milliliters of this solution from a 100% acetic acid solution?

_____

_____

_____

16. You have a 2.75% otic boric acid solution. How many grams of boric acid would be contained in 200 milliliters? _____

17. A patient has an accumulation of ear wax (cerumen) in the ear canal. A 6.5% solution of carbamide peroxide (Debrox), which is an otic solution, is prescribed. How many milligrams of Debrox will be contained in 75 milliliters? _____

18. The prescriber has ordered a 15 mL IV push of a 10% solution of magnesium sulfate. How many grams of magnesium sulfate will the patient receive? _____

19. How many grams of sodium chloride are in 1000 milliliters of 0.45% normal saline? _____

20. An order requests that 250 milligrams of 2% lidocaine solution be added to an infusion of 5% D/W. How many milliliters of this solution contain 250 milligrams of lidocaine? _____

CUMULATIVE REVIEW EXERCISES

Review your mastery of earlier chapters.

1. How do you prepare 250 milliliters of 2.5% boric acid solution (an antiseptic) from a 10% stock solution?

_____

_____

_____

2. The pharmacist must prepare a $2\frac{1}{2}$% magnesium sulfate solution (an electrolyte). How many grams of pure magnesium sulfate are contained in 100 milliliters of this solution? _____

3. The prescriber ordered 1 g lidocaine added to 250 mL of 5% D/W. How many milliliters of a 2% lidocaine solution would be added?

_____

_____

_____

4. The order is 0.25 milligram of the anti-anxiety drug alprazolam (Xanax); the tablets on hand are grain $\frac{1}{120}$. How many tablets would you administer?

_____

5. The physician orders 900 milligrams of clindamycin hydrochloride (Cleocin). The bottle label states that 1 tablet equals 0.15 gram. How many tablets are equal to 900 milligrams? _____

6. ORDER: gr $\frac{1}{200}$ atropine sulfate. How many tablets would you administer when the tablets are 0.3 milligram each? _____

7. The order is dram 1 of Robitussin. How many minims are contained in dram 1 of this drug, which has an antitussive action? _____

8. The order reads: Zithromax 0.25 g po qd. How many milligrams are contained in this dosage? _____

9. 400 mg = _____ g   10. 1500 mg = _____ g

11. 80 mg = gr _____

12. The order is for 4 milligrams po of benztropine mesylate (Cogentin). Each tablet contains 0.5 milligram. How many tablets of this antiparkinsonian drug would you administer? _____

13. The prescriber ordered 0.0006 gram sc of scopolamine hydrobromide, an anticholinergic drug. Convert this amount to milligrams. _____

14. gr IV = _____ mg   15. $3\frac{1}{2}$ qt = _____ pt

Parenteral Medications

Parenteral medications are supplied in sterile liquid form in vials and ampules (Figure 9.1). They can also be supplied in powdered form in a sealed vial or ampule. Powdered drugs must be dissolved in sterile water or 0.9% sodium chloride (normal saline) prior to injection. This chapter introduces you to the calculations you will use to prepare and administer parenteral medications safely.

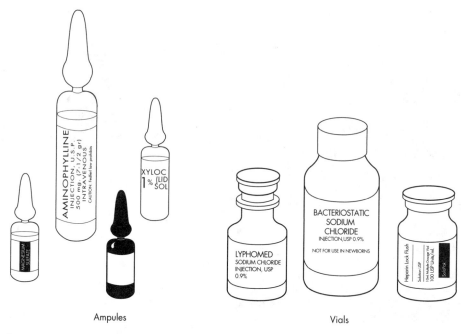

Ampules   Vials

▶ **FIGURE 9.1 Ampules and vials**

PARENTERAL MEDICATIONS SUPPLIED AS LIQUIDS

When parenteral medications are supplied in liquid form, you need to calculate the volume of liquid that contains the prescribed amount of the drug. To do this, you will use the dimensional analysis method you have been using for all other calculations.

▶ **EXAMPLE 9.1**

The prescriber ordered 3 milligrams of methadone hydrochloride (Dolophine) sc. Study the label in Figure 9.2. How many milliliters would you administer to the patient?

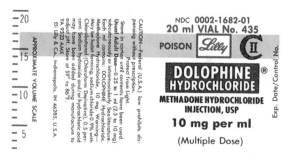

▶ **FIGURE 9.2 Drug label for methadone hydrochloride**

Begin by finding out how many milliliters of the liquid in the vial contains the prescribed quantity of the drug (3 milligrams of methadone hydrochloride). That is, you want to convert 3 milligrams to an equivalent in milliliters.

3 mg = ? mL

You cancel the milligrams and obtain the equivalent quantity in milliliters.

$$3 \text{ mg} \times \frac{? \text{ mL}}{? \text{ mg}} = ? \text{ mL}$$

The label reads 10 milligrams per milliliter, which means 10 mg = 1 mL. So, the equivalent fraction is $\frac{1 \text{ mL}}{10 \text{ mg}}$.

$$3 \cancel{\text{ mg}} \times \frac{1 \text{ mL}}{10 \cancel{\text{ mg}}} = 0.3 \text{ mL}$$

So, 0.3 milliliter contains 3 milligrams of methadone, and you would administer 0.3 milliliter of the drug to your patient.

___

▶ **EXAMPLE 9.2**

A drug vial reads 2500 milligrams per minims 150. How many minims would you administer if the medication order reads 1500 milligrams IM of the drug?

You want to convert the order (1500 milligrams) to its equivalent in minims.

1500 mg = ℳ ?

You cancel the milligrams and obtain the equivalent amount in minims.

$$1500 \text{ mg} \times \frac{\text{ℳ} ?}{? \text{ mg}} = \text{ℳ} ?$$

The label reads 2500 milligrams per minims 150. So, the equivalent fraction is $\frac{\text{ℳ} 150}{2500 \text{ mg}}$.

$$\overset{3}{\cancel{1500 \text{ mg}}} \times \frac{\text{ℳ} 150}{\underset{5}{\cancel{2500 \text{ mg}}}} = \text{ℳ} \frac{450}{5} = \text{ℳ} 90$$

So, minims 90 contain 1500 milligrams, and you would administer minims 90 IM of the drug to your patient.

___

▶ **EXAMPLE 9.3**

The prescriber ordered 0.002 gram of naloxone HCL (Narcan) IM. Read the label in Figure 9.3, and calculate how many milliliters of this narcotic antagonist you would administer.

NDC 0590-0368-05

NARCAN® **1** mg/ml
(naloxone HCl) injection

10 ml VIAL

Each ml contains 1.0 mg naloxone HCl*,
8.35 mg sodium chloride, 2.0 mg methyl-
paraben and propylparaben as preservatives in a ratio of 9:1. pH is adjusted with
hydrochloric acid.
*(-)-17-Allyl-4,5 α-epoxy-3,14-dihydroxy-
morphinan-6-one hydrochloride

FOR IM, SC OR IV USE
DOSAGE: Read accompanying product
information.
CAUTION: Federal law prohibits dispen-
sing without prescription.
Store at controlled room temperature
(59°-86°F, 15°-30°C). **PROTECT FROM
LIGHT. STORE IN CARTON UNTIL CON-
TENTS HAVE BEEN USED.**

Du Pont Pharmaceuticals, Inc.
Subsidiary of
E.I. du Pont de Nemours & Co. (Inc.)
P.O. Box 363, Manati, Puerto Rico 00701 YO

Lot:

Exp:

▶ F I G U R E   9 . 3   **Drug label for Narcan**

The label shows Narcan in milligrams per milliliter, so you want to convert 0.002 gram to its equivalent in milligrams and then change milligrams to milliliters.

$$0.002 \text{ g} \longrightarrow ? \text{ mg} \longrightarrow ? \text{ mL}$$

Do this on one line as follows:

$$0.002 \text{ g} \times \frac{? \text{ mg}}{? \text{ g}} \times \frac{? \text{ mL}}{? \text{ mg}} = ? \text{ mL}$$

The first equivalent fraction is $\frac{1000 \text{ mg}}{1 \text{ g}}$.

The label reads 1 milligram per milliliter, which means 1 mg = 1 mL. So, the second fraction is $\frac{1 \text{ mL}}{1 \text{ mg}}$.

$$0.002 \text{ g} \times \frac{1000 \text{ mg}}{1 \text{ g}} \times \frac{1 \text{ mL}}{1 \text{ mg}} = 2 \text{ mL}$$

You would administer 2 milliliters of naloxone HCL IM, which would contain 0.002 gram of naloxone HCL.

E X A M P L E   9 . 4

The medication order reads 75 milligrams of oxytetracycline (Terramycin) IM. Read the label in Figure 9.4, and calculate how much of this antibiotic you would administer.

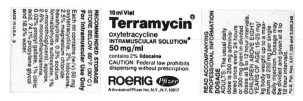

▶ F I G U R E   9 . 4   **Drug label for Terramycin**

Because this drug is available in milligrams per milliliter, you want to convert the order (75 milligrams) to its equivalent in milliliters.

75 mg = ? mL

You cancel the milligrams and obtain the equivalent amount in milliliters.

$$75 \text{ mg} \times \frac{? \text{ mL}}{? \text{ mg}} = ? \text{ mL}$$

Because the label reads 50 milligrams per milliliter, you use the equivalent fraction $\frac{1 \text{ mL}}{50 \text{ mg}}$.

$$\overset{3}{\cancel{75 \text{ mg}}} \times \frac{1 \text{ mL}}{\underset{2}{\cancel{50 \text{ mg}}}} = \frac{3}{2} \text{ mL} = 1.5 \text{ mL}$$

So, 1.5 milliliters contain 75 milligrams of Terramycin, and you would administer 1.5 milliliters IM to your patient.

▶ **EXAMPLE 9.5**

Mr. Jones is to receive grain $\frac{1}{600}$ of atropine sulfate sc. The ampule of liquid is labeled grain $\frac{1}{150}$ per minims 15. How many minims of this anticholinergic drug should be administered to the patient?

You want to convert the order of grain $\frac{1}{600}$ to its equivalent in minims.

$$\text{gr } \frac{1}{600} = ℳ \text{ ?}$$

You cancel the grains and obtain the equivalent amount in minims.

$$\text{gr } \frac{1}{600} \times \frac{ℳ \text{ ?}}{\text{gr ?}} = ℳ \text{ ?}$$

Because the label on the ampule reads grain $\frac{1}{150}$ per minims 15, the equivalent fraction is $\frac{ℳ \, 15}{\text{gr } \frac{1}{150}}$.

$$\cancel{\text{gr}} \frac{1}{600} \times \frac{ℳ \, 15}{\cancel{\text{gr}} \dfrac{1}{150}} = ℳ \frac{1 \times 15}{\dfrac{600}{150}} = ℳ \frac{15}{4} = ℳ \, 3\frac{3}{4}$$

So, minims $3\frac{3}{4}$ of this solution contains grain $\frac{1}{600}$ of atropine sulfate. Normally, you would give the patient minims 4, since three-fourths of a minim is too small to measure into the syringe (Figure 9.5).

Parenteral Medications Supplied as Liquids   187

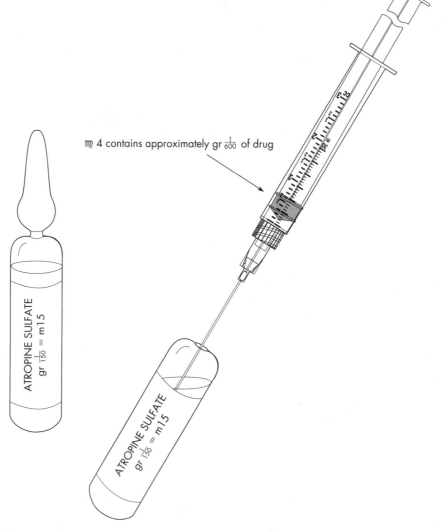

m 4 contains approximately gr $\frac{1}{600}$ of drug

ATROPINE SULFATE
gr $\frac{1}{150}$ = m15

ATROPINE SULFATE
gr $\frac{1}{150}$ = m15

▶ FIGURE 9.5 Preparing atropine sulfate gr $\frac{1}{600}$ from an ampule

▶ EXAMPLE 9.6

The prescriber ordered: Kantrex 0.4 g IM. Read the information on the label in Figure 9.6, and explain how to prepare the medication for administration to the patient.

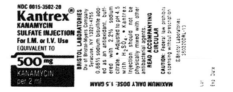

▶ FIGURE 9.6 Drug label for Kantrex

Because the vial contains medication measured in milligrams per milliliter, you want to convert 0.4 gram to milligrams and then find the amount in milliliters.

$$0.4 \text{ g} \longrightarrow ? \text{ mg} \longrightarrow ? \text{ mL}$$

$$0.4 \text{ g} \times \frac{? \text{ mg}}{? \text{ g}} \times \frac{? \text{ mL}}{? \text{ mg}} = ? \text{ mL}$$

The first equivalent fraction is $\frac{1000 \text{ mg}}{1 \text{ g}}$.

The label reads 500 milligrams per 2 milliliters, so the second equivalent fraction is $\frac{2 \text{ mL}}{500 \text{ mg}}$.

$$0.4 \text{ \cancel{g}} \times \frac{\overset{2}{\cancel{1000 \text{ mg}}}}{1 \text{ \cancel{g}}} \times \frac{2 \text{ mL}}{\underset{1}{\cancel{500 \text{ mg}}}} = 1.6 \text{ mL}$$

So, 1.6 milliliters contains 0.4 gram of Kantrex, and you would administer 1.6 milliliters IM to your patient.

▶ **E X A M P L E 9 . 7**

Examine the label in Figure 9.7, and determine the quantity of solution to be withdrawn from the vial if the medication order reads 250 milligrams of 10% calcium chloride.

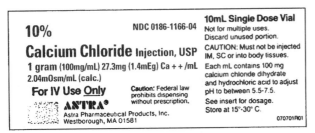

10%

NDC 0186-1166-04

Calcium Chloride Injection, USP

1 gram (100mg/mL) 27.3mg (1.4mEg) Ca + + /mL
2.04mOsm/mL (calc.)

For IV Use Only

Caution: Federal law prohibits dispensing without prescription.

ASTRA®
Astra Pharmaceutical Products, Inc.
Westborough, MA 01581

10mL Single Dose Vial
Not for multiple uses.
Discard unused portion.
CAUTION: Must not be injected IM, SC or into body tissues.
Each mL contains 100 mg calcium chloride dihydrate and hydrochloric acid to adjust pH to between 5.5-7.5.
See insert for dosage.
Store at 15°-30° C.

070701R01

▶ **FIGURE 9.7 Drug label for calcium chloride**

You want to convert milligrams to milliliters.

$$250 \text{ mg} \longrightarrow ? \text{ mL}$$

$$250 \text{ mg} \times \frac{? \text{ mL}}{? \text{ mg}} = ? \text{ mL}$$

The label "10% calcium chloride" means that 10 grams of calcium chloride are in 100 milliliters, or 100 milligrams of calcium chloride are in 1 milliliter. So, the equivalent fraction is $\frac{1 \text{ mL}}{100 \text{ mg}}$.

$$\overset{5}{\cancel{250 \text{ mg}}} \times \frac{1 \text{ mL}}{\underset{2}{\cancel{100 \text{ mg}}}} = 2.5 \text{ mL}$$

So you would withdraw 2.5 milliliters from the vial.

▶ **E X A M P L E   9 . 8**

The prescriber ordered 40 units of NPH insulin (Humulin N) sc for a patient, and you must use a standard syringe because no insulin syringe is available. What would the dose be in milliliters? The label on the vial is shown in Figure 9.8.

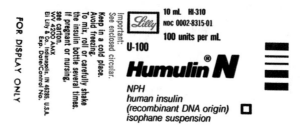

▶ **FIGURE 9.8 Drug label for Humulin N**

You want to convert 40 units to milliliters.

40 u = ? mL

You cancel the units and obtain the equivalent amount in milliliters.

$$40 \text{ u} \times \frac{? \text{ mL}}{? \text{ u}} = ? \text{ mL}$$

The label reads 100 units per milliliter, which means 100 u = 1 mL. So, the equivalent fraction is $\frac{1 \text{ mL}}{100 \text{ u}}$.

$$\overset{4}{\cancel{40}} \text{ u} \times \frac{1 \text{ mL}}{\underset{10}{\cancel{100}} \text{ u}} = 0.4 \text{ mL}$$

So, 40 units would be contained in 0.4 milliliter, and you would draw 0.4 milliliter into the standard syringe.

HEPARIN

Heparin is an anticoagulant (clot-preventing) medication that can be administered to a patient by subcutaneous injection, intermittent intravenous injection, and by continuous intravenous infusion. Like insulin, penicillin, and some other medications, heparin is supplied in *USP units,* which are often shortened (as noted in Chapter 7) to *units* and abbreviated u. Vials of heparin are prepared by the manufacturer in a variety of strengths. Some examples of heparin preparations are shown in Table 9.1.

TABLE 9.1

USP Unit Potencies of Heparin

Supplied Form	Potency per mL
Vials	1000 units
	5000 units
	20,000 units
	40,000 units
Ampules	1000 units
	5000 units
	10,000 units

NOTES/WORKSPACE

Heparin is also available in premixed intravenous solutions—for example, 12,500 units in 250 milliliters of 5% D/W; 25,000 units in 500 milliliters of 0.45% saline solution. With a premixed parenteral solution, the nurse has to convert the physician's order to the volume of solution that contains the amount of heparin ordered.

EXAMPLE 9.9

The prescriber ordered:

Fragmin 5000 u sc q12h

The label on the vial (Figure 9.9) reads 10,000 units per milliliter. How many milliliters will you administer to the patient?

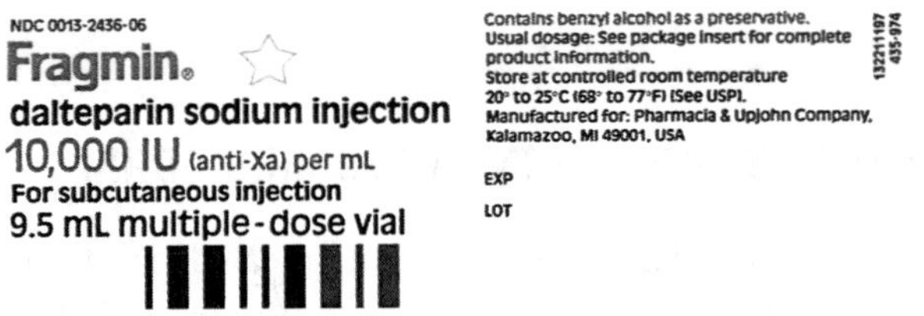
NDC 0013-2436-06
Fragmin®
dalteparin sodium injection
10,000 IU (anti-Xa) per mL
For subcutaneous injection
9.5 mL multiple-dose vial
Contains benzyl alcohol as a preservative.
Usual dosage: See package insert for complete product information.
Store at controlled room temperature 20° to 25°C (68° to 77°F) [See USP].
Manufactured for: Pharmacia & Upjohn Company, Kalamazoo, MI 49001, USA
EXP
LOT
132211197
435-974

FIGURE 9.9 Drug label for Fragmin

You want to convert units to milliliters.

$$5000 \text{ u} = ? \text{ mL}$$

You cancel the units and obtain the equivalent amount in milliliters.

$$5000 \text{ u} \times \frac{? \text{ mL}}{? \text{ u}} = ? \text{ mL}$$

The label on the vial reads 10,000 units per milliliter, so the equivalent fraction is $\frac{1 \text{ mL}}{10{,}000 \text{ u}}$.

$$\overset{1}{\cancel{5000}} \cancel{\text{u}} \times \frac{1 \text{ mL}}{\underset{2}{\cancel{10{,}000}} \cancel{\text{u}}} = 0.5 \text{ mL}$$

So, 0.5 milliliter contains 10,000 units of heparin, and you would administer 0.5 milliliter of Fragmin, which is a low molecular weight heparin, to the patient sc.

▶ **EXAMPLE 9.10**

The prescriber ordered:

heparin 8000 u sc q8h

If the label on the drug vial reads 10,000 units per minims 15, how many minims equal 8000 units?

You want to convert 8000 units to minims.

$$8000 \text{ u} = \text{m} \text{?}$$

You cancel the units and obtain the equivalent amount in minims.

$$8000 \text{ u} \times \frac{\text{m} \text{ ?}}{\text{? u}} = \text{m} \text{ ?}$$

The label on the vial reads 10,000 units per minims 15, so the fraction is $\frac{\text{m} \, 15}{10,000 \text{ u}}$.

$$\overset{8}{\cancel{8000}} \text{ u} \times \frac{\text{m} \, 15}{\underset{10}{\cancel{10,000}} \text{ u}} = \frac{\text{m} \, 120}{10} = \text{m} \, 12$$

So, minims 12 contain 8000 units of heparin, and you would administer minims 12 sc to your patient.

PARENTERAL MEDICATIONS SUPPLIED IN POWDERED FORM

Some parenteral medications are supplied in powdered form in sealed vials (Figure 9.10). The powder cannot be removed from these vials. You must add sterile water or saline to the vial and dissolve the powder to form a solution. You then inject the liquid volume of prepared solution that contains the proper amount of the drug.

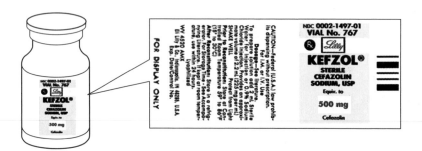

▶ **FIGURE 9.10 A sealed vial of Kefzol in powdered form with label detail**

The pharmaceutical manufacturer provides instructions that specify the amount of sterile liquid that must be injected into the vial of powder to make a solution of a given strength. After preparing the solution, you need to calculate the volume that contains the prescribed amount of the drug.

▶ **EXAMPLE 9.11**

The prescriber ordered 112.5 milligrams of cefazolin (Kefzol) IV. Read the label shown in Figure 9.10. How would you prepare this dose?

First prepare the solution. Inject 2 milliliters of sterile water into the vial. Now the vial contains a solution in which

$$1 \text{ mL} = 225 \text{ mg}$$

To calculate the amount of this solution, you need to convert milligrams to milliliters.

$$112.5 \text{ mg} \times \frac{? \text{ mL}}{? \text{ mg}} = ? \text{ mL}$$

The vial now contains 225 milligrams per 1 milliliter, so the equivalent fraction is $\frac{1 \text{ mL}}{225 \text{ mg}}$.

$$112.5 \text{ mg} \times \frac{1 \text{ mL}}{225 \text{ mg}} = 0.5 \text{ mL}$$

So, you would add 2 mL of sterile water to the vial, then withdraw 0.5 milliliters from the vial and administer it to the patient.

▶ **EXAMPLE 9.12**

The prescriber has ordered 0.25 gram of the antibiotic ceftazidime (Fortaz). The label on the vial reads 500 milligrams per milliliter. How many milliliters of the solution would contain the prescribed dose?

You want to convert 0.25 gram to milliliters. This is a two-step problem.

$$0.25 \text{ g} \longrightarrow ? \text{ mg} \longrightarrow ? \text{ mL}$$

$$0.25 \text{ g} \times \frac{? \text{ mg}}{? \text{ g}} \times \frac{? \text{ mL}}{? \text{ mg}} = ? \text{ mL}$$

The first equivalent fraction is $\frac{1000 \text{ mg}}{1 \text{ g}}$.

Because the prepared solution is 1 mL = 500 mg, the second equivalent fraction is $\frac{1 \text{ mL}}{500 \text{ mg}}$.

$$0.25 \text{ g} \times \frac{\overset{2}{\cancel{1000 \text{ mg}}}}{1 \text{ g}} \times \frac{1 \text{ mL}}{\underset{1}{\cancel{500 \text{ mg}}}} = 0.5 \text{ mL}$$

So, 0.5 milliliter of the solution contains 0.25 gram of Fortaz.

▶ **E X A M P L E   9 . 1 3**

The prescriber ordered: cefoxitin sodium 0.75 g IM q12h. The vial of cefoxitin sodium, an antibiotic, contains 5 grams of powder. The instructions are as follows: Add 13.2 mL of sterile water to the vial, 3 mL = 1 g. How many milliliters of the solution would contain the prescribed dose?

You want to change 0.75 gram to milliliters.

$$0.75 \text{ g} \times \frac{? \text{ mL}}{? \text{ g}} = ? \text{ mL}$$

Because the prepared solution is 3 mL = 1 g, the equivalent fraction is $\frac{3 \text{ mL}}{1 \text{ g}}$.

$$0.75 \text{ g} \times \frac{3 \text{ mL}}{1 \text{ g}} = 2.25 \text{ mL}$$

So, 2.25 milliliters of the prepared solution contain 0.75 gram of cefoxitin sodium.

C A S E   S T U D Y   9

A patient was admitted to the hospital with a diagnosis of type II diabetes Mellitus, congestive heart failure, hypertension, and a urinary tract infection.

Her vital signs are as follows: BP, 168/102; P, 92; R, 30; T, 101F. The patient responded well to her treatment and was discharged with the following orders:

- Visiting nurse qd × 3 with follow-up
- NPH insulin 44 units ac breakfast daily sc
- Blood glucose levels q6h
- Diabenese 0.2 g bid po
- Doxazosin 0.004 g qd hs po
- Lasix 60 mg po qd
- K-Lor 30 mEq po qd
- Vistaril 20 mg hs qd prn
- Antivert 0.025 g 4h prn for nausea
- Zoloft 0.1 g qd po

1. Place an arrow at the appropriate measurement on the correct syringe to indicate the amount of subcutaneous medication to be administered.

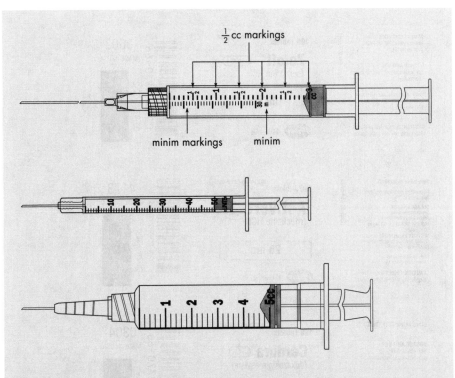

$\frac{1}{2}$ cc markings

minim markings   minim

2. Lasix is supplied in 20, 40, and 80 mg tablets. Which strength tablets and how many would you administer to the patient? _____

3. You have K-Lor tablets 10 mEq each. How many of these tablets equal the prescribed dose? _____

Read the appropriate labels at the end of this case study and answer questions 4 through 8.

4. How many tablets of chlorpropamide will you prepare for this patient? _____

5. How many tablets of Cardura will you give to the patient? _____

6. Calculate the number of milliliters that equals the prescribed dose of hydroxyzine. _____

7. How many tablets of meclizine per day would be given to the patient? _____

8. Calculate the number of tablets of sertraline that equals the prescribed dose. _____

Answers to Case Studies appear in Appendix A.

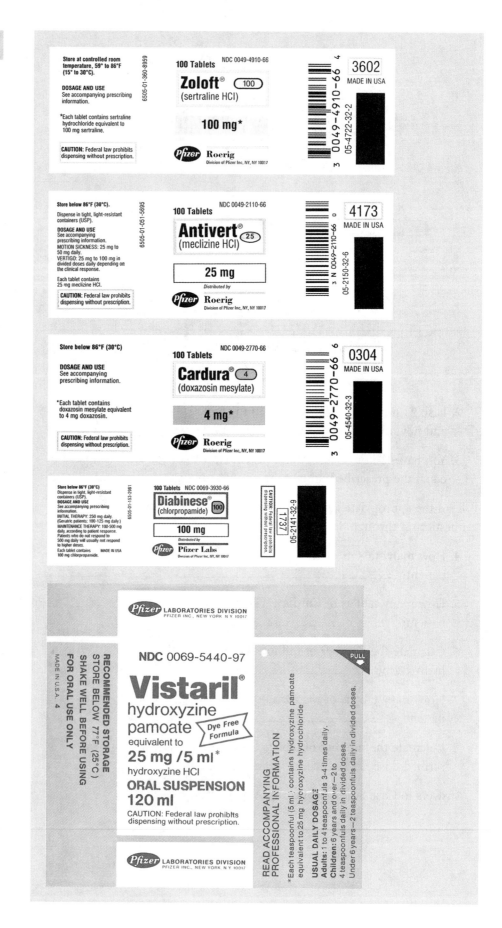

You will find the answers to the *Try These for Practice* below. Answers to *Exercises* and *Cumulative Review* appear in Appendix A at the back of the book. Your instructor has the answers to the *Additional Exercises*.

Try These for Practice

Test your comprehension after reading the chapter.

1. The prescriber ordered cefazolin sodium 0.44 g IM q8h. The directions state: Add 2.5 mL of sterile water to a vial labeled 1 g, 1 mL = 330 mg. How many milliliters equal 0.44 gram? _____

2. The prescriber ordered low-dose insulin 0.54 u/kg sc qd. The label on the vial reads 100 units per milliliter. How many milliliters will you give your patient, whose weight is 50 kilograms? _____

3. Your patient is to receive grain $\frac{1}{400}$ of atropine sulfate. The label on the vial reads 0.1 milligram per milliliter. How many milliliters equal grain $\frac{1}{400}$?

_____

4. An ampule of digoxin is labeled 0.125 milligram per milliliter. How many milliliters equal 0.25 milligram? _____

5. If your patient's medication order is for 5000 units of heparin and the vial is labeled 10,000 units per milliliter, how many minims equal 5000 units? _____

Answers 1. 1.3 mL   2. 0.3 mL   3. 1.5 mL   4. 2 mL   5. ℥ 8

Exercises

Reinforce your understanding in class or at home.

1. A patient is to receive 25 units of the hormonal drug vasopressin (Pitressin) IM. If the label reads 50 units per 2 milliliters, how many milliliters will you administer to the patient? _____

2. The order reads: calcitonin 2.5 u/kg sc daily. The label reads: 100 units per milliliter. How many milliliters will you administer to the patient if the the weight of the patient is 62 kilograms? _____

3. The order reads: amitriptyline 0.025 g IM tid. If the drug vial is labeled 10 milligrams per milliliter, how many milliliters will you prepare for the patient? _____

4. The prescriber ordered clindamycin 200 mg IM q6h. The label reads: 1 mL = 150 mg. How many milliliters will equal 200 milligrams?

_____

5. Read the first medication order in Figure 9.11. The vial of furosemide is labeled 10 milligrams per milliliter. How many milliliters would you prepare for a patient who weighs 45 kilograms? _____

✚ GENERAL HOSPITAL ✚

PRESS HARD WITH BALLPOINT PEN. WRITE DATE & TIME AND SIGN EACH ORDER

DATE	TIME	A.M.
12/5/01	4	(P.M.)

1. furosemide 0.1 mg/kg IV

2. diphenhydramine 0.05 g IM stat

3. Premarin 0.25 mg q12h for 4 doses

IMPRINT
605432   12/5/01
Julie Jones   5/16/37
316 E. Main St, Apt 20   Prot
Puyallup, WA 97054   Medicare

Dr. Leon Ablon

ORDERS NOTED
DATE _12/5/01_ TIME _4:05_ (A.M. / P.M.)

❑ MEDEX   ❑ KARDEX

NURSE'S SIG. _J. Olsen_

SIGNATURE
L. Ablon   M.D.

FILLED BY   DATE

PHYSICIAN'S ORDERS

▶ **FIGURE 9.11 Physician's order sheet**

6. In the second medication order in Figure 9.11, the patient must receive 0.05 gram of the antihistamine diphenhydramine (Benadryl) IM stat. The vial is labeled 50 milligrams per milliliter. How many milliliters will you administer to this patient? _____

7. Read the information in the third medication order in Figure 9.11. If the vial of Premarin is labeled 0.025 gram per 5 milliliters, how many milliliters equal the prescribed single dose? _____

8. The dose of dobutamine (Dobutrex) ordered by the prescriber is 100 micrograms per kilogram. If the patient weighs 75 kilograms and the vial is labeled 12.5 milligrams per milliliter, how many milliliters would you prepare? _____

9. The order reads: nitroglycerine 0.3 mg IV once only. The vial is labeled 50 milligrams per 10 milliliters. Calculate the amount in milliliters required for this dose. _____

10. The label on the vial of verapamil HCl reads: 10 milligrams per 4 milliliters. If the medication order is 2.5 milligrams, calculate the amount in milliliters you would prepare for this patient. _____

11. The label on a vial reads: penicillin G 1,000,000 u. The instructions are as follows: Add 19.6 mL of sterile diluent to vial, 1 mL = 50,000 u. How many milliliters contain 100,000 units? _____

12. The prescriber ordered: Dolophine HCl 0.015 g IM q4h prn. Read the label in Figure 9.12. How many milliliters will you prepare for this patient? _____

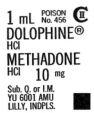

POISON No. 456 C II
1 mL
DOLOPHINE®
HCl
METHADONE
HCl   **10** mg
Sub. Q. or I.M.
YU 6001 AMU
LILLY, INDPLS.

▶ **FIGURE 9.12 Drug label for Dolophine HCl**

13. Read the label in Figure 9.13. Calculate how many milliliters of insulin you will prepare if the order reads: NPH insulin 40 u sc at breakfast.

_____

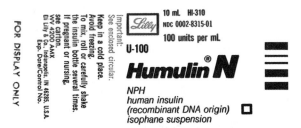

▶ **FIGURE 9.13 Drug label for Humulin N**

14. The order reads: Terramycin 10 mg/kg IM q12h. Read the label in Figure 9-14. How many milliliters will you prepare for a patient who weighs 25 kilograms? _____

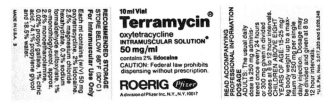

▶ **FIGURE 9.14 Drug label for Terramycin**

15. The patient must receive 190 milligrams of ceftizoxime (Cefizox) IM. The 1 g vial has the following directions: Add 10 mL of sterile water, 1 mL = 95 mg. How many minims of this antibiotic will you administer to the patient? _____

16. Your patient is to receive 75 milligrams of dexamethasone (Dalalone), injected into a joint by the physician. If the vial is labeled 20 milligrams per milliliters, how many milliliters will you prepare? _____

17. The order reads: phenytoin 0.2 g IM stat. The drug label reads 200 milligrams per 2 milliliters. How many milliliters of this anticonvulsant will you administer to your patient? _____

18. Your patient has been prescribed 1.3 milliliters of the antineoplastic drug methotrexate sodium (Folex) IM per day. The recommended dose is 3.3 milligrams per square meter per day. The label on the vial reads 25 milligrams per milliliter. If this patient's body surface area (BSA) is 1.42 square meters, is this an appropriate dose? _____

19. Prepare 1550 milligrams of ticarcillin (Ticar) from a vial that has the following directions: Add 13 mL of sterile water to the vial, 200 mg = 1 mL. How many milliliters contain this dose? _____

20. The order reads: methylergonovine maleate (Methergine) 0.0002 g IM q4h for three doses. The drug label reads 0.2 milligram per milliliter. How many milliliters will you administer in one dose? What is the total number of milligrams this patient will receive in three doses of this oxytocic drug? _____

Additional Exercises

Now, on your own, test yourself! Ask your instructor to check your answers.

1. Describe how to prepare 6500 units sc of heparin from a vial labeled 10,000 units per milliliter.

_____

_____

2. The prescriber ordered: epinephrine HCL 0.5 mg IM stat. The label on the vial reads 1:1000. How many milliliters will you administer to the patient? _____

3. The medication order reads: atropine sulfate gr $\frac{1}{150}$ sc @ 7 A.M. The drug ampule reads 0.5 milligram per milliliter. How many milliliters will you administer to the patient? _____

4. The prescriber ordered: diltiazem 17.5 mg IV. The label on the vial reads 5 milligrams per milliliter. How many milliliters will you prepare of this drug? _____

5. Read the first medication order in Figure 9.15. The ampule for this medication reads 1 mL = 25 mg meperidine HCL and 25 mg promethazine. How many milliliters will you administer to your patient? _____

⊕ GENERAL HOSPITAL ⊕

PRESS HARD WITH BALLPOINT PEN. WRITE DATE & TIME AND SIGN EACH ORDER

DATE 9/9/01	TIME 12 noon

1. meperidine HCL 50mg } IM stat
   promethazine 50 mg
2. Irrigate PICC (peripherally inserted central catheter) q12h with 5000 u of urokinase
3. estrone 0.001 g IM qd × 5

SIGNATURE   J. Olsen   M.D.

IMPRINT
407553   9/9/01
Joshua Kelley   3/21/48
1505M. Street   Jewish
Los Angeles, CA 93120   BC
Dr. J. Olsen

ORDERS NOTED
DATE 9/9/01 TIME 12:10 A.M./P.M.
❏ MEDEX ❏ KARDEX
NURSE'S SIG. A.Giangrasso

FILLED BY   DATE

PHYSICIAN'S ORDERS

▶ **FIGURE 9.15** Physician's order sheet

6. The second medication order in Figure 9.15 is for 5000 units of urokinase. If the label on the drug vial reads 5000 units per milliliter, how many milliliters of this thrombolytic drug will you use in 48 hours? _____

7. The third medication order in Figure 9.15 is prepackaged in a vial labeled 2 milligrams per milliliter. How many milliliters of this hormone will you administer to your patient? _____

8. The patient must receive 900 milligrams of clindamycin phosphate. The label reads: Add 4.8 mL of sterile water to vial, 0.4 g = 1 mL. How many milliliters equal the prescribed dose? _____

9. The order reads: digoxin 0.25 mg IM qd. The label reads 0.5 milligrams per 2 milliliters. How many milliliters of this cardiotonic drug will you administer to the patient? _____

NOTES/WORKSPACE

Practice Sets 201

10. The medication order reads: compazine 0.01 g IM. How many milliliters would equal this dose if the label on the vial reads 5 mg per milliliter? _____

11. The order reads: vitamin B$_{12}$ 800 mcg IM stat. The drug vial is labeled 1 milligram per milliliter. How many milliliters will you administer to your patient? _____

12. The order reads: Kantrex 275 mg IM stat. Read the information on the drug label in Figure 9.16, and calculate the amount of medication in milliliters you will administer to your patient. _____

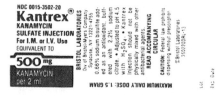

▶ FIGURE 9.16 Drug label for Kantrex

13. The prescriber ordered: Humulin BR insulin 45 u sc 7 A.M. Read the label in Figure 9.17, and calculate the amount in minims you would prepare for this order. _____

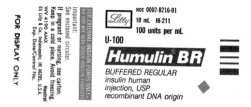

▶ FIGURE 9.17 Drug label for Humulin BR

14. Your patient has an order for 0.5 unit per kilogram of Semilente Iletin I. The patient weighs 110 kilograms. According to the label in Figure 9.18, how many cubic centimeters will you administer to your patient? _____

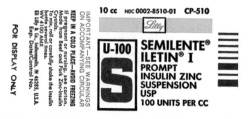

▶ FIGURE 9.18 Drug label for Semilente Iletin I

15. The patient is to receive 25 milligrams of furosemide IM. Read the information on the label in Figure 9.19, and determine the amount in milliliters you will give your patient. _____

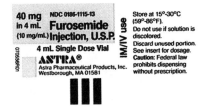

▶ **FIGURE 9.19 Drug label for furosemide**

16. Your client must receive grain $\frac{1}{500}$ of atropine sulfate sc. The ampule reads 1 milligram per 10 milliliters. How may milliliters contain grain $\frac{1}{500}$?

_____

17. If the order for magnesium sulfate is 1200 milligrams IM, how many milliliters would you administer from a vial labeled 50% magnesium sulfate?

_____

18. The prescriber has ordered 100 units per kilogram of erythropoietin sc tiw for a patient in end-stage renal disease. The patient weighs 60 kilograms, and the label on the vial reads 6000 units per milliliter. How many minims will you administer? _____

19. If you were to prepare grain $\frac{1}{400}$ atropine sulfate from a vial labeled 0.2 milligram per milliliter, how many minims would equal this dose?

_____

20. The order reads: sumatriptan 0.006 g sc stat. The label on the vial reads 6 milligrams per 0.5 milliliter. How may milliliters contain this dose?

_____

CUMULATIVE REVIEW EXERCISES

Review your mastery of earlier chapters.

1. The medication order is for 5 milligrams per kilogram of ritonavir (Norvir). Read the label in Figure 9.20, and determine how many milliliters are contained in this dose if the patient weighs 48 kilograms?

_____

NDC 0074-1940-63
240 mL

NORVIR®

(RITONAVIR ORAL SOLUTION)

80 mg per mL

Shake well before each use.

DO NOT REFRIGERATE

Use within 30 days from dispensing.

▶ **FIGURE 9.20 Drug label for Norvir**

2. The medication order is for grain $\frac{1}{3}$ po of dicyclomine HCl (Bentyl), an antispasmodic drug. The tablets on hand are 10 milligrams. How many tablets would you administer? _____

3. The medication order reads 0.12 gram qd of propranolol (Inderal SL), an antihypertensive drug. Each capsule contains 60 milligrams. How many capsules would you administer? _____

4. The medication order reads: Viagra 0.05 g po. How many tablets would you administer if each tablet contains 50 mg? _____

5. A vial is labeled meperidine HCl (Demerol), 50 milligrams per milliliter. The prescriber orders 12.5 milligrams IM. How many minims of this analgesic narcotic would you administer? _____

6. The order is for K-Lor 60 mEq po stat. Read the label in Figure 9.21, and determine the number of packets you would need and the number of ounces of liquid the patient would receive. _____

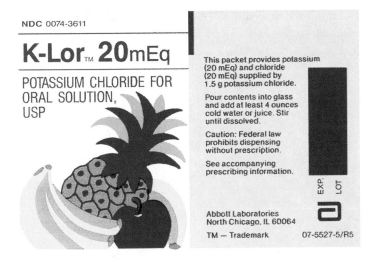

NDC 0074-3611

K-Lor™ 20mEq

POTASSIUM CHLORIDE FOR
ORAL SOLUTION,
USP

This packet provides potassium
(20 mEq) and chloride
(20 mEq) supplied by
1.5 g potassium chloride.

Pour contents into glass
and add at least 4 ounces
cold water or juice. Stir
until dissolved.

Caution: Federal law
prohibits dispensing
without prescription.

See accompanying
prescribing information.

EXP.
LOT

Abbott Laboratories
North Chicago, IL 60064

TM — Trademark   07-5527-5/R5

▶ **FIGURE 9.21 Drug label for K-Lor**

7. The prescriber ordered: norfloxacin 0.4 g po. The drug label reads
   1 tab = 400 mg. How many tablets of this oral antibiotic would you
   administer? _____

8. The medication order is for 150 mg IM of cimetidine (Tagamet), an anti-
   ulcer agent. The drug label reads 300 milligrams per 2 milliliters. How
   many milliliters would you administer to the patient? _____

9. The medication order is for 0.3 gram po of rifabutin (Mycobutin), an antibiotic. Read the label in Figure 9.22. How many capsules would you administer to the patient? _____

NDC 0013-5301-17

MYCOBUTIN®
(Rifabutin Capsules, USP)

Keep tightly closed.
Store at controlled room
temperature, 15° to 30°C
(59° to 86°F).
Dispense in a tight
container as defined in the
USP.
Lot No./Expires

150 mg

Each capsule contains:
Rifabutin, USP 150 mg.

CAUTION: Federal law
prohibits dispensing without
prescription.

100 CAPSULES

Pharmacia

USUAL DOSAGE: Two
capsules in a single daily
administration. For
additional prescribing
information read package
insert.
Manufactured by:
PHARMACIA S.p.A.
ASCOLI PICENO, ITALY
For:
Pharmacia Inc.
Kalamazoo, MI 49001, USA

057070496

▶ **FIGURE 9.22 Drug label for Mycobutin**

10. The drug vial contains 1,000,000 units of penicillin G. The label directions state: Add 2.3 mL of sterile water to the vial, 1.2 mL = 500,000 u. How many milliliters equal 200,000 units? _____

11. gr $\dfrac{1}{200}$ = _____ g

12. 0.003 g = _____ mg

13. 90 mg = gr _____

14. $2\dfrac{1}{2}$ t = _____ gtt

15. 0.06 mg = gr _____

Specialized Medication Preparations

CHAPTER TEN

Calculating Flow Rates for Enteral Solutions and Intravenous Infusions

▶ **Objectives**

After completing this chapter, you will be able to

- Understand the basic concepts and standard equipment involved in the delivery of intravenous (IV) and enteral infusions.
- Calculate the flow rate of IV solutions.
- Calculate the flow rate of enteral solutions.

This chapter introduces the basic concepts and standard equipment involved in intravenous and enteral therapy. You will also learn how to use dimensional analysis to calculate flow rates for these infusions.

INTRODUCTION TO INTRAVENOUS AND ENTERAL SOLUTIONS

Fluids can be given to a patient slowly over a period of time through a vein (*intravenous*) or through a tube inserted into the alimentary tract (*enteral*).

Enteral Solutions

When a patient needs nutrients, fluid, or medications and cannot swallow, the prescriber may write an order for an enteral feeding. Enteral feedings provide nutrients by way of a tube into the alimentary tract.

There are various methods for tube feeding. The feeding tube is inserted into the stomach either indirectly (through the nares and esophagus) or directly (through an incision in the abdomen and the stomach).

A tube inserted directly into the stomach and sutured in place is called a ***gastrotomy tube.*** The ***percutaneous endoscopic gastrotomy (PEG)*** tube is another type of feeding tube inserted directly into the stomach.

Currently available enteral feeding solutions include Isocal, Ensure, and Sustacal.

An enteral solution order might read:

Isocal 50 mL/hr via nasogastric tube

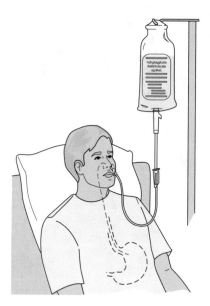

▶ **FIGURE 10.1 Using a calibrated plastic bag to administer a tube feeding.**

Intravenous Fluids

Intravenous means through the veins. Fluids are administered intravenously to provide fluid, nutrients, electrolytes, minerals, and specific medications to the patient.

Intravenous Solutions

The most commonly prescribed intravenous solutions are listed in Table 10.1.

Intravenous Solutions

Name of Solution	Common Abbreviation
0.45% sodium chloride injection USP	1/2 NS, 0.45% NS
0.9% sodium chloride injection USP	0.9% NS
5% dextrose in 0.22% sodium chloride injection USP	5% D/0.22% NS
5% dextrose injection USP	5% D/W, D/5/W
5% dextrose in 0.45% sodium chloride injection USP	5% D/0.45% NS D/5/0.45% NS
5% dextrose in 0.9% sodium chloride injection USP	5% D/0.9% NS D/5/09% NS
Lactated Ringer's injection USP	LR, RL, RLS
Lactated Ringer's and 5% dextrose injection USP	5% D/RL, D/5/RL

Intravenous fluids generally contain dextrose, sodium chloride, and/or electrolytes:

- D/5/W (or 5% D/W) is a 5% dextrose solution, which means that 5 milliliters or 5 grams of dextrose are dissolved in water to make each 100 milliliters of this solution.

- 0.9% NS stands for a solution in which each 100 milliliters contains 0.9 gram of sodium chloride.

- 5% D/0.45% NS stands for a solution containing 5 milliliters or 5 grams of dextrose in each 100 milliliters of 0.45% normal saline solution.

- Ringer's lactate (RL), also called lactated Ringer's solution (LRS), is a solution containing electrolytes.

Additional information on IV fluids can be found in nursing and pharmacology textbooks.

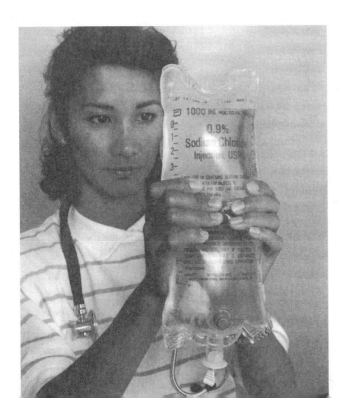

An order for intravenous fluids must include the name of the solution, medication (if required), and the length of time the solution is to infuse.
For example, an intravenous order might read:

1000 mL 5% D/W IV for 8 hr

The registered professional nurse, vocational nurse, or licensed practical nurse must perform the necessary calculations to determine the correct rate at which the enteral or intravenous solutions will enter the body (**flow rate**). The flow rate will be measured in drops per minute, milliliters per minute, or milliliters per hour.

EQUIPMENT FOR IV INFUSIONS

The equipment that must be used for the administration of IV infusions includes the IV solution, the package of tubing, and the drop chamber (Figure 10.2).

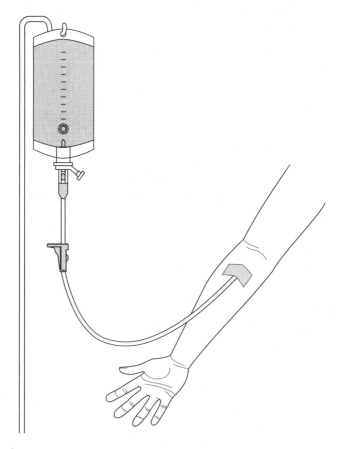

▶ **FIGURE 10.2 Primary intravenous line**

Figure 10.3 shows packaging of IV tubing.

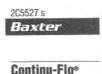

2C5527 s

Baxter

Continu-Flo®
Solution Set

3 Injection Sites

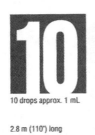

10 drops approx. 1 mL

2.8 m (110") long

▶ **FIGURE 10.3 Box of IV tubing calibrated at 10 drops approximately 1mL**

The drip chamber (Figure 10.4) is located at the site of the entrance of the tubing into the container of intravenous solution. It allows you to count the number of drops per minute that the client is receiving (flow rate).

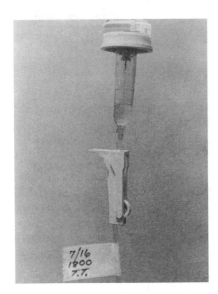

▶ **FIGURE 10.4 Tubing labeled with date, time of attachment, and nurse's initials**

A roll valve clamp or clip (Figure 10.4) is connected to the tubing and can be manipulated to increase or decrease the flow rate.

The size of the drop that IV tubing delivers is not standard; it depends on the way the tubing is designed. Manufacturers specify the number of drops that equal 1 milliliter for their particular tubing. This equivalent is called the tubing's **drop factor;** see Table 10.2. You must know the tubing's drop factor when calculating the flow rate of solutions in drops per minute (gtt/min) or microdrops per minute (μgtt/min).

▶ TABLE 10.2

Common Drop Factors		
10 gtt	=	1 mL
15 gtt	=	1 mL
20 gtt	=	1 mL
60 μgtt	=	1 mL

NOTE: 60 microdrops = 1 milliliter is a universal equivalent for IV tubing calibrated in microdrops.

Intravenous infusions can also be controlled by electronic devices called **infusion pumps.** These pumps are operated by electricity or by battery and can be set to deliver the IV solution in either milliliters per minute or milliliters per hour. There are many different types of infusion pumps. These include syringe pumps, controller pumps, volumetric pumps, and burettes.

The burette and syringe pumps are generally used for smaller amounts of solution and are not electronic.

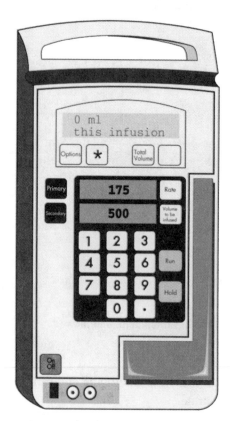
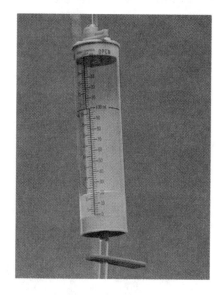

▶ FIGURE 10.5 (a) Typical infusion pump; (b) A volume-control set below the drip chamber of an intravenous infusion

Pumps have many advantages over traditional tubing. On the newer pumps, the amount of fluid, the amount of medication, and the flow rate can easily be coded on the pump panel. If there is an interruption in the flow, an alarm sounds to alert the nursing staff and the patient.

CALCULATING THE FLOW RATE OF INFUSIONS

▶ **EXAMPLE 10.1**

The order is 240 cc per 10 hours of D/5/W. Using the tubing in Figure 10.3, calculate the number of drops per minute that you would administer.

In Figure 10.3, the drop factor is 10 drops per milliliter. The notation "240 cubic centimeters in a 10-hour period" means $\frac{240 \text{ cc}}{10 \text{ hr}}$. You want to convert cubic centimeters per hour to drops per minute.

$$\frac{240 \text{ cc}}{10 \text{ hr}} \longrightarrow \frac{? \text{ gtt}}{? \text{ min}}$$

This is a two-step problem, which you do in one line as follows:

$$\frac{240 \text{ cc}}{10 \text{ hr}} \times \frac{? \text{ gtt}}{? \text{ cc}} \times \frac{? \text{ hr}}{? \text{ min}} = ? \frac{\text{gtt}}{\text{min}}$$

Because 10 gtt = 1 cc, the first equivalent fraction is $\frac{10 \text{ gtt}}{1 \text{ cc}}$. Because 60 min = 1 hr, the second equivalent fraction is $\frac{1 \text{ hr}}{60 \text{ min}}$.

$$\frac{240 \cancel{\text{cc}}}{\cancel{10} \cancel{\text{hr}}} \times \frac{\cancel{10} \text{ gtt}}{1 \cancel{\text{cc}}} \times \frac{\cancel{1} \text{ hr}}{60 \text{ min}} = \frac{4 \text{ gtt}}{\text{min}}$$

So, 240 cubic centimeters given over a 10-hour period would be administered at the rate of 4 drops per minute.

▶ **EXAMPLE 10.2**

The medication order reads:

250 mL 0.9% NS in 16 h IV

The drop factor is 60 microdrops per milliliter. How many microdrops per minute would you administer?

The notation "250 milliliters in a 16-hour period" means $\frac{250 \text{ mL}}{16 \text{ hr}}$. You want to convert milliliters per hour to microdrops per minute:

$$\frac{250 \text{ mL}}{16 \text{ hr}} \longrightarrow \frac{? \mu\text{gtt}}{? \text{ min}}$$

This is a two-step problem, which you do on one line, as follows:

$$\frac{250 \text{ mL}}{16 \text{ hr}} \times \frac{? \text{ }\mu\text{gtt}}{? \text{ mL}} \times \frac{? \text{ hr}}{? \text{ min}} = ? \frac{\text{gtt}}{\text{min}}$$

Because 60 μgtt = 1 mL, the first equivalent fraction is $\frac{60 \text{ }\mu\text{gtt}}{1 \text{ mL}}$. Because 60 min = 1 hr, the second equivalent fraction is $\frac{1 \text{ hr}}{60 \text{ min}}$.

$$\frac{250 \text{ mL}}{16 \text{ hr}} \times \frac{\overset{1}{60} \text{ }\mu\text{gtt}}{1 \text{ mL}} \times \frac{1 \text{ hr}}{\underset{1}{60} \text{ min}} = \frac{250 \text{ }\mu\text{gtt}}{16 \text{ min}} = 15.6 \frac{\mu\text{gtt}}{\text{min}}$$

So, 16 microdrops per minute would be administered.

EXAMPLE 10.3

The prescriber ordered:

750 mL of 0.9% NS IV in 8 hr

The label on the box containing the intravenous set to be used for this infusion is shown in Figure 10.6. Calculate the flow rate in drops per minute.

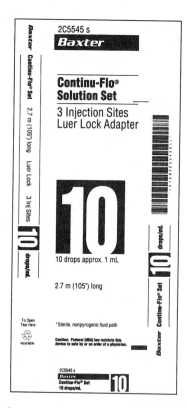

▶ FIGURE 10.6 Continu-Flo Solution Set box label

You want to convert the flow rate from milliliters per hour to drops per minute.

$$\frac{750 \text{ mL}}{8 \text{ hr}} \longrightarrow ? \frac{\text{gtt}}{\text{min}}$$

Do this on one line as follows:

$$\frac{750 \text{ mL}}{8 \text{ hr}} \times \frac{1 \text{ hr}}{60 \text{ min}} \times \frac{\overset{1}{10} \text{ gtt}}{1 \text{ mL}} = \frac{750 \text{ gtt}}{48 \text{ min}} = 15.6 \frac{\text{gtt}}{\text{min}}$$

So, the flow rate will be 16 drops per minute.

Sometimes, the infusion flow rate can change for a variety of reasons. A change will affect the prescribed duration of time in which the solution will be administered. Therefore, the nurse must assess the flow rate periodically and make any necessary adjustments.

▶ **E X A M P L E   10.4**

The medication order is for 500 milliliters of 5% D/W to infuse in 5 hours. Calculate the flow rate in drops per minute if the drop factor is 15 drops per milliliter.

To calculate the original flow rate, you want to convert milliliters per hour to drops per minute.

$$\frac{500 \text{ mL}}{5 \text{ hr}} \longrightarrow \frac{? \text{ gtt}}{\text{min}}$$

You can do this in one line as follows:

$$\frac{\overset{100}{500} \text{ mL}}{5 \text{ hr}} \times \frac{15 \text{ gtt}}{1 \text{ mL}} \times \frac{1 \text{ hr}}{60 \text{ min}} = \frac{1500 \text{ gtt}}{60 \text{ min}} = 25 \text{ gtt/min}$$

So, the original flow rate was 25 gtt/min.

When the nurse later checks the infusion, 400 milliliters remain to be absorbed in 3 hours. Now you must recalculate the flow rate for the remaining 400 milliliters.

You want to convert milliliters per hour to drops per minute.

$$\frac{400 \text{ mL}}{3 \text{ hr}} \longrightarrow ? \frac{\text{gtt}}{\text{min}}$$

Do this on one line as follows:

$$\frac{400 \text{ mL}}{3 \text{ hr}} \times \frac{? \text{ gtt}}{? \text{ mL}} \times \frac{? \text{ hr}}{? \text{ min}}$$

Because 15 gtt = 1 mL, the first equivalent fraction is $\frac{15 \text{ gtt}}{1 \text{ mL}}$. Because 60 min = 1 hr, the second equivalent fraction is $\frac{1 \text{ hr}}{60 \text{ min}}$.

$$\frac{400 \text{ mL}}{3 \text{ hr}} \times \frac{\overset{1}{15} \text{ gtt}}{1 \text{ mL}} \times \frac{1 \text{ hr}}{60 \text{ min}} = \frac{400 \text{ gtt}}{12 \text{ min}} = 33.3 \frac{\text{gtt}}{\text{min}}$$

So, the new flow rate would be 33 drops per minute.

► **EXAMPLE 10.5**

The order is 775 mL of 5% D/W in 6 hours. The flow rate was set at 26 drops per minute. You assess the infusion flow 3 hours later, and the patient has received 500 mL IV with 275 mL remaining to be infused. Recalculate the flow rate with a drop factor of 12 drops per milliliter.

You want to convert milliliters per hour to drops per minute.

$$\frac{275 \text{ mL}}{3 \text{ hr}} \longrightarrow \frac{? \text{ gtt}}{\text{min}}$$

Do this on one line as follows:

$$\frac{275 \text{ mL}}{3 \text{ hr}} \times \frac{? \text{ gtt}}{? \text{ mL}} \times \frac{? \text{ hr}}{? \text{ min}}$$

Because 12 gtt = 1 mL, the first equivalent fraction is $\frac{12 \text{ gtt}}{1 \text{ mL}}$. Because 60 min = 1 hr, the second equivalent fraction is $\frac{1 \text{ hr}}{60 \text{ min}}$.

$$\frac{275 \cancel{\text{ mL}}}{3 \cancel{\text{ hr}}} \times \frac{\overset{1}{\cancel{12}} \text{ gtt}}{\cancel{\text{mL}}} \times \frac{\cancel{1} \text{ hr}}{\underset{5}{\cancel{60}} \text{ min}} = \frac{275 \text{ gtt}}{15 \text{ min}} = 18.3 \frac{\text{gtt}}{\text{min}}$$

So, the new flow rate would be 18 drops per minute.

Notice that if you had realized that 3 hours is equivalent to 180 minutes, Example 10.5 could have been done more simply as follows:

$$\frac{275 \cancel{\text{ mL}}}{\underset{15}{\cancel{180}} \text{ min}} \times \frac{\overset{1}{\cancel{12}} \text{ gtt}}{\cancel{\text{mL}}} = 18.3 \frac{\text{gtt}}{\text{min}}$$

► **EXAMPLE 10.6**

The prescriber ordered 500 milliliters of 5% D/W. It has been calculated that the flow rate is 21 drops per minute. The drop factor is 10 drops per mL. What is the flow rate in milliliters per hour?

You want to convert drops per minute to milliliters per hour.

$$\frac{21 \text{ gtt}}{1 \text{ min}} \longrightarrow ? \frac{\text{mL}}{\text{hr}}$$

Do this on one line as follows:

$$\frac{21 \text{ gtt}}{1 \text{ min}} \times \frac{? \text{ mL}}{? \text{ gtt}} \times \frac{? \text{ min}}{? \text{ hr}} = ? \frac{\text{mL}}{\text{hr}}$$

Because 10 gtt = 1 mL and 60 min = 1 hr, the two equivalent fractions are $\frac{1 \text{ mL}}{10 \text{ gtt}}$ and $\frac{60 \text{ min}}{1 \text{ hr}}$.

$$\frac{21 \ \cancel{gtt}}{1 \ \cancel{min}} \times \frac{1 \ mL}{\cancel{10} \ \cancel{gtt}}_{1} \times \frac{\overset{6}{\cancel{60} \ \cancel{min}}}{1 \ hr} = 126 \ \frac{mL}{hr}$$

So, the patient would receive 126 milliliters per hour.

EXAMPLE 10.7

The prescribers ordered 850 mL of D/5/.45% NS to infuse at 17 drops per minute. If the drop factor is 15 drops per milliliter, how many milliliters per hour will the patient receive?

You want to convert drops per minute to milliliters per hour.

$$\frac{17 \ gtt}{1 \ min} \longrightarrow \frac{mL}{hr}$$

Do this on one line as follows:

$$\frac{17 \ gtt}{1 \ min} \times \frac{? \ mL}{? \ gtt} \times \frac{? \ min}{? \ hr} = \frac{? \ mL}{? \ hr}$$

Because 15 gtt = 1 mL and 60 min = 1 hr, the two equivalent fractions are $\frac{1 \ mL}{15 \ gtt}$ and $\frac{60 \ min}{1 \ hr}$.

$$\frac{17 \ \cancel{gtt}}{1 \ \cancel{min}} \times \frac{1 \ mL}{\cancel{15} \ gtt}_{1} \times \frac{\overset{4}{\cancel{60} \ \cancel{min}}}{1 \ hr} = \frac{68 \ mL}{hr}$$

So, the patient would receive 68 milliliters per hour.

EXAMPLE 10.8

The order reads:

125 mL 5% D/W in 1 hour

The drop factor is 60 microdrops per milliliter. What is the flow rate in micro-drops per minute?

You want to change the flow rate from milliliters per hour to microdrops per minute.

$$\frac{125 \ mL}{1 \ hr} = \frac{? \ \mu gtt}{? \ min}$$

Do this in one line as follows:

$$\frac{125 \ \cancel{mL}}{1 \ \cancel{hr}} \times \frac{1 \ \cancel{hr}}{\cancel{60} \ min} \times \frac{\cancel{60} \ \mu gtt}{1 \ \cancel{mL}} = \frac{125 \ \mu gtt}{min}$$

So, you would administer 125 microdrops per minute.

> **NOTE**
>
> In Example 10.8, it was shown that 125 milliliters per hour is the same flow rate as 125 microdrops per minute. Therefore, the flow rates of milliliters per hour and microdrops per minute are equivalent. So, for example, calculations are not necessary to change 137 mL/hr to 137 μgtt/min.

CALCULATING THE FLOW RATE OF ENTERAL SOLUTIONS

▶ **E X A M P L E   10.9**

A patient must receive a tube-feeding of Ensure, 240 milliliters in 60 minutes. The calibration of the tubing is 20 drops per milliliter. Calculate the flow rate in drops per minute.

You want to convert milliliters per minute to drops per minute.

$$\frac{240 \text{ mL}}{60 \text{ min}} \longrightarrow ? \frac{\text{gtt}}{\text{min}}$$

Do this on one line as follows:

$$\frac{\overset{4}{\cancel{240 \text{ mL}}}}{\underset{1}{\cancel{60 \text{ min}}}} \times \frac{20 \text{ gtt}}{1 \cancel{\text{ mL}}} = 80 \frac{\text{gtt}}{\text{min}}$$

So, the flow rate is 80 drops per minute.

▶ **E X A M P L E   10.10**

A patient has an order for Sustacal 240 milliliters in 2 hours via feeding tube. The calibration of the tubing is 18 drops per milliliter. Calculate the rate of flow in drops per minute.

You want to convert the milliliters per hour into drops per minute.

$$\frac{240 \text{ mL}}{2 \text{ hr}} \longrightarrow \frac{? \text{ gtt}}{? \text{ min}}$$

Do this in one line as follows

$$\frac{\overset{4}{\cancel{240 \text{ mL}}}}{2 \cancel{\text{ hr}}} \times \frac{1 \cancel{\text{ h}}}{\underset{1}{\cancel{60 \text{ min}}}} \times \frac{18 \text{ gtt}}{1 \cancel{\text{ mL}}} = 36 \frac{\text{gtt}}{\text{min}}$$

So, the patient would receive 36 drops per minute.

A patient has been admitted to the hospital with a diagnosis of right upper lobe pneumonia, dehydration, and left-sided hemiparesis. Patient has a nasogastric tube in place for tube feedings. Vital signs are as follows: T 101F, P 128, R 30, BP 140/102. The attending physician wrote the following orders:

- Enteral feeding q 3 h, Sustacal 240 mL followed by 50 milliliters of sterile water.
- 400 mL 5% D$\frac{1}{2}$ NS q 6 h IV (continuous)
- Colace 100 mg oral suspension bid vial enteral tube
- Azithromycin in oral suspension 750 mg q.d. via enteral tube
- Tylenol oral suspension 600 mg q 4 h prn for temperature above 101.8F via enteral tube
- Lasix 40 mg bid via enteral tube, oral suspension
- K-lor 40 meq packet dissolved in 40 milliliters of H$_2$O bid.

1. Calculate the flow rate of the Sustocal. The drop factor is 18 drops per milliliter. _____

2. Calculate the flow rate for the 5% D$\frac{1}{2}$ NS. The drop factor is 60 micro drops per milliliter. _____

3. Colace oral suspension is prepared 150 milligram per 15 mL. How many milliliters will you administer to your patient? _____

4. The label for the azithromycin reads 125 milligrams = 5 milliliters. How many milliliters will you administer to this patient? _____

5. Calculate the amount of Lasix you will administer to your patient if the label reads 0.04 g in 5 milliliters. _____

6. Your patient has a temperature of 102F. How many milliliters of Tylenol will you administer if the label reads 100 milligrams per milliliter? _____

7. Calculate the total amount of fluid this patient will receive in 24 hours (enteral and intravenous only). _____

Answers to Case Studies appear in Appendix A.

You will find the answers to *Try These for Practice* below. Answers to *Exercises* and *Cumulative Review* appear in Appendix A at the back of the book. Your instructor has the answers to the *Additional Exercises*.

Try These for Practice

Test your comprehension after reading the chapter.

1. The prescriber ordered:

     500 mL 5% D/W in 4 hr IV

   Calculate the flow rate when the drop factor is 10 drops per milliliter.

   _____

2. The prescriber ordered:

     1000 mL 0.9% NS in 8 hr IV

   The flow rate is 21 drops per minute. When the nurse assessed the infusion, 400 milliliters had infused in 4 hours. Calculate the new flow rate if the drop factor is 15 drops per milliliter. _____

3. The prescriber ordered:

     850 mL 5% D/W IV in 8 hr.

   Calculate the flow rate in milliliters per hour. _____

4. The physician ordered 500 mL D/5/0.45% N/S to infuse in 5 hours. One hour later, 300 mL remained. Recalculate the flow rate in drops per minute if the drop factor is 15 gtt/mL. _____

5. An IV solution is infusing at the rate of 60 milliliters per hour. How many microdrops per minute is this flow rate? _____

Answers: 1. 21 gtt/min 2. 38 gtt/min 3. 106.3 mL/hr 4. 19 gtt/min 5. 60 μgtt/min

Exercises

1. The prescriber ordered 1800 milliliters of 5% D/W in 24 hours IV. The patient was receiving 75 microdrops per minute. After 12 hours, the patient had received 1240 milliliters. Recalculate the flow rate.

   _____

2. An intravenous solution of 5% D/W was infusing at a flow rate of 42 drops per minute. The drop factor was 10 drops per milliliter. How many milliliters per hour will the patient receive? _____

3. The flow rate of an intravenous solution was 16 drops per minute. The drop factor was 15 drops per milliliter. How many milliliters per hour is the patient receiving? _____

4. The prescriber ordered 500 milliliters of 5% D/W to infuse in 10 hours. After 4 hours, 400 milliliters of the infusion remained to be infused. Recalculate the flow rate when the drop factor is 10 drops per milliliter.

_____

5. An infusion of 5% D/W has a flow rate of 36 drops per minute. The drop factor is 15 drops per milliliter. What is the flow rate in milliliters per hour? _____

6. An infusion of 1100 milliliters of 5% D/W is infusing at a rate of 31 drops per minute. The drop factor is 20 drops per milliliter. How many milliliters per hour is the patient receiving? _____

7. A patient is receiving 10% D/W via a peripheral line at a rate of 40 milliliters per hour. How many microdrops per minute is this?

_____

8. The prescriber ordered:

   250 mL 5% D/W IV in 2.5 hr.

   Calculate the flow rate when the drop factor is 15 drops per minute.

_____

9. The physician ordered tube feedings of Ensure 240 milliliters per four hours. Calculate the flow rate in milliliters per hour. _____

10. The prescriber ordered a tube feeding of Sustacal 480 milliliters in 2 hours. The drop factor is 20 drops per milliliter. Calculate the flow rate.

_____

11. A patient has an order for total parenteral nutrition (TPN), 3000 milliliters of 20% D/W in 24 hours. Calculate the flow rate in milliliters per hour. _____

12. The prescriber ordered:

   2500 mL 5% D/W in 24 hr IV.

   The drop factor is 10 drops per milliliter. Calculate the flow rate.

_____

13. 125 μgtt/min = ? mL/hr. _____

14. The physician's order reads:

400 mL Ensure via PEG in 4.4 hr.

Calculate the flow rate in milliliters per hour. _____

15. The patient has an order for PEG. What is the meaning of this abbreviation? _____

16. The order is 1250 milliliters of 5% D/W IV in 12 hours. The flow rate is 25 drops per minute; the drop factor is 15 drops per milliliter. How many milliliters per hour is the patient receiving? _____

17. An infusion of 15% D/0.22% NS has been prepared for a patient. The flow rate is 26 drops per minute. The drop factor is 15 drops per milliliter. How many milliliters per hour is this patient receiving?

_____

18. The order reads:

900 mL 5% D/0.45% NS IV 5 hr.

Calculate the flow rate when the drop factor is 10 drops per milliliter.

_____

19. Calculate the flow rate in milliliters for the order in the previous problem. _____

20. Recalculate the flow rate for an intravenous infusion of 500 milliliters of 5% D/W that is infusing at 100 microdrops per minute in 5 hours. The new flow rate ordered by the physician is 80 microdrops per minute. How many milliliters per hour will this patient receive? _____

Additional Exercises

1. The order reads:

360 mL 5% D/0.45% NS for 24 hr.

Calculate the flow rate in microdrops per minute. _____

2. 50 mL 5% D/W in 20 min IV = ? μgtt/min. _____

3. A patient has an intravenous infusion of 500 milliliters of 5% D/W. The flow rate is 21 drops per minute. The drop factor is 10 gtt/mL. Is the flow rate correct if the intravenous infusion must be completed in 4 hours?

_____

4. The prescriber ordered an infusion of 125 milliliters per hour. Calculate the flow rate when the drop factor is 15 drops per milliliter. _____

5. The order reads:

   1000 mL 5% D/W q24h IV.

   The drop factor is 20 drops per milliliter. Calculate the flow rate.

   _____

6. The order reads:

   1000 mL to infuse in 10 hours IV.

   The flow rate is 25 drops per minute. Three hours later, 850 milliliters remained in the IV bag. Recalculate the flow rate. The drop factor is 15 drops per milliliter. _____

7. The order reads:

   2000 mL 5% D/W for 16 hr IV.

   The flow rate is 17 drops per minute. When the nurse assessed the infusion, 400 milliliters had infused in 4 hours. Recalculate the flow rate. The drop factor is 15 drops per milliliter. _____

8. A patient has an intravenous infusion of 850 milliliters of 5% D/W infusing at 24 drops per minute. The drop factor is 20 drops per milliliter. How many milliliters per hour is this patient receiving? _____

9. The order reads:

   500 mL 5% D/W in 2 hour fluid challenge IV.

   Calculate the flow rate in drops per minute. The drop factor is 10 drops per milliliter. _____

10. An intravenous solution is infusing at a rate of 42 drops per minute, with a drop factor of 15 drops per milliliter. How many milliliters per hour is the patient receiving? _____

11. The physician's order reads:

    1250 mL 5% D/0.9% NS IV q12h.

    The drop factor is 60 microdrops per milliliter. Calculate the flow rate in microdrops per minute.

    _____

12. The prescriber ordered 250 milliliters of 0.9% NS IV in 1 hour. Calculate the flow rate in drops per minute. The drop factor is 10 drops per milliliter.

    _____

13. An intravenous solution of 5% D/W is infusing at 17 drops per minute. The drop factor is 15 drops per milliliter. Calculate the flow rate in milliliters per hour. _____

14. The order reads:

    120 mL 5% D/W IV in 30 min.

    Calculate the flow rate in drops per minute. The drop factor is 10 drops per milliliter. _____

15. The order reads:

    850 mL IV 5% D/W in 8.5 hr.

    Calculate flow rate in milliliters per hour. _____

16. The physician's order reads:

    1000 mL 0.9% NS IV, infuse at rate of 2.5 mL/min.

    Calculate the flow rate in milliliters per hour. _____

17. A patient is to receive 750 milliliters of 5% D/W in 15 hours IV. The flow rate is 8 drops per minute. Four hours later, 600 milliliters remain in IV bag. Recalculate the flow rate. The drop factor is 10 drops per milliliter.

    _____

18. 100 μgtt/min = ? mL/hr _____

19. The order reads:

    1750 mL 5% D/W in 16 hr IV.

    The drop factor 15 drops per milliliter. Calculate the flow rate. _____

20. The prescriber wrote the following order:

    750 mL 5% D/W @ 17 gtt/min IV.

The drop factor is 15 drops per milliliter. How many milliliters per hour will the patient receive? _____

CUMULATIVE REVIEW EXERCISES

1. An intravenous solution is infusing at 40 microdrops per minute. How many milliliters per hour is the patient receiving? _____

2. The order reads:

   2000 mL lactated Ringer's solution IV over a 12-hr period postoperative.

   How many milliliters per hour will the patient receive? _____

3. The prescriber orders TPN, 2500 milliliters of 20% D/W to infuse in 16 hours. How many microdrops per minute should the patient receive?

   _____

4. An infusion of 1000 milliliters of 5% D/W was to infuse at a rate of 25 drops per minute for 10 hours. After 4 hours the patient had received 600 milliliters. The drop factor is 15 drops per milliliter. Recalculate the flow rate. _____

5. A patient has an order for gr 1/150 of atropine sulfate s/c. Convert gr 1/150 to mg. _____

6. The patient has a BSA of 1.6 m^2. The medication order is 0.8 mg per m^2. The capsule is labeled 1.2 mg. How many capsules will you prepare?

   _____

7. You have a sodium chloride solution with a concentration of 23.4%. How many milligrams of sodium chloride are in 1 milliliter? _____

8. You are to prepare 0.02 g of gentamicin IM for your patient. The label reads 40 mg/mL. How many milliliters will you prepare for your patient?

   _____

9. Your patient weighs 200 pounds. The prescriber has ordered 6.6 milligrams per kilogram of lithium. You have lithium capsules labeled 300 milligrams each. How many capsules will you prepare? _____

Cumulative Review Exercises   227

10. The order reads:

Phenobarbital 120 mg IM.

The label reads 100 mg/2 mL. How many milliliters will you prepare?

_____

11. 2 T = ? tsp _____   **12.** 8 mg = gr ? _____

13. 5 mL = ? gtt _____   **14.** gr 1/100 = ? g _____

15. 1 oz = ? mL _____

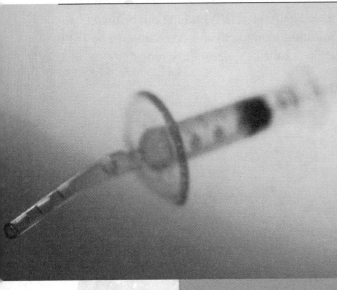

CHAPTER ELEVEN

Calculating Flow Rates for Intravenous Medications and Duration of Flow

> ## Objectives

After completing this chapter, you will be able to

- Understand intravenous piggyback medication administration.
- Calculate the rate of flow of intravenous piggyback medications.
- Calculate the flow rate of intravenous solutions based on the amount of drug per minute or per hour.
- Determine the amount of drug a patient will receive IV per minute or per hour.
- Calculate IV flow rates based on weight.
- Calculate IV flow rates based on body surface area.
- Calculate the infusion time of an IV solution.

This chapter extends the discussion of intravenous infusions to include intravenous piggyback (IVPB) infusions. You will also learn how to calculate the infusion time of an IV as well as how to determine flow rates for IVs based on weight or BSA.

INTRAVENOUS PIGGYBACK INFUSIONS

Patients can receive a drug through a port in an existing IV line. This is called *intravenous piggyback (IVPB);* see Figure 11.1. IVPB tubing can be used to administer small amounts of medication along with the IV solution. The IVPB tubing that delivers the medication is called the *secondary set.*

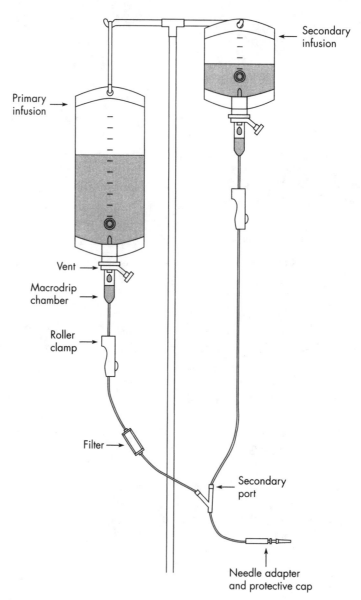

Primary
infusion

Secondary
infusion

Vent

Macrodrip
chamber

Roller
clamp

Filter

Secondary
port

Needle adapter
and protective cap

▶ **FIGURE 11.1 Primary and secondary (IVPB) infusion setup**

Notice in Figure 11.1 that the secondary bag is higher than the primary bag so that the pressure in the secondary line will be greater than the pressure in the primary line. Therefore, the secondary medication infuses first. Once the secondary infusion is completed, the primary line begins to flow. Remember to maintain the patency of both systems. If you close the primary line, when the secondary IVPB is completed the primary line will not flow into the vein.

The box in Figure 11.2 is an example of a secondary medication set.

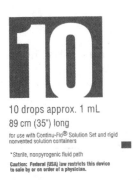

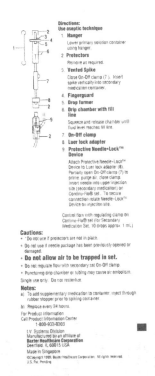

▶ **FIGURE 11.2** **Box of secondary IV tubing**

Let's look at some examples involving IVPB or secondary IV medications. Keep in mind that some medications for intermittent infusion are premixed by the manufacturer in 50 milliliters or 100 milliliters of D/5/W or 0.9% NS.

INTRAVENOUS PIGGYBACK MEDICATIONS

A patient who is already receiving 5% D/W via an IV line is to receive 1 gram of cefazolin (Ancef) every 4 hours. The prescriber's order reads:

Ancef 1 g IVPB q4h

This indicates that your patient will receive 1 gram of Ancef in solution via a secondary IV line that is attached to a port (piggyback) on the primary line.

▶ **EXAMPLE 11.1**

The prescriber ordered:

Ancef 1 g IVPB q4h

The package insert information is as follows: Add 50 mL sterile water to the bag of Ancef 1 g and infuse in 30 min. The tubing is labeled 20 drops per milliliter. Calculate the flow rate for this antibiotic.

You want to change the flow rate from milliliters per minute to drops per minute.

$$\frac{50 \text{ mL}}{30 \text{ min}} \longrightarrow ? \frac{\text{gtt}}{\text{min}}$$

Do this on one line as follows:

$$\frac{\overset{5}{\cancel{50}} \text{ mL}}{\underset{3}{\cancel{30}} \text{ min}} \times \frac{20 \text{ gtt}}{1 \text{ mL}} = \frac{100 \text{ gtt}}{3 \text{ min}} = 33.3 \frac{\text{gtt}}{\text{min}}$$

So, the flow rate is 33 drops per minute.

> ### E X A M P L E   1 1 . 2

The prescriber ordered:

Kefzol 500 mg IVPB q8h.

Read the information for this antibiotic medication in Figure 11.3. Follow the directions on the label, and infuse in 1 hour. The tubing is labeled 60 microdrops per milliliter. Calculate the flow rate.

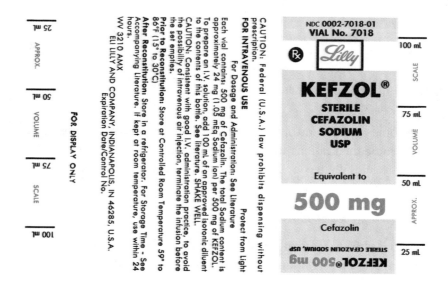

▶ **FIGURE 11.3 Kefzol 500 mg**

Because 1 hour equals 60 minutes, you want to change the flow rate from milliliters per minute to microdrops per minute.

$$\frac{100 \text{ mL}}{60 \text{ min}} \longrightarrow ? \frac{\mu\text{gtt}}{\text{min}}$$

Do this on one line as follows:

$$\frac{100 \text{ mL}}{\cancel{60} \text{ min}} \times \frac{\cancel{60} \text{ } \mu\text{gtt}}{1 \text{ mL}} = 100 \frac{\mu\text{gtt}}{\text{min}}$$

So, the flow rate is 100 microdrops per minute.

▶ **EXAMPLE 11.3**

The medication order reads:

1000 mL 5% D/W with 500 mg lidocaine at 1 mg/min

Calculate the flow rate if the drop factor is 15 drops per milliliter. In this example, the prescriber has specified the solution (1000 milliliters of 5% D/W containing 500 milligrams of the drug lidocaine) and also the amount of lidocaine per minute (1 milligram per minute) that the patient is to receive.

You want to change the flow rate from milligrams per minute to drops per minute.

$$1 \frac{mg}{min} \longrightarrow ? \frac{gtt}{min}$$

Do this on one line as follows:

$$\frac{1\ mg}{1\ min} \times \frac{?\ mL}{?\ mg} \times ? \frac{gtt}{mL} = ? \frac{gtt}{min}$$

Because 1000 milliliters contain 500 milligrams and because 15 gtt = 1 mL, the equivalent fractions are

$$\frac{1\ mg}{1\ min} \times \frac{\overset{2}{\cancel{1000\ mL}}}{\underset{1}{\cancel{500\ mg}}} \times \frac{15\ gtt}{1\ \cancel{mL}} = 30 \frac{gtt}{min}$$

So, you would administer 30 drops per minute.

▶ **EXAMPLE 11.4**

The prescriber writes an order for 1000 milliliters of 5% D/W with 10 units of synthetic oxytocin (Pitocin). Your patient must receive 10 milliunits of this drug per minute. The drop factor is 60 microdrops per milliliter. Calculate the flow rate in microdrops per minute.

You want to change the flow rate from milliunits per minute to microdrops per minute.

$$10 \frac{mU}{min} \longrightarrow ? \frac{\mu gtt}{min}$$

NOTE

1000 milliunits (mU) = 1 unit (u)

Do this on one line as follows:

$$\frac{10\ mU}{1\ min} \times \frac{?\ u}{?\ mU} \times \frac{?\ mL}{?\ u} \times \frac{?\ \mu gtt}{?\ mL} = ? \frac{\mu gtt}{min}$$

Because 1000 mU = 1 u, 1000 mL = 10 u, and 60 μgtt = 1 mL, the equivalent fractions are

$$\frac{\overset{1}{\cancel{10 \text{ mU}}}}{1 \text{ min}} \times \frac{1 \text{ u}}{\underset{1}{\cancel{1000 \text{ mU}}}} \times \frac{\overset{1}{\cancel{1000 \text{ mL}}}}{\underset{1}{\cancel{10 \text{ u}}}} \times \frac{60 \text{ }\mu\text{gtt}}{1 \text{ }\cancel{\text{mL}}} = 60 \text{ } \frac{\mu\text{gtt}}{\text{min}}$$

So, you will administer 60 microdrops per minute.

> **E X A M P L E   11.5**

Calculate the flow rate in milliliters per hour if the medication order reads: Add 10,000 u of heparin to 1000 mL 5% D/W IV. Your patient is to receive 250 units of this anticoagulant per hour via an infusion pump.

You want to change the flow rate from units per hour to milliliters per hour.

$$\frac{250 \text{ u}}{1 \text{ hr}} \longrightarrow ? \text{ } \frac{\text{mL}}{\text{hr}}$$

Do this on one line as follows:

$$\frac{250 \text{ }\cancel{\text{u}}}{1 \text{ hr}} \times \frac{\overset{1}{\cancel{1000}} \text{ mL}}{\underset{10}{\cancel{10,000}} \text{ }\cancel{\text{u}}} = \frac{250 \text{ mL}}{10 \text{ hr}} = 25 \text{ } \frac{\text{mL}}{\text{hr}}$$

So, your patient will receive 25 milliliters per hour.

In Examples 11.6 and 11.7, you are given the flow rate in milliliters per hour, and you need to determine the amount of medication the patient will receive per hour.

> **E X A M P L E   11.6**

The medication order reads:

500 mL 5% D/W with 24,000 u of heparin, infuse at rate of 10 milliliters per hour

How many units is your patient receiving per hour?

You want to convert the flow rate from milliliters per hour to units per hour.

$$\frac{10 \text{ mL}}{1 \text{ hr}} \longrightarrow ? \text{ } \frac{\text{u}}{\text{hr}}$$

Do this on one line as follows:

$$\frac{10 \; \cancel{mL}}{1 \; hr} \times \frac{24{,}000 \; u}{500 \; \cancel{mL}} = 480 \; \frac{u}{hr}$$

So, your patient is receiving 480 units of heparin per hour.

▶ **EXAMPLE 11.7**

Your patient is receiving an IV of 1000 milliliters of 0.9% NS with 1000 milligrams of the bronchodilator aminophylline (somophyllin). The flow rate is 35 milliliters per hour. How many milligrams per hour is your patient receiving?

You want to convert the flow rate from milliliters per hour to milligrams per hour.

$$\frac{35 \; mL}{1 \; hr} \longrightarrow ? \; \frac{mg}{hr}$$

Do this on one line as follows:

$$\frac{35 \; \cancel{mL}}{1 \; hr} \times \frac{\overset{1}{\cancel{1000}} \; mg}{\underset{1}{\cancel{1000}} \; \cancel{mL}} = 35 \; \frac{mg}{hr}$$

So your patient is receiving 35 milligrams of aminophylline per hour.

CALCULATING FLOW RATES BASED ON BODY WEIGHT

Some IV and enteral medications are prescribed based on your patient's weight. For example, the medication order might read:

0.001 mg/kg/min

This means that each minute, your patient is to receive 0.001 milligram of the drug for every kilogram of body weight. This can also be written as $\frac{0.001 \; mg}{kg \times min}$.

▶ **EXAMPLE 11.8**

The prescriber ordered:

250 mL 5% D/W with 90 mg Aredia, 0.001 mg/kg/min IV.

The patient weighs 80 kilograms, and the drop factor is 20 drops per milliliter. Calculate the flow rate.

Because the amount of drug ordered is based on the weight of the patient (kilograms), the weight will determine the flow rate (drops per minute). You want to convert kilograms to drops per minute. You have the following information:

- The patient weighs 80 kg
- The order is 0.001 mg/kg/min
- 90 mg = 250 mL
- 20 gtt = 1 mL

Do this problem on one line as follows:

$$80 \; \cancel{kg} \times \frac{0.001 \; \cancel{mg}}{\cancel{kg} \times min} \times \frac{250 \; \cancel{mL}}{90 \; \cancel{mg}} \times \frac{20 \; gtt}{1 \; \cancel{mL}} = 4.4 \; \frac{gtt}{min}$$

So, the flow rate is 4 drops per minute.

▶ EXAMPLE 11.9

The medication order reads:

Vibramycin 0.012 mg/kg/min in 200 mL 5% D/W IV.

Read the directions on the label in Figure 11.4. How many milliliters will you add to the vial? The patient weighs 60 kilograms. How many milliliters per hour will your patient receive?

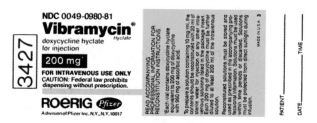

▶ **FIGURE 11.4 Vibramycin 200 mg**

If 20 mL of sterile water are added to the vial, and this drug is then added to the 200 mL of 5% D/W, the total infusion will be 200 mL. You have the following information:

- The patient weighs 60 kg
- The order is 0.012 mg/kg/min
- 220 mL = 200 mg

Do this problem on one line as follows:

$$60 \; \cancel{kg} \times \frac{0.012 \; \cancel{mg}}{\cancel{kg} \times \cancel{min}} \times \frac{220 \; mL}{200 \; \cancel{mg}} \times \frac{60 \; \cancel{min}}{1 \; hr} = 47.5 \; \frac{mL}{hr}$$

So, your patient will receive 47.5 milliliters per hour.

CALCULATING FLOW RATES BASED ON BODY SURFACE AREA

As you know, certain medications are ordered based on body surface area (BSA). Chapter 6 discusses how to determine BSA, and you will find a nomogram, the chart that enables you to do this, in Appendix F.

The following examples show how to calculate flow rates for this type of medication order.

EXAMPLE 11.10

The prescriber ordered 2 grams of oxacillin (Prostaphlin), an antibiotic drug, in 1000 milliliters 0.9% NS, to be infused at a rate of 200 milligrams per square meter per hour (see the label in Figure 11.5 for drug information). Your patient's BSA is 1.5 square meters. How many milliliters per hour should your patient receive?

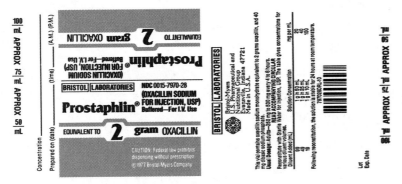

▶ **FIGURE 11.5 Drug label for Oxacillin**

Because the medication order is based on the BSA of the patient, the BSA will determine the flow rate (milliliters per hour). You have the following information:

- The BSA of the patient is 1.5 m^2
- The order is 200 mg/m^2/hr
- 1000 mL = 2 g of Prostaphlin

Do this problem on one line as follows:

$$1.5 \text{ m}^2 \times \frac{200 \text{ mg}}{\text{m}^2 \times \text{h}} \times \frac{1000 \text{ mL}}{2000 \text{ mg}} = \frac{150 \text{ mL}}{\text{h}}$$

So, your patient should receive 150 milliliters per hour.

EXAMPLE 11.11

The prescriber ordered:

Cefobid 1200 mg/m²/h IV.

Read the label in Fig. 11.6, and use 40 milliliters per 2 grams for reconstitution. Calculate the flow rate in milliliters per hour if the patient's BSA is 1.6 square meters.

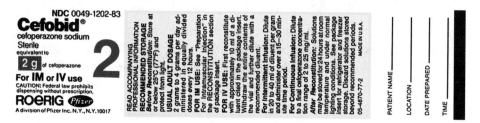

▶ FIGURE 11.6 Cefobid 2g

You have the following information:

- The BSA of the patient is 1.6 m²
- The order is 1200 mg/m²/min
- Because 2 g = 40 mL, 2000 mg = 40 mL

Do this problem on one line as follows:

$$1.6 \; m^2 \times \frac{1200 \; mg}{m^2 \times hr} \times \frac{40 \; mL}{2000 \; mg} = 38.4 \; \frac{mL}{hr}$$

So, the flow rate is 38.4 milliliters per hour.

CALCULATING THE DURATION OF FLOW FOR IV AND ENTERAL SOLUTIONS

In the following examples, you will determine the length of time it will take to complete an infusion.

EXAMPLE 11.12

An infusion of 5% D/W has solution remaining in the bag (Figure 11.7). It is infusing at a rate of 20 drops per minute. If the drop factor is 12 drops per milliliter, how many hours will it take for the remaining solution in the bag to infuse?

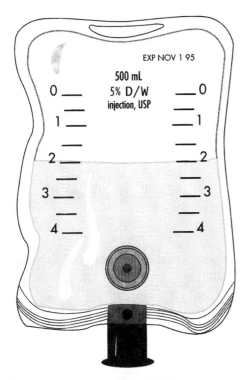

▶ **FIGURE 11.7 5% D/W intravenous solution (300 milliliters remaining in bag)**

You can see that 500 milliliters of solution were originally in the bag and that the patient has received 200 milliliters. Therefore, 300 milliliters remain to be infused.

You want to convert milliliters to hours.

$$300 \text{ mL} \longrightarrow \text{? gtt} \longrightarrow \text{? min} \longrightarrow \text{? hr}$$

Do this on one line as follows:

$$300 \text{ mL} \times \frac{\text{? gtt}}{\text{? mL}} \times \frac{\text{? min}}{\text{? gtt}} \times \frac{\text{? hr}}{\text{? min}} = \text{? hr}$$

Because 12 gtt = 1 mL, 20 gtt = 1 min, and 60 min = 1 hr, these become the equivalent fractions.

$$\overset{15}{\cancel{300 \text{ mL}}} \times \frac{\overset{1}{\cancel{12 \text{ gtt}}}}{1 \text{ mL}} \times \frac{1 \cancel{\text{ min}}}{\underset{1}{\cancel{20 \text{ gtt}}}} \times \frac{1 \text{ hr}}{\underset{5}{\cancel{60 \text{ min}}}} = 3 \text{ hr}$$

So, it will take 3 hours to infuse this solution.

▶ **EXAMPLE 11.13**

A patient is receiving an IV of 1000 milliliters of 5% D/W. The flow rate is 32 drops per minute. If the drop factor is 10 drops per milliliter, how many hours will it take for this infusion to finish?

You want to convert milliliters to hours.

$$1000 \text{ mL} \longrightarrow \text{? gtt} \longrightarrow \text{? min} \longrightarrow \text{? hr}$$

Do this on one line as follows:

$$1000 \text{ mL} \times \frac{\text{? gtt}}{\text{? mL}} \times \frac{\text{? min}}{\text{? gtt}} \times \frac{\text{? hr}}{\text{? min}} = \text{? hr}$$

Because 10 gtt = 1 mL, 32 gtt = 1 min, and 60 min = 1 hr, these become the equivalent fractions.

$$1000 \text{ mL} \times \frac{\overset{1}{\cancel{10} \text{ gtt}}}{1 \text{ mL}} \times \frac{1 \text{ min}}{32 \text{ gtt}} \times \frac{1 \text{ hr}}{\underset{6}{\cancel{60} \text{ min}}} = 5.2 \text{ hr}$$

Convert the portion of an hour to minutes — that is, convert 0.2 hour to minutes.

$$0.2 \text{ hr} \times \frac{60 \text{ min}}{1 \text{ hr}} = 12 \text{ min}$$

So, the infusion will take 5 hours and 12 minutes.

> **EXAMPLE 11.14**

An IV of 1000 milliliters of 5% D/W 0.9% NS is started at 1 P.M. The flow rate is 17 drops per minute, and the drop factor is 10 drops per milliliter. At what time will this infusion finish?

You want to convert milliliters to hours.

$$1000 \text{ mL} \longrightarrow \text{? gtt} \longrightarrow \text{? min} \longrightarrow \text{? hr}$$

Do this on one line as follows:

$$1000 \text{ mL} \times \frac{\text{? gtt}}{\text{? mL}} \times \frac{\text{? min}}{\text{? gtt}} \times \frac{\text{? hr}}{\text{? min}} = \text{? hr}$$

Because 10 gtt = 1 mL, 17 gtt = 1 min, and 60 min = 1 hr, these become the equivalent fractions.

$$1000 \text{ mL} \times \frac{\overset{1}{\cancel{10} \text{ gtt}}}{1 \text{ mL}} \times \frac{1 \text{ min}}{17 \text{ gtt}} \times \frac{1 \text{ hr}}{\underset{6}{\cancel{60} \text{ min}}} = 9.8 \text{ hr}$$

You then convert 0.8 hour to minutes.

$$0.8 \text{ hr} \times \frac{60 \text{ min}}{1 \text{ hr}} = 48 \text{ min}$$

So, the IV will infuse for 9 hours and 48 minutes. Because the infusion started at 1 P.M., it will finish at 10:48 P.M.

An IV of 1500 milliliters of 10% D/W is to infuse at a rate of 40 drop per minute. The drop factor is 15 drops per milliliter. If this IV solution begins to infuse at 10:15 A.M., at what time will it finish?

You want to convert milliliters to hours.

$$1500 \text{ mL} \longrightarrow ? \text{ gtt} \longrightarrow ? \text{ min} \longrightarrow ? \text{ hr}$$

Do this on one line as follows:

$$1500 \text{ mL} \times \frac{? \text{ gtt}}{? \text{ mL}} \times \frac{? \text{ min}}{? \text{ gtt}} \times \frac{? \text{ hr}}{? \text{ min}} = ? \text{ hr}$$

Because 15 gtt = 1 mL, 40 gtt = 1 min, and 60 min = 1 hr, these become the equivalent fractions.

$$1500 \text{ mL} \times \frac{\overset{1}{\cancel{15} \text{ gtt}}}{1 \text{ mL}} \times \frac{1 \text{ min}}{40 \text{ gtt}} \times \frac{1 \text{ hr}}{\underset{4}{\cancel{60} \text{ min}}} = 9.4 \text{ hr}$$

You then convert 0.4 hour to minutes.

$$0.4 \text{ hr} \times \frac{60 \text{ min}}{1 \text{ hr}} = 24 \text{ min}$$

So, the IV will infuse for 9 hours and 24 minutes. Because the infusion started at 10:15 A.M., it will finish at 7:39 P.M.

A 45-year-old man is admitted to the hospital for a closure of a colostomy. His original surgery took place 3 months ago. At that time, his diagnosis was intestinal obstruction. A colostomy was performed. His admission vital signs are as follows: T, 98.6F; P, 88; R, 18; and BP, 132/82. He weighs 70 kilograms. His surgeon has written the following orders:

Orders for the Day of Surgery:

- Demerol 50 mg and Versed 0.005 g IM at 7 A.M.
- gr $\frac{1}{100}$ atropine sulfate IM at 7 A.M.

Postoperative Orders:

- Antivert 25 mg po q6h prn
- Demerol 50 mg and Vistaril 0.8 mg/kg IM q4h prn for relief of pain
- Unasyn 1.5 g in 100 mL 5% D/W IVPB q8h; infuse in 60 min
- Pepcid 50 mg in 100 mL 5% D/W IVPB q8h; infuse in 30 min
- Clear fluids po
- D/5 $\frac{1}{2}$ NS 125 mL qh
- The drop factor for all IV solutions is 10 gtt per mL

The drop factor for all IV solutions and medications is 10 drops per milliliter.

1. Calculate the flow rate for all IVPB solutions. _____

2. How many milliliters equal the prescribed dose of atropine sulfate if the ampule reads 0.4 milligram per milliliter? _____

3. If the label for Demerol reads 50 milligrams per milliliter and the label for Versed reads 0.005 gram per milliliter, how many milliliters of each will you administer to this patient? _____

4. What is the total amount of fluid the patient will receive from the IVPB medications in 24 hours and the solution of 5% D/0.45% NS?

_____

5. Calculate the amount of Versed the patient will receive with 50 milligrams of Demerol if the ampule of Versed reads 1 milligram per milliliter. _____

6. Read the label below. How many tablets of Antivert would you administer? _____

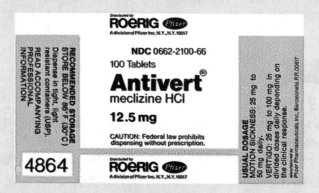

7. Read the label below. The directions for Unasyn are as follows: Add drug to 100 mL 5% D/W. How many milligrams of Unasyn will the patient receive in $\frac{1}{2}$ hour? _____

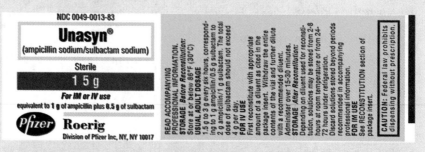

The answers to the Case Studies appear in Appendix A.

You will find the answers to the *Try These for Practice* below. Answers to *Exercises* and *Cumulative Review Exercises* appear in Appendix A at the back of the book. Your instructor has the answers to the *Additional Exercises*.

Try These for Practice

Test your comprehension after reading the chapter.

1. The patient must receive 2 grams of Mefoxin IVPB at 6 A.M. The label reads:

    Add 2 g Mefoxin to 200 mL 5% D/W; infuse in 2 hours.

    The drop factor is 60 microdrops per milliliter. Calculate the flow rate.

    _____

2. The order reads:

    Pitocin 10 u in 1000 mL of 0.9% NS IV. Infuse at rate of 3 mU/min.

    Calculate the flow rate in mL/hr. _____

3. The patient is to receive 1400 units of heparin q1h IV. If the order is 250 milliliters of 5% D/W with 25,000 units of heparin, how many milliliters per hour will your patient receive of this drug? See Figure 11.8.

    _____

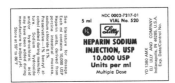

► **FIGURE 11.8**

4. A patient has an IV of 250 milliliters of 5% D/W. The flow rate is 19 microdrops per minute. If the drop factor is 60 microdrops per milliliter, how many hours will it take for this infusion to finish? _____

5. Read the first medication order in Figure 11.9. The label for this drug reads:

clindamycin phosphate 900 mg/2 mL

a. How many milliliters of clindamycin phosphate would you add to a 50 mL bag of 5% D/W? _____

b. Calculate the infusion rate in microdrops per minute when the total time of this infusion is 1 hour. _____

⊕ GENERAL HOSPITAL ⊕

PRESS HARD WITH BALLPOINT PEN. WRITE DATE & TIME AND SIGN EACH ORDER

DATE	TIME	**A.M.**
9/30/01	10	**P.M.**

1. *clindamycin phosphate 600 mg IVPB q6h x 5 days*

2. *solu-Medrol 1 g in 250 mL 5% D/W,*

   infuse 20 mg/hr

3. *aminophylline 1 g in 250 mL 5% D/W,*

   infuse 0.15 g/hr

SIGNATURE

A. Giangrasso   M.D.

IMPRINT
506713   9/30/01
Jason Vuu   6/22/40
26 Marin Dr.   RC
Thousand Oaks, Ore.   Aetna
80413

Dr. A. Giangrasso

ORDERS NOTED   **A.M.**
DATE _9/30/01_   TIME __10__   **P.M.**

❑ MEDEX   ❑ KARDEX

NURSE'S SIG. _L. Ablon_

FILLED BY   DATE

PHYSICIAN'S ORDERS

▶ **FIGURE 11.9 Physician's order sheet**

Answers: 1. 100 μgtt/min   2. 18 mL/hr   3. 14 mL/hr   4. 13h 10 min   5. (a) 1.3 mL; (b) 51 μgtt/min

---

Exercises

Reinforce your understanding in class or at home.

1. Read the information in the third medication order in Figure 11.9. Calculate the rate of flow in drops per minute when the drop factor is 10 drops per milliliter. _____

2. The prescriber has ordered 3.1 grams of ticarcillin disodium (Timentin), an antibiotic, IVPB in 100 milliliters of 5% D/W. The directions are as follows: Add 13 mL to vial, 15 mL = 3.1 g. (Total amount of fluid IV: 115 milliliters.) This IV is to be infused in 60 minutes; the drop factor is 15 drops per milliliter. Calculate the flow rate. _____

3. A patient is to receive 500 milliliters of 5% D/W with 20 units of synthetic oxytocin (Pitocin) IV at a rate of 0.002 unit per minute. How many milliliters per hour will your patient receive? _____

4. The order reads: Cefizox 18 mg/kg IVPB q8h. The patient weighs 120 pounds. The directions read: Add 100 mL 0.9% NS to vial (1 g). How many milligrams will equal the ordered dose? How many milliliters will you administer? _____

5. The order reads: 500 mg of lidocaine in 250 mL 5% D/W. Infuse at 25 μgtt/min. Read the label in Figure 11.10, and (a) calculate the amount of lidocaine you will add to the 250 milliliters of 5% D/W; (b) calculate the flow rate in milliliters per hour; and (c) if the IV order is changed to infuse in 5 hours, determine the flow rate in milliliters per hour.

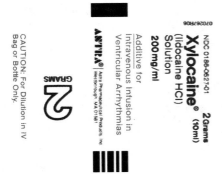

▶ **FIGURE 11.10 Lidocaine 2g**

6. The physician ordered cisplatin 20 mg/m^2 IV for a patient with a BSA of 1.7 m^2. The label of Cisplatin reads 10 mg = 10 mL. (a) How many milligrams should the patient receive? (b) How many milliliters contain the prescribed dose? (c) Add the correct amount of cisplatin to 1000 mL 0.22% N.S., and calculate the rate of flow in milliliters per hour if you infuse in 8 hours. _____

7. Calculate the flow rate in milliliters per hour for a patient receiving an IV of 250 milliliters of 5% D/W with 250 milligrams of aminophylline. The medication order is 0.006 milligram per kilogram per minute and the patient weighs 66 kilograms. _____

8. The prescriber has ordered 250 milliliters of 5% D/W with 2500 units of heparin; the patient is to receive 50 milliliters per hour IV. How many units per hour will your patient receive? _____

9. The order states that 200 milligrams of morphine are to be added to 250 milliliters of 5% D/W, and this solution is to be infused at a rate of 10 milligrams per hour. How many milliliters per hour will your patient receive? _____

10. The medication order is for 180 milligrams of morphine sulfate to be added to 250 milliliters of 5% D/W. If your patient is to receive 0.005 milligram per kilogram per minute IV, how many milligrams per hour should a patient who weighs 100 pounds receive? _____

11. The antifungal drug Diflucan has been prescribed for a 70 kg patient at 4.8 micrograms per kilogram per minute IV. Read the label in Figure 11.11. Calculate the flow rate in milliliters per hour. _____

*Each 100 mL unit contains 200 mg of fluconazole, 900 mg of sodium chloride (USP) and water for injection (USP). The solution is sterile and iso-osmotic (approximately 300 mOsmol/L).

DOSAGE AND USE
See accompanying prescribing information.

03-4532-00-2

MADE IN USA

CAUTION: Federal law prohibits dispensing without prescription.

6 Units x 100 mL NDC 0049-3371-26

DIFLUCAN® | **1206**

(Fluconazole Injection)
(for intravenous infusion only)

Sterile Solution in 0.9% Sodium Chloride Injection

200 mg/100 mL*

(2 mg/mL)

Store between 41° and 86°F (5° and 30°C)
PROTECT FROM FREEZING

Pfizer **Roerig**
Division of Pfizer Inc, NY, NY 10017

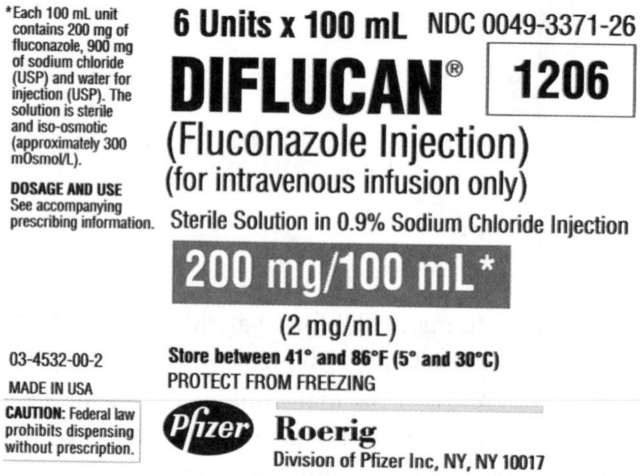

▶ FIGURE 11.11 Drug label for Diflucan

12. The prescriber ordered dopamine hydrochloride (Intropin) at a rate of 0.003 milligram per kilogram per minute; the patient weighs 122 pounds. The directions are as follows: Add 160 mg (1 mL) to 250 mL of 5% D/W. Calculate the flow rate in milliliters per hour for this infusion.

_____

13. A medication order states that 50 milliliters of asparaginase (Elspar) are to be added to 100 milliliters of 5% D/W (total 150 milliliters). Calculate the flow rate in microdrops so that your patient, who weighs 60 kilograms, receives 1 milliliter per kilogram per hour of this antineoplastic drug. _____

14. The prescriber has ordered 500 milliliters of 5% D/W with 100 units of Humulin R insulin (1 milliliter). Infuse at a rate of 0.7 milliliter per minute. How many hours will it take to complete this infusion?

_____

15. The order reads:

500 mL of D/5/W with 2 g of lidocaine.

Read the label in Figure 11.12. The flow rate is 15 mL/h. How many mg/min will the patient receive? _____

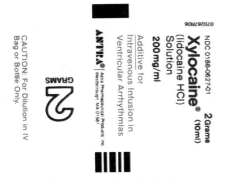

▶ **FIGURE 11.12 Drug label for lidocaine**

16. An infusion of 1000 milliliters of 5% D/W is started at 11 A.M. The flow rate is 20 drops per minute, and the drop factor is 20 drops per milliliter. At what time will this infusion finish? _____

17. The prescriber ordered Vibramycin 200 mg in 50 milliliters of lactated Ringer's solution, 0.08 mg/kg/min. The patient weighs 74 kilograms, and the drop factor is 10 drops per milliliter. Calculate the flow rate in drops per minute IV. _____

18. Calculate the flow rate in milliliters per hour for a patient receiving an IV of 250 milliliters of 5% D/W with 200 milligrams of methyldopa (Aldomet), 0.005 milligram per kilogram per minute. The patient weighs 200 pounds. _____

19. The medication order states that 12,000 units of heparin are to be added to 250 milliliters of 5% D/W. The patient is to receive 1200 units per hour IV. How many milliliters per hour will your patient receive?

_____

20. The prescriber ordered: amikacin sulfate 120 mg/m^2/hr IV. The package insert directions are as follows: Add 250 mg to 100 mL 5% D/W. Calculate the flow rate in milliliters per hour if the patient's BSA is 0.9 square meter. _____

Additional Exercises

Now, on your own, test yourself! Ask your instructor to check your answers.

1. The prescriber ordered acyclovir sodium 5 mg/kg/hr IV. The directions are as follows: Add 500 mg (10 mL) to 100 mL 5% D/W. Calculate the flow rate in milliliters per hour for a patient who weighs 160 pounds.

_____

2. Read the first medication order in Figure 11.13. How many milliliters per hour will this IV infuse if your patient weighs 80 kilograms? _____

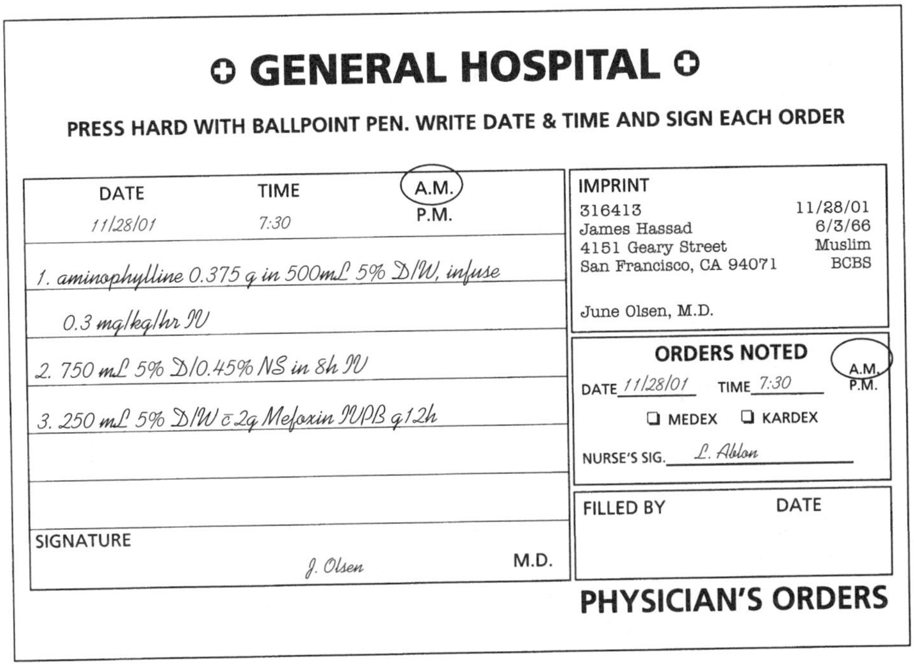

✚ GENERAL HOSPITAL ✚

PRESS HARD WITH BALLPOINT PEN. WRITE DATE & TIME AND SIGN EACH ORDER

DATE	TIME	A.M. P.M.
11/28/01	7:30	

1. aminophylline 0.375 g in 500ml 5% D/W, infuse

   0.3 mg/kg/hr IV

2. 750 ml 5% D/0.45% NS in 8h IV

3. 250 ml 5% D/W c̄ 2g Mefoxin IVPB q 12h

SIGNATURE
        J. Olsen   M.D.

IMPRINT
316413   11/28/01
James Hassad   6/3/66
4151 Geary Street   Muslim
San Francisco, CA 94071   BCBS

June Olsen, M.D.

ORDERS NOTED   A.M. P.M.
DATE _11/28/01_   TIME _7:30_
☐ MEDEX   ☐ KARDEX
NURSE'S SIG. _L. Ablon_

FILLED BY   DATE

PHYSICIAN'S ORDERS

▶ **FIGURE 11.13 Physician's order sheet**

3. Read the second medication order in Figure 11.13. Calculate the flow rate for the infusion ordered. The drop factor is 10 drops per milliliter.

4. Read the third medication order in Figure 11.13. How would you administer the medication if the drop factor is 15 drops per milliliter to infuse in two hours? _____

5. A patient is to receive 600 units of heparin per hour. The drop factor is 60 microdrops per milliliter. The order states that 12,500 units of heparin are to be added to 250 milliliters of 5% D/W. How many microdrops per minute will you infuse? _____

6. A patient has an IV of 1000 milliliters of 5% D/W. The flow rate is 36 drops per minute. If the drop factor is 10 drops per milliliter, how many hours will it take this IV to finish? _____

7. An infusion of 1000 milliliters of lactated Ringer's solution is infusing at a rate of 17 drops per minute. What time will it be completed if the drop factor is 15 drops per milliliter and this infusion started at 7 A.M.?

_____

8. How many hours will an IV of 1000 milliliters of 5% D/W infuse if the order is for 125 milliliters per hour? _____

9. The thrombolytic enzyme streptokinase (Streptase) has been ordered intravenously, 1,500,000 units over 60 minutes in 50 milliliters of 0.9% NS. What will the flow rate be in microdrops per minute? _____

10. The prescriber has ordered 250 milliliters of 5% D/W with 250 milligrams of esmolol hydrochloride (Brevibloc) at a rate of 10 micrograms per kilogram per minute IV. What will the flow rate be in milliliters per hour if the patient weighs 75 kilograms? _____

11. If an IV is infusing at a rate of 80 microdrops per minute, how many milliliters per hour will your patient receive? _____

12. Read the mixing information on the label in Figure 11.14. The medication order reads: Solu-Medrol 1 g in 250 mL 5% D/W, 50 mg/hr. How many milliliters per hour will your patient receive IV? _____

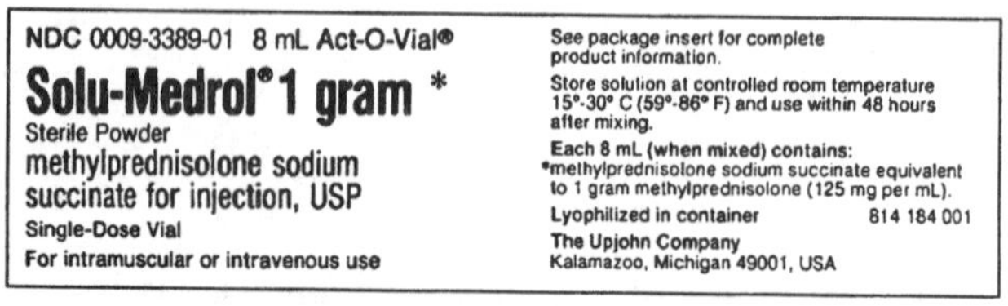

NDC 0009-3389-01 8 mL Act-O-Vial®	See package insert for complete product information.
Solu-Medrol® 1 gram * Sterile Powder methylprednisolone sodium succinate for injection, USP Single-Dose Vial For intramuscular or intravenous use	Store solution at controlled room temperature 15°-30° C (59°-86° F) and use within 48 hours after mixing. Each 8 mL (when mixed) contains: *methylprednisolone sodium succinate equivalent to 1 gram methylprednisolone (125 mg per mL). Lyophilized in container 814 184 001 The Upjohn Company Kalamazoo, Michigan 49001, USA

▶ **FIGURE 11.14 Drug label for Solu-Medrol**

13. The prescriber has ordered 500 milliliters of 5% D/W with 500 milligrams of lidocaine IV and your patient, who weighs 80 kilograms, must receive 20 micrograms per kilogram per minute. What will the flow rate be in milliliters per hour? _____

14. The prescriber ordered 250 mL 5% D/W with 12,500 u heparin. This is to be infused at a rate of 900 units per hour. Calculate the flow rate in milliliters per hour. _____

15. Read the information on the label in Figure 11.15

    a. How many milliliters will you add to the bottle if you want 1,000,000 units per milliliter? _____

    b. Using the solution in part (a), add 5,000,000 units of penicillin to 50 milliliters of 5% D/W; infuse in 30 minutes. The drop factor is 15 drops per milliliter. Calculate the flow rate. _____

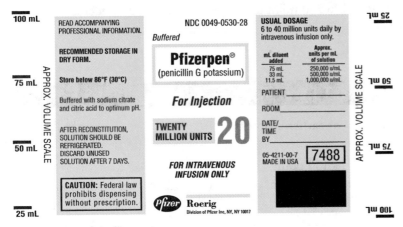

▶ FIGURE 11.15 Drug label for Pfizerpen

16. You have an order for pentamidine isethionate (Pentam 300), 300 milligrams in 250 milliliters of 5% D/W at a rate of 2.5 milligrams per minute IV. What is the flow rate in drops per minute if the drop factor is 15 drops per milliliter? _____

17. The prescriber ordered amphotericin B 150 mg IVPB. The directions are as follows: Add 150 mg to 250 mL; infuse in 6 hr. Calculate the flow rate in drops per minute when the drop factor is 10 drops per milliliter. If

medication order is changed to 20 milligrams per hour, what would the new flow rate be in drops per minute? _____

18. You have an order for 250 milliliters of 0.9% sodium chloride IV. Calculate the flow rate in drops per minute. The drop factor is 10 drops per milliliter, and the infusion time is 2 hours. _____

19. An infusion of 500 milliliters of lactated Ringer's solution was started at 1 P.M. The flow rate is 25 drops per minute, and the drop factor is 15 drops per milliliter. At what time will this IV finish? _____

20. A loading dose of the bronchodilator aminophylline (Aminophyllin) is ordered at 0.18 milligram per kilogram per minute IV. The patient weighs 70 kilograms. What will the flow rate be if 500 milligrams of aminophylline is added to 250 milliliters of 5% D/W? The drop factor is 10 drops per milliliter. _____

CUMULATIVE REVIEW EXERCISES

Review your mastery of earlier chapters.

1. The patient weighs 130 pounds. The medication order for a drug is for 200 micrograms per kilogram of body weight. The label read 2 milligrams per milliliter. How many milliliters of solution is equal to the medication order? _____

2. The prescriber ordered 0.06 g ketorolac IM. How many milliliters of this NSAID are equal to 0.06 gram of this drug if the label reads 30 milligrams per milliliter? _____

3. The patient must receive 1,500,000 units of penicillin IM, and the vial contains 20,000,000 units (in powdered form). The directions are as follows: Add 38.7 mL to vial, 1 mL = 500,000 u. How many milliliters will equal 1,500,000 units? _____

4. A patient must receive grain $\frac{1}{120}$ of scopolamine, a parasympathetic depressant. The label on the ampule reads 0.6 milligram per milliliter. How many minims will you administer to this client? _____

5. The prescriber ordered cefprozil 0.3 g po q12h. The bottle is labeled 125 mg = 5 mL. How many milliliters of this antibiotic will you give your patient? _____

6. If you have a vial labeled 80 milligrams per milliliter, how many milliliters would equal 0.08 grams? _____

7. The physician has ordered 0.5 gram of clarithromycin (Biaxin). The tablets are 250 milligrams each. How many tablets equal 0.5 gram of this antibiotic? _____

8. The prescriber has requested that you give 20 milliequivalents of potassium chloride (K-Lor) po to a patient from a bottle labeled 10 milliequivalents per 5 milliliters. How many milliliters are needed? _____

9. gr $\frac{1}{3000}$ = _____ mg

10. 0.4 mg = gr _____

11. 12.5 g = gr _____

12. gr $\frac{1}{150}$ = _____ g

13. 1 mL = _____ gtt

14. 1 T = _____ t

15. 30 mL = ʒ _____

CHAPTER TWELVE

Calculating Pediatric Dosages

▶ **Objectives**

After completing this chapter, you will be able to

- Calculate pediatric dosages based on body weight.
- Calculate pediatric dosages based on body surface area.
- Determine body surface area using a pediatric nomogram.
- Calculate pediatric intravenous dosages.

T he prescriber must determine the proper kind and amount of medication for a patient. However, the dosage for infants and children is usually less than the adult dosage because their body mass is smaller and their metabolism different from that of adults. In this chapter, you will be introduced to methods of calculating pediatric dosages.

For many years, pediatric dosage calculations used pediatric formulas such as Fried's rule, Young's rule, and Clark's rule (see Appendix G). These formulas are based on the weight of the child in pounds, or on the age of the child in months, and the normal adult dose of a specific drug. By using these formulas, one could determine how much should be prescribed for a particular child.

At the present time, the most accurate methods of determining an appropriate pediatric dose are by weight and body surface area (see Appendix F). You **must** know whether the amount of a prescribed pediatric dosage is the safe or appropriate amount for a particular patient. If this information is not on the drug label, it can be found on the package insert, in the hospital formulary, *Physician's Desk Reference* (PDR), *United States Pharmacopeia*, or in pharmacology texts.

CALCULATING DRUG DOSAGES BY BODY WEIGHT

Drug manufacturers sometimes recommend a dosage based on the weight of the patient. You were introduced to this idea in Chapter 6.

▶ **EXAMPLE 12.1**

The medication order reads:

erythromycin 30 mg/kg po

Read the label in Figure 12.1. The child weighs 38 kilograms. How many milliliters of the drug will you administer to this child?

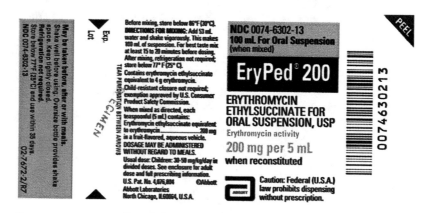

▶ **FIGURE 12.1 Drug label for Erythromycin**

You want to convert body weight to dose in milliliters.

$$38 \text{ kg} \longrightarrow ? \text{ mL}$$

Do this problem on one line as follows:

$$38 \text{ kg} \times \frac{? \text{ mg}}{? \text{ kg}} \times \frac{? \text{ mL}}{? \text{ mg}} = ? \text{ mL}$$

Because 30 mg = 1 kg, the first equivalent fraction is $\frac{30\ \text{mg}}{1\ \text{kg}}$. Because 5 mL = 200 mg, the second equivalent fraction is $\frac{5\ \text{mL}}{200\ \text{mg}}$. You cancel the kilograms and milligrams and obtain the dose in milliliters.

$$38\ \cancel{\text{kg}} \times \frac{30\ \cancel{\text{mg}}}{1\ \cancel{\text{kg}}} \times \frac{5\ \text{mL}}{200\ \cancel{\text{mg}}} = 28.5\ \text{mL}$$

So, the child should receive 28.5 milliliters of Erythromycin.

▶ EXAMPLE 12.2

How many milligrams of the antibiotic ceftazidime (Fortaz) would you administer to a child with a body weight of 25 kilograms if the order is 50 milligrams per kilogram?

You want to convert body weight to dose in milligrams.

$$25\ \text{kg} \longrightarrow ?\ \text{mg}$$

$$25\ \text{kg} \times \frac{?\ \text{mg}}{?\ \text{kg}} = ?\ \text{mg}$$

Because 50 mg = 1 kg, the equivalent fraction is $\frac{50\ \text{mg}}{1\ \text{kg}}$. You cancel the kilograms and obtain the dose in milligrams.

$$25\ \cancel{\text{kg}} \times \frac{50\ \text{mg}}{\cancel{\text{kg}}} = 1250\ \text{mg}$$

So, the child would receive 1250 milligrams of ceftazidime.

▶ EXAMPLE 12.3

Compute the dose of the drug vancomycin hydrochloride (Vancocin), an antibiotic drug, for a child who weighs 48 kilograms and for a prescribed order of 40 milligrams per kilogram in divided doses per day.

You want to convert body weight to dose in milligrams.

$$48\ \text{kg} \longrightarrow ?\ \text{mg}$$

$$48\ \text{kg} \times \frac{?\ \text{mg}}{?\ \text{kg}} = ?\ \text{mg}$$

Because 40 mg = 1 kg, the equivalent fraction is $\frac{40\ \text{mg}}{1\ \text{kg}}$. You cancel the kilograms and obtain the dose in milligrams.

$$48\ \cancel{\text{kg}} \times \frac{40\ \text{mg}}{\cancel{\text{kg}}} = 1920\ \text{mg}$$

So, the child should receive 1920 milligrams of vancomycin hydrochloride in divided doses per day.

▶ E X A M P L E   1 2 . 4

Read the information on the label in Figure 12.2. The prescriber ordered:

cefaclor 20 mg/kg po bid

The child weighs 14 kilograms. How many milliliters of this antibiotic will you prepare?

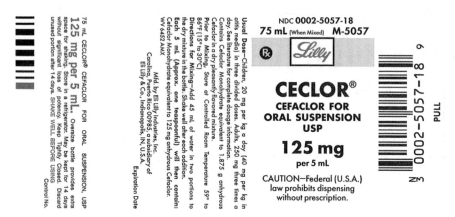

▶ F I G U R E 1 2 . 2 Drug label for Ceclor

You want to convert body weight to dose in milliliters.

$$14 \text{ kg} \longrightarrow \text{? mL}$$

Do this on one line as follows:

$$14 \text{ kg} \times \frac{\text{? mg}}{\text{? kg}} \times \frac{\text{? mL}}{\text{? mg}} = \text{? mL}$$

Because 20 mg = 1 kg, the first equivalent fraction is $\frac{20 \text{ mg}}{1 \text{ kg}}$. Because 125 mg = 5 mL, the second equivalent fraction is $\frac{5 \text{ mL}}{125 \text{ mg}}$.

$$14 \text{ kg} \times \frac{20 \text{ mg}}{\text{kg}} \times \frac{5 \text{ mL}}{125 \text{ mg}} = 11.2 \text{ mL}$$

So, you would prepare 11.2 milliliters of cefaclor.

▶ E X A M P L E   1 2 . 5

You have an order for 5 milligrams per kilogram of acetaminophen (Tylenol). How many grains would you administer to a child who weighs 15 kilograms?

You want to convert body weight to dose in grains.

$$15 \text{ kg} \longrightarrow \text{gr ?}$$

Do this on one line as follows:

$$15 \text{ kg} \times \frac{\text{? mg}}{\text{? kg}} \times \frac{\text{gr ?}}{\text{? mg}} = \text{gr ?}$$

Because 5 mg = 1 kg, the first equivalent fraction is $\frac{5 \text{ mg}}{1 \text{ kg}}$. Because 60 mg = gr 1, the second equivalent fraction is $\frac{\text{gr } 1}{60 \text{ mg}}$.

$$15 \text{ kg} \times \frac{5 \text{ mg}}{\text{kg}} \times \frac{\text{gr } 1}{60 \text{ mg}} = \text{gr } 1\frac{1}{4}$$

So, the dose of this analgesic drug should be grains $1\frac{1}{4}$.

▶ **E X A M P L E   12.6**

The order reads:

> *atropine sulfate 0.04 mg IM stat*

The child weighs 40 kilograms, and the recommended dose is 0.001 milligram per kilogram. Is this a safe dose for this child?

Again, you want to convert body weight to dose in milligrams.

$$40 \text{ kg} \longrightarrow ? \text{ mg}$$

$$40 \text{ kg} \times \frac{? \text{ mg}}{? \text{ kg}} = ? \text{ mg}$$

You cancel the kilograms and obtain the dose in milligrams.

$$40 \text{ kg} \times \frac{0.001 \text{ mg}}{1 \text{ kg}} = 0.04 \text{ mg}$$

So, 0.04 milligram is a safe dose for this child.

▶ **E X A M P L E   12.7**

The prescriber ordered 0.068 milligram po of digoxin (Lanoxin). The child weighs 45 pounds, and the recommended dose is 0.0015 milligram per pound. Is this a safe dose?

You want to convert body weight to dose in milligrams.

$$45 \text{ lb} \longrightarrow ? \text{ mg}$$

$$45 \text{ lb} \times \frac{? \text{ mg}}{? \text{ lb}} = ? \text{ mg}$$

You cancel the pounds and obtain the dose in milligrams.

$$45 \text{ lb} \times \frac{0.0015 \text{ mg}}{1 \text{ lb}} = 0.0675 \text{ mg}$$

Therefore, 0.0675 or 0.068 milligram is the correct dose, so the prescribed dose (0.068 milligrams) is correct.

> ## EXAMPLE 12.8

The prescriber ordered:

digoxin 0.01 mg/kg po qd

The infant weighs 18 kilograms. How many milliliters would you prepare if the label reads 0.05 mg/mL?

You want to convert body weight to dose in milliliters.

$$18 \text{ kg} \longrightarrow ? \text{ mL}$$

$$18 \text{ kg} \times \frac{? \text{ mg}}{? \text{ kg}} \times \frac{? \text{ mL}}{? \text{ mg}} = ? \text{ mL}$$

You cancel the kilograms and milligrams and obtain the dose in milliliters.

$$18 \text{ kg} \times \frac{0.01 \text{ mg}}{\text{kg}} \times \frac{1 \text{ mL}}{0.05 \text{ mg}} = 3.6 \text{ mL}$$

So, the infant should receive 3.6 milliliters of digoxin.

> ## EXAMPLE 12.9

The prescriber ordered the antibiotic cefpodoxime (Vantin) for a child with a weight of 25 kilograms. The label reads 50 milligrams per 5 milliliters (Figure 12.3). The order is 4 milligrams per kilogram. What would be the dose in milliliters?

See package insert for dosage and complete product information.

Warning: Not for injection

Store unconstituted product at controlled room temperature 20° to 25°C (68° to 77°F) [see USP]. Store constituted suspension in a refrigerator 2° to 8°C (36° to 46°F). Shake well before using. Keep container tightly closed. The mixture may be used for 14 days. Discard unused portion after 14 days.

Directions for mixing: Shake bottle to loosen granules. Add approximately 1/2 the total amount of distilled water required for constitution (total water = 58 mL). Shake vigorously to wet the granules. Add remaining water and shake vigorously.

Each 5 mL of suspension contains cefpodoxime proxetil equivalent to 50 mg cefpodoxime.

U.S. Patent Nos. 4,486,425; 4,409,215
815 119 103

Licensed from Sankyo Company, Ltd., Japan
Manufactured by
Pharmacia & Upjohn S.A.-N.V., Puurs - Belgium
for
Pharmacia & Upjohn Company
Kalamazoo, MI 49001, USA

5Q4990/1

NDC 0009-3531-01
100 mL
(when mixed)

Pharmacia
&Upjohn

Vantin®For Oral Suspension

cefpodoxime proxetil
for oral suspension

 50 mg per 5 mL

Equivalent to 50 mg per 5 mL
cefpodoxime when constituted

Caution: Federal law prohibits
dispensing without prescription.

> **FIGURE 12.3 Drug label for Vantin**

You want to convert the body weight to dose in milliliters.

$$25 \text{ kg} \longrightarrow ? \text{ mL}$$

Do this on one line as follows:

$$25 \text{ kg} \times \frac{? \text{ mg}}{? \text{ kg}} \times \frac{? \text{ mL}}{? \text{ mg}} = ? \text{ mL}$$

You cancel the kilograms and milligrams and obtain the dose in milliliters.

$$25 \text{ kg} \times \frac{4 \text{ mg}}{1 \text{ kg}} \times \frac{\overset{1}{\cancel{5}} \text{ mL}}{\underset{10}{\cancel{50}} \text{ mg}} = 10 \text{ mL}$$

So, the prescribed dose is 10 milliliters of Vantin.

▶ **E X A M P L E 1 2 . 1 0**

The prescriber ordered:

Norvir 4 mg/kg po.

The child weighs 42 kilograms. Read the information on the label in Figure 12.4, and calculate the dose in milliliters for this antiviral drug.

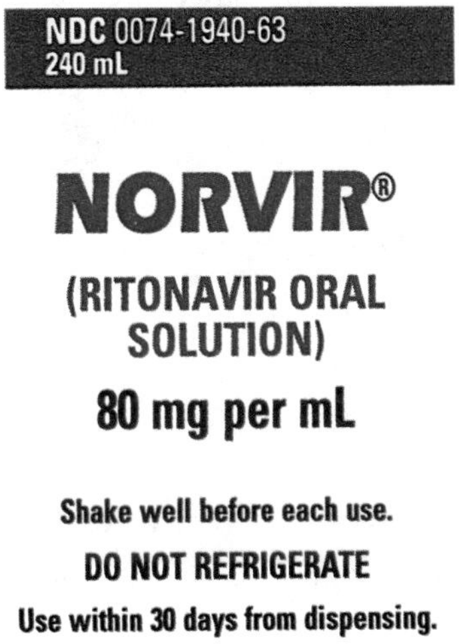

NDC 0074-1940-63
240 mL

NORVIR®

(RITONAVIR ORAL SOLUTION)

80 mg per mL

Shake well before each use.

DO NOT REFRIGERATE

Use within 30 days from dispensing.

▶ **FIGURE 12.4 Drug label for Norvir**

You want to convert the body weight to dose in milliliters.

42 kg ⟶ ? mL

Do this on one line as follows:

$$42 \text{ kg} \times \frac{? \text{ mg}}{? \text{ kg}} \times \frac{? \text{ mL}}{? \text{ mg}} = ? \text{ mL}$$

The order is 4 milligrams per kilogram, so the first equivalent fraction is $\frac{4 \text{ mg}}{1 \text{ kg}}$. Because 80 mg = 1 mL, the second equivalent fraction is $\frac{1 \text{ mL}}{80 \text{ mg}}$.

$$42 \text{ kg} \times \frac{\overset{1}{\cancel{4}} \text{ mg}}{1 \text{ kg}} \times \frac{1 \text{ mL}}{\underset{20}{\cancel{80}} \text{ mg}} = 2.1 \text{ mL}$$

So, the prescribed dose is 2.1 milliliters of Norvir.

CALCULATING DRUG DOSAGES BY BODY SURFACE AREA

Drug manufacturers often recommend a pediatric dosage based on body surface area (BSA). You have already been introduced to this idea in Chapters 2 and 6.

▶ **EXAMPLE 12.11**

The prescriber ordered: digoxin 0.72 mg/m^2 po qd. The child's BSA is 0.9 square meter. How many milligrams would you administer to this child of this loading dose?

You want to convert body surface area to dose in milligrams.

$$0.9 \text{ m}^2 \longrightarrow ? \text{ mg}$$

$$0.9 \text{ m}^2 \times \frac{? \text{ mg}}{? \text{ m}^2} = ? \text{ mg}$$

Because 0.72 mg = 1 m^2, the equivalent fraction is $\frac{0.72 \text{ mg}}{1 \text{ m}^2}$. You cancel the square meter and obtain the dose in milligrams.

$$0.9 \text{ m}^2 \times \frac{0.72 \text{ mg}}{1 \text{ m}^2} = 0.648 \text{ or } 0.65 \text{ mg}$$

So, the child should receive 0.65 milligram of digoxin.

▶ **EXAMPLE 12.12**

If a child has a BSA of 0.5 square meter and the medication order is for 1.25 milligrams per square meter of vinblastine sulfate (Velban), then how many milligrams of this antineoplastic drug should the child receive?

You want to convert body surface area to dose in milligrams.

$$0.5 \text{ m}^2 \longrightarrow ? \text{ mg}$$

$$0.5 \text{ m}^2 \times \frac{? \text{ mg}}{? \text{ m}^2} = ? \text{ mg}$$

Because the order is for 1.25 mg = 1 m^2, the equivalent fraction is $\frac{1.25 \text{ mg}}{1 \text{ m}^2}$. You cancel the square meters and obtain the dose in milligrams.

$$0.5 \text{ m}^2 \times \frac{1.25 \text{ mg}}{1 \text{ m}^2} = 0.625 \text{ mg}$$

So, the child should receive 0.625 milligram of vinblastine sulfate.

BSA PEDIATRIC NOMOGRAM

In Chapter 6, you used the adult nomogram to determine BSA. For children, you can use the pediatric nomogram (Figure 12.5).

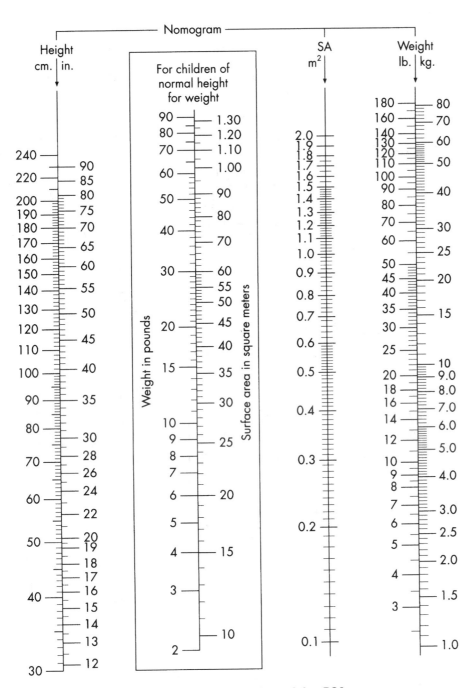

▶ **FIGURE 12.5 Pediatric nomogram for determining BSA**

The body surface area is shown in the column labeled SA in Figure 12.5. A straight line is drawn between the child's height (first column) and the child's weight (last column). The point at which the line crosses the SA column is the estimated *BSA in square meters*. The boxed column listing weight on the left and surface in square meters on the right can be used when a child is of normal height for his or her weight. For additional information concerning a BSA nomogram, see a text of pediatrics.

EXAMPLE 12.13

Estimate the BSA of a child who weighs 40 pounds and is 90 centimeters tall.

Using the nomogram in Figure 12.6, connect the 90 cm mark in the left col-

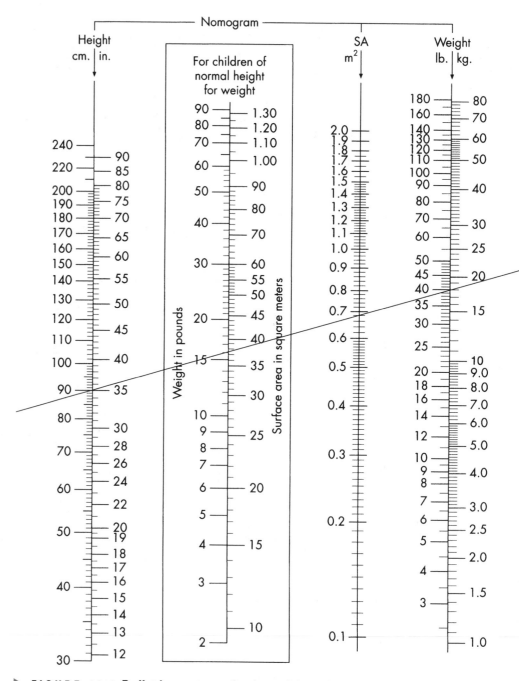

▶ FIGURE 12.6 Pediatric nomogram for determining BSA for Examples 12.13

umn and the 40 lb mark in the right column with a straight line. This line crosses the SA column at 0.68 square meter.

So, the child's estimated BSA is 0.68 square meter.

> **EXAMPLE 12.14**

The prescriber has ordered 30 milligrams per square meter of Cortef. The child weighs 40 kilograms and is 45 inches tall. Read the label in Figure 12.7, and determine how many milliliters this child should receive.

NDC 0009-0142-01
4 Fl Oz

Pharmacia
&Upjohn

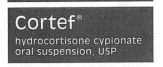

Cortef®
hydrocortisone cypionate
oral suspension, USP

10 mg/5 mL*

Caution: Federal law prohibits dispensing without prescription.
810 322 506

> **FIGURE 12.7 Drug label for Cortef**

You want to find the body surface area and convert it to dose in milliliters.

$$\text{BSA} \longrightarrow ? \text{ mL}$$

$$\text{m}^2 \times \frac{? \text{ mg}}{? \text{ m}^2} \times \frac{? \text{ mL}}{? \text{ mg}} = ? \text{ mL}$$

Using the nomogram, the child has a BSA of approximately 1.16 square meter. The equivalent fraction is $\frac{30\,\text{mg}}{1\,\text{m}^2}$. You cancel the square meter and milligrams to obtain the dose in milliliters.

$$1.16\ \cancel{\text{m}^2} \times \frac{30\ \cancel{\text{mg}}}{1\ \cancel{\text{m}^2}} \times \frac{\overset{1}{\cancel{5}}\,\text{mL}}{\underset{2}{\cancel{10}}\,\cancel{\text{mg}}} = 17.4 \text{ mL}$$

So, the dose should be 17.4 milliliters.

> **EXAMPLE 12.15**

Methylphenidate (Ritalin HCL), a CNS stimulant, has been ordered for a child. How many tablets will you administer to a child 50 inches tall weighing 75 pounds if the order is for 10 milligrams per square meter po? Read the label in Figure 12.8, and use the formula to calculate the BSA.

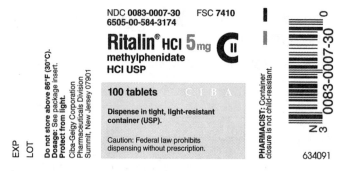

▶ **FIGURE 12.8 Drug label for Ritalin**

The formulas for calculating pediatric BSA are the same as for adults (see Chapter 6). So, in this problem you use the household formula:

$$BSA = \sqrt{\frac{Weight \times Height}{3131}}$$

$$BSA = \sqrt{\frac{75 \times 50}{3131}}$$

$$BSA = \sqrt{1.1977}$$

$$BSA = 1.09 \ m^2$$

You want to convert body surface area to dose in tablets. According to the formula, the child's BSA is 1.09 square meters.

$$1.09 \ m^2 = ? \ tab$$

Do this on one line as follows:

$$1.09 \ m^2 \times \frac{? \ mg}{? \ m^2} \times \frac{? \ tab}{? \ mg} = ? \ tab$$

$$1.09 \ m^2 \times \frac{10 \ mg}{m^2} \times \frac{1 \ tab}{5 \ mg} = 2.18 \ tab$$

So, you will administer 2 tablets of Ritalin to the child.

<hr>

▶ **EXAMPLE 12.16**

The prescriber has ordered 250 milligrams po qid of the antiviral drug zidovudine (AZT, Retrovir). Is this a safe dose for a child whose BSA is 1.11 square meter and the recommended dose for the drug is 100 to 180 milligrams per square meter?

You want to convert body surface area to dose in milligrams.

$$11.2 \ m^2 \longrightarrow ? \ mg$$

First, use the *minimum* recommended dose of 100 milligrams per square meter.

$$1.11 \text{ m}^2 \times \frac{100 \text{ mg}}{1 \text{ m}^2} = 111 \text{ mg}$$

Second, use the *maximum* recommended dose of 180 milligrams per square meter.

$$1.11 \text{ m}^2 \times \frac{180 \text{ mg}}{1 \text{ m}^2} = 199.8 \text{ or } 200 \text{ mg}$$

Therefore, any prescribed amount in the range of 111 to 200 milligrams would be acceptable. So, 250 milligrams is not a safe dose.

PEDIATRIC INTRAVENOUS DOSAGES

▶ **E X A M P L E   12.17**

The prescriber ordered 300 mg/m²/hr of Keflex IV. The label reads: Add 1 g of Keflex to 100 mL of 5% D/W. How many milliliters per hour would be given to a child who weighs 15 kilograms and is 77 centimeters tall?

The BSA can be estimated using either the pediatric nomogram or the formula. Using the metric BSA formula yields

$$\begin{aligned} \text{BSA} &= \sqrt{\frac{\text{WT} \times \text{HT}}{3600}} \\ &= \sqrt{\frac{15 \times 77}{3600}} \\ &= \sqrt{0.3208} \\ &= 0.57 \text{ m}^2 \end{aligned}$$

You want to convert the BSA of 0.57 square meter to a dose in milliliters per hour.

$$0.57 \text{ m}^2 = ? \frac{\text{mL}}{\text{hr}}$$

Do this in one line as follows:

$$0.57 \text{ m}^2 \times \frac{300 \text{ mg}}{\text{m}^2 \times \text{hr}} \times \frac{\overset{1}{100} \text{ mL}}{1 \text{ g}} \times \frac{1 \text{ g}}{\underset{10}{1000} \text{ mg}} = 17.1 \frac{\text{mL}}{\text{hr}}$$

So, you would administer 17.1 milliliters per hour of Keflex to the child.

▶ **E X A M P L E   12.18**

The prescriber ordered the antibiotic chloramphenicol (Chloromycetin) 250 mg in 100 mL of D/5W IV for a child who weighs 34.6 kilograms. The dose is 0.2 mg/kg/min. The drop factor is 15 drops per milliliter. Calculate the flow rate.

You want to change the weight (34.6 kg) to the flow rate (gtt/min).

$$34.6 \text{ kg} \times \frac{0.2 \text{ mg}}{\text{kg} \times \text{min}} \times \frac{100 \text{ mL}}{250 \text{ mg}} \times \frac{15 \text{ gtt}}{\text{mL}} = 41.5 \frac{\text{gtt}}{\text{min}}$$

So, the flow rate is 42 drops per minute.

CASE STUDY 12

A child, age 8, has been admitted to the hospital with a diagnosis of acute lymphocytic leukemia. The child weighs 35 kilograms and is 112 centimeters tall.

Orders include the following:

- 50 mL 5% D/W q1h IV
- vincristine 2 mg/m² IV weekly for 4 doses on Monday; add to 50 mL D/5W, IVPB infuse in 15 minutes, start at 12 noon
- prednisone 40 mg/m² po in divided doses q8h for 21 days; use oral solution 5 mg/5 mL
- asparaginase 1000 international units (IU) per kg; add to 50 mL 5% D/W, IVPB in 30 minutes, begin at 12 noon every Tuesday

Maintenance standby when order is activated:

- methotrexate 3.3 mg/m²/day IVPB, add to 25 mL of 0.9% NaCl and infuse in 20 minutes × 42 days
- acetaminophen 650 mg by rectal suppository q1/2h prior to administration of IV medication

1. How many milliliters of the 5% D/W q1h will the patient receive in the 12 hour period from 1 pm to 1 am? _____

2. (a) How many milligrams of vincristine will the patient receive each week? (b) The label on the vial reads 1 mg/mL. How many milliliters will be added to 50 milliliters of 5% D/W? Calculate the flow rate in milliliters per minute. _____

3. The dose of asparaginase is 1000 IU/kg IV (a) How many international units will this patient receive? (b) If each 10,000 unit vial is dissolved in 5 milliliters of sterile H₂O, how many milliliters will you prepare? (c) Add to 50 milliliters of 5% D/W. This drug must infuse in 30 minutes. Calculate the flow rate. _____

4. (a) Calculate the current amount of prednisone for this patient daily. (b) Divide into three doses. (c) How many milliliters po will the patient receive in each dose? (d) How many milligrams of prednisone will the patient receive in 21 days? _____

5. The physician initiates the order for methotrexate. The vial is labeled 2.5 mg/mL. (a) How many milliliters will you add to 25 mL of D5W? (b) Calculate IV rates in milliliters per minute. (c) How many milligrams will the patient receive in 6 weeks?

_____

6. What is the total amount of IV fluid the child will receive in 24 hours on Monday? _____

7. How many grams of acetaminophen will you administer if the physician writes an order for 650 mg? _____

8. The physician has written an additional order to be given if child develops urticaria and pruritus: Benadryl 2.5 mg/kg added to 200 mL 5% D/W; infuse in 6 h. The drop factor is 10 drops per milliliter. Each vial of Benadryl is labeled 50 mg = 1 mL. Calculate the flow rate in drops per minute. _____

The answers to the Case Studies appear in Appendix A.

NOTES/WORKSPACE

PRACTICE SETS

You will find the answers to *Try These for Practice* below. Answers to *Exercises* and *Cumulative Review Exercises* appear in Appendix A at the back of the book. Your instructor has the answers to the *Additional Exercises.*

Try These for Practice

Test your comprehension after reading this chapter.

1. The following order has been given for a child with a weight of 35 kilograms:

   Humulin R insulin 0.14 u/kg sc bid ac breakfast and dinner

   How many units will this child receive of this low-dose insulin?

   ____

2. Read the information on the label in Figure 12.9. What would the prescribed dose in milliliters of cephalexin be for a patient who weighs 20 pounds if the order is for 7.5 milligrams per kilogram? ________

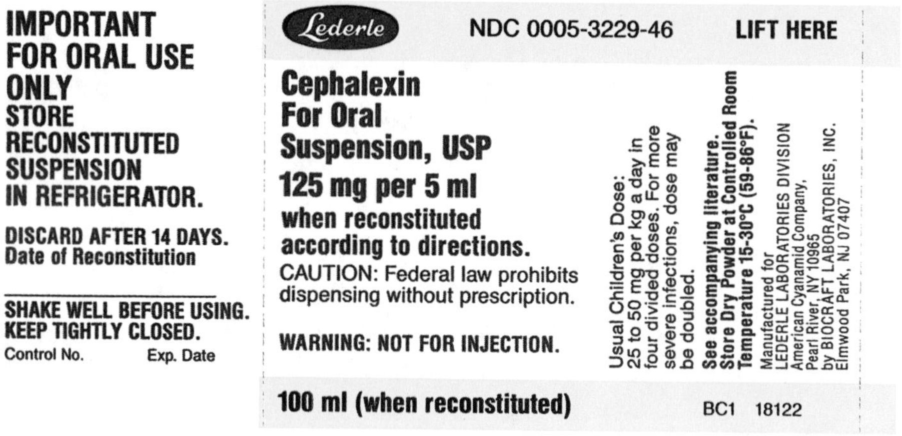

▶ **FIGURE 12.9 Drug label for Cephalexin**

3. A child must receive meperidine hydrochloride (Demerol). The child's BSA is 0.8 square meter. How many milliliters will you administer to the child if the order is for 30 milligrams per square meter and the label reads 50 milligrams per milliliter? ________

4. Read the information on the label in Figure 12.10. How many milliliters of Spectrobid would you administer in divided doses to a child who weighs 40 kilograms when the order is for 25 milligrams per kilogram?

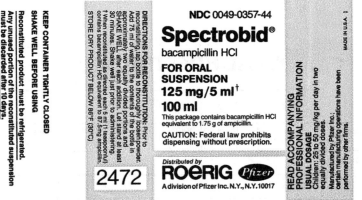

▶ **FIGURE 12.10 Drug label for pediatric Spectrobid**

5. The order reads: zidovudine 180 mg/m² po q6h. The label reads 50 mg = 5 mL. How many milliliters would you administer to a child whose BSA is 0.9 square meter? _____

Answers: 1. 5 u   2. 2.7 mL   3. 0.5 mL   4. 40 mL   5. 16.2 mL

Exercises

Reinforce your understanding in class or at home.

1. Read the first order in the medication administration record shown in Figure 12.11. The label reads 25 milligrams per 5 milliliters. How many teaspoons will you administer? _____

⊕ GENERAL HOSPITAL ⊕

Year 2001 Month 11	Day	.24	.25	.26			
Medication Dosage and Interval		Initials* and Hours	Initials and Hours	Initials and Hours	Initials and Hours	Initials and Hours	Initials and Hours
Date started: *11/24/01* *Vistaril 0.025 g qid*	I	*JO*	*JO*	*JO*			
	AM	10	10	10			
	I	*LD LD LD*	*LD LD LD*	*LD LD LD*			
Discontinued: *11/30/01*	PM	2 6 10	2 6 10	2 6 10			
Date started: *11/24/01* *aspirin 162 mg* *po q4h prn*	I	*JO*	*AG JO*	*AG JO*			
	AM	10	1 9	7 11			
	I	*JO LD*	*JO LD LD*	*LD LD*			
Discontinued: *11/30/01*	PM	2 8	2 6 10	3 12			
Date started: *11/24/01* *Keflex 6.25 mg/kg* *po qid*	I	*JO*	*JO*	*JO*			
	AM	10	10	10			
	I	*LD LD LD*	*LD LD LD*	*LD LD LD*			
Discontinued: *11/30/01*	PM	2 6 10	2 6 10	2 6 10			

Allergies: (Specify)

Init*	Signature
JO	*June Olsen*
LD	*Larissa Dingman*
AG	*Anthony Giangrasso*

PATIENT IDENTIFICATION

```
0312578                          11/24/01
Mary Johnson
2183 Avantlar Ave               6/21/79
Phoenix, AR                         Prot
10357                              Aetna

Leon Ablon, M.D.
```

MEDICATION ADMINISTRATION RECORD

▶ **FIGURE 12.11 Medication administration record**

2. Read the second order in the MAR shown in Figure 12.11. The label on the bottle of aspirin reads 81 milligrams per tablet. How many tablets will you administer to this patient? _____

3. Read the third order in Figure 12.11. The child weighs 40 kilograms. How many milliliters of Keflex will you give the child if the label reads 125 milligrams per 5 milliliters? _____

4. The prescriber has ordered 3.3 micrograms per kilogram IM of fentanyl citrate (Sublimaze) as a pre-operative medication. The label on the vial reads 50 micrograms per milliliter. How many milliliters will you administer to this child whose weight is 30 kilograms? _____

5. The normal dose of a drug for a child is 0.3 milligram per square meter. If the child's BSA is 0.6 square meter, how many milligrams should this child receive? _____

6. A child's BSA is 0.93 square meters, and 100 milligrams per square meter of the antineoplastic drug procarbazine HCl (Matulane) has been ordered. How many milligrams should this child receive? _____

7. If a child's BSA is 1.1 square meters, how many milligrams of the antibiotic gentamicin sulfate (Garamycin) should the child receive if the prescribed amount is 45 milligrams per square meter? _____

8. A long-acting anti-inflammatory medication, dexamethasone (Decadron), has been ordered for a child with a BSA of 1.04 square meters. How many milligrams should this child receive if the prescribed amount is 50 milligrams per square meter? _____

9. The anticholinergic medication scopolamine (Triptone) has been ordered for a child with a BSA of 0.8 square meter. How many milliliters will you prepare if the order is for 0.2 milligram per square meter and the ampule reads 0.2 milligram per milliliter? _____

10. Atropine sulfate has been ordered for a child who weighs 35 kilograms. The prescribed dose is 0.01 milligram per kilogram. Read the medication label in Figure 12.12. How many milliliters equal the prescribed dose?

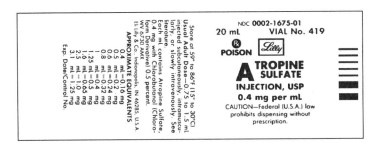

▶ FIGURE 12.12 Drug label for atropine sulfate

11. The anticonvulsant medication phenytoin sodium (Dilantin) is ordered for a child with a BSA of 1.25 square meters. The prescribed dose is 250 milligrams per square meter. How many milliliters should this child receive if the oral suspension is 125 milligrams per milliliter? _____

12. The order states that a child is to receive 1% lidocaine 0.5 mg/kg IV bolus. How many milliliters will you prepare for this child whose weight is 45 kilograms? _____

13. The prescriber orders 0.54 unit per kilogram of NPH insulin (Humulin N). If the child weighs 44 kilograms, how many milliliters will you prepare of the insulin in Figure 12.13. _____

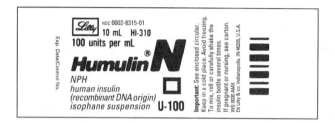

▶ **FIGURE 12.13 Drug label for Humulin N insulin**

14. The prescriber ordered Lasix 2 mg/kg po. If the child weighs 42 kilograms and the label reads 10 milligrams per milliliter, how many milliliters will you give to the child? _____

15. A 10-year-old child has a fever of 101F, and 0.4 gram po of the antipyretic acetaminophen (Tylenol) has been ordered. If the elixir is labeled 160 milligrams per 5 milliliters, how many teaspoons will you give to the child? _____

16. A child has to receive an IV bolus of 2% lidocaine, 1 milligram per kilogram. How many milliliters will you prepare for a child with a weight of 50 kilograms? _____

17. Read the information on the label in Figure 12.14. The prescriber has ordered Terramycin IM for a child. If the child weighs 42 kilograms and the prescribed dose is 1.2 milligrams per kilogram, how many milliliters will you administer to this child? _____

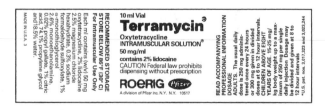

▶ **FIGURE 12.14 Drug label for Terramycin**

18. The prescriber has ordered a stat dose of the gastrointestinal stimulant metoclopramide HCl (Reglan) IV, 0.1 milligram per kilogram direct IV push. If the vial is labeled 5 milligrams per milliliter and the child weighs 38 kilograms, how many milliliters will you prepare? _____

19. Meperidine HCl (Demerol) has been prescribed for a child whose weight is 75 pounds. The label on the vial reads 100 milligrams per milliliter. How many milliliters would you prepare of this narcotic analgesic if the prescribed amount is 1.04 milligrams per kilogram? _____

20. A child must receive the antineoplastic drug melphalan (Alkeran). The scored tablets are 2 milligrams each. What would be the correct dose if the order is 3 milligrams per square meter and the child's BSA is 1.02 square meters? _____

Additional Exercises

Now, on your own, test yourself! Ask your instructor to check your answers.

1. The order reads: furosemide 0.2 mg/kg IV g12h. The child weighs 48 kilograms. Read the information in Figure 12.15 and calculate the milliliters in this prescribed dose. _____

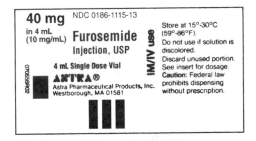

▶ **FIGURE 12.15 Drug label for furosemide**

2. The prescribed order for a child is 12 milligrams per kilogram of the sulfonamide sulfasalazine (Azulfidine), and the medication is available in 500 mg tablets. How many tablets would you give a child with a weight of 88 pounds? _____

3. Cyanocobalamin (vitamin B$_{12}$) is available in vials labeled 1 milligram per milliliter. How many micrograms would you give a child if the order is 2 micrograms per kilogram and the child's weight is 25 kilograms? How many milliliters would you administer to this child IM? _____

4. The order reads: diphenhydramine 125 mcg/kg IM stat. The child weighs 31 kilograms, and the medication label reads 5 milligrams per milliliter. How many milliliters will you administer to this child? _____

5. The antispasmodic drug tincture of belladonna has been prescribed for a child with nocturnal enuresis; the child is to receive 0.033 milligram per kilogram at bedtime. The label reads 0.3 milligram per milliliter. How many milliliters will you administer to this child, whose weight is 70 pounds? _____

6. Read the information in Figure 12.16, and calculate the amount of atropine sulfate you would administer to a child if the order is 0.2 milligram per square meter and the child's BSA is 1 square meter. _____

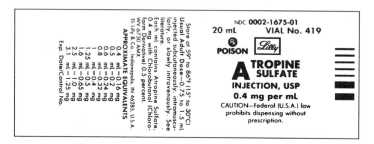

▶ **FIGURE 12.16 Drug label for atropine sulfate**

7. The thiazide diuretic chlorothiazide (Diuril) has been prescribed for a child, 0.005 gram per kilogram qd. The label reads 50 milligrams per 5 milliliters. How many milliliters would the child receive if the child's weight is 34 kilograms? _____

8. The prescriber has written an order for the anti-inflammatory medication dexamethasone (Decadron) for a child with a BSA of 0.64 square meter. How many milligrams should the child receive if the order is for 0.05 gram per square meter? _____

9. The order reads: ibuprofen (Motrin) 5 mg/kg po q6h prn. Each 5 milliliters contain 100 milligrams. If the child weighs 20 pounds, how many milliliters will you administer to this child? _____

10. A prescriber orders erythromycin (EryPed) for a child who has a BSA of 0.9 square meter. Read the label in Figure 12.17. If the recommended dose is 100 milligrams per square meter, how many milliliters will the child receive of this broad-spectrum antibiotic? _____

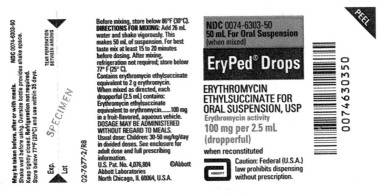

▶ **FIGURE 12.17** Drug label for EryPed

11. A prescriber orders ketamine hydrochloride (Ketalar), a drug that causes disassociative anesthesia. The label reads 10 milligrams per milliliter, and the child weighs 35 kilograms. The order is for 0.35 milligrams per kilogram. How many milliliters will the child receive IV from the anesthesiologist? _____

12. The order reads: digoxin 0.01 mg/kg po qd. The label on the vial reads 0.25 milligram per milliliter. How many minims will you administer to a child who weighs 18 kilograms? _____

13. The prescriber has ordered methohexital sodium (Brevital Sodium) IV, a general anesthetic for a short-term procedure. If 70 milligrams are prepared and the label reads 50 milligrams per 5 milliliters, how many milliliters equal the prescribed dose? _____

14. Digitoxin (Crystodigin), a cardiac glycoside, has been prescribed. The child weighs 36 kilograms and each tablet contains 0.2 milligram. How many tablets will you prepare if the order is for 0.011 milligram per kilogram? _____

15. The order reads:

    0.14 units/kg of Humulin U.

    If the child weighs 57 kilograms, how many milliliters will you prepare of the insulin in Figure 12.18? _____

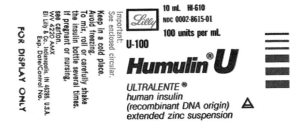

▶ **FIGURE 12.18** Drug label for Humulin

16. The order reads: demeclocycline hydrochloride 0.15 g po tid. The recommended dose for children is 6 milligrams per pound. If the child's weight is 25.5 kilograms, would this be a safe dose? ________

17. Read the label in Figure 12.19 for Cylert. If the prescriber gave the child 2 tablets, how many milligrams of Cylert will the child receive?

____

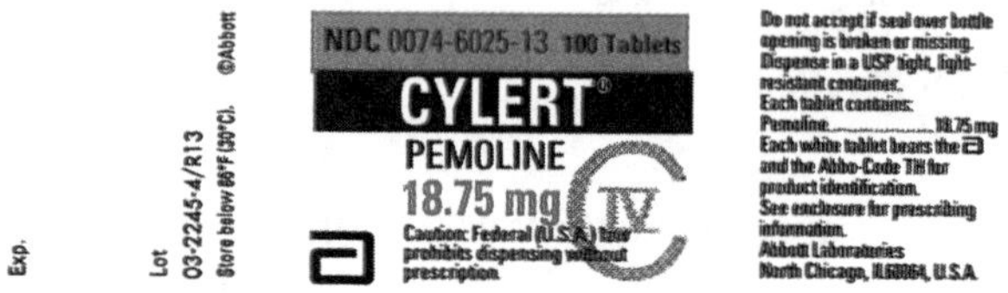

FIGURE 12.19 Drug label for Cylert

18. Read the first order in Figure 12.20. If the label reads 10 milligrams per milliliter, how many milliliters will you prepare for a child who weighs 75 pounds? ________

GENERAL HOSPITAL

Year 2001 Month April Day		10	11	12	13	14	15
Medication Dosage and Interval		Initials* and Hours	Initials and Hours	Initials and Hours	Initials and Hours	Initials and Hours	Initials and Hours
Date started: 4/10/01 chlorpromazine 0.25 mg/kg q6h Im 12 noon, 6 P.M., 12 mid, 6 A.M. Discontinued: 4/13/01	I	LD LD	LD LD	LD LD	LD LD		
	AM	12 6	12 6	12 6	12 6		
	I	JO JO	JO JO	JO JO	JO JO		
	PM	12 6	12 6	12 6	12 6		
Date started: 4/10/01 Alkeran 3 mg/m² qd po x 14 doses, start at 10 A.M. Discontinued: 4/13/01 after 2 P.M.	I	LD	LD	LD	LD		
	AM	10	10	10	10		
	I						
	PM						

Allergies: (Specify)

Init*	Signature
LD	L. Dingman
JO	June Olsen

MEDICATION ADMINISTRATION RECORD

PATIENT IDENTIFICATION

1077854 4/10/01
Johnny Davis 12/4/82
1622 Alki Dr. #43 RC
Seattle, WA 94032 US Health Care
L.Ablon, M.D.

FIGURE 12.20 Medication administration record

19. Read the second order in Figure 12.20 for the antineoplastic drug Alkeran. The child's BSA is 0.8 square meter. How many milligrams will you prepare of this drug? _____

20. The initial dose of dextrothyroxine (Choloxin), a drug used for the treatment of hyperlipidemia in euthyroid patients, is 0.05 milligram per kilogram. How many milligrams should be given to a child who weighs 42 kg? _____

CUMULATIVE REVIEW EXERCISES

Review your mastery of earlier chapters.

1. How many milligrams of ethambutol HCl (Myambutal), an antitubercular drug, would you administer if the prescribed dose po is 15 milligrams per kilogram and the child weighs 35 kilograms? _____

2. How many milligrams of the antibiotic penicillin would you prepare for a child who weighs 40 kilograms if the order is 7.5 milligrams per kilogram? _____

3. The order reads: cefixime 8 mg/kg po. How many milligrams of this antibiotic would you administer to a child whose weight is 20 kilograms?

    _____

4. The order reads: 50 u Lente insulin sc. The vial is labeled 100 units per milliliter. How many minims would you administer to the patient?

    _____

5. The prescriber has ordered 1,200,000 units of penicillin G IM. The 5,000,000 u vial of powder has these instructions: Add 8 mL of sterile water, 1 mL = 500,000 u. How many milliliters equals 1,200,000 units?

    _____

6. The order is for 0.125 gram of Depakote. Read the label in Figure 12.21. How many capsules equal the prescribed dose of this anticonvulsant drug? _____

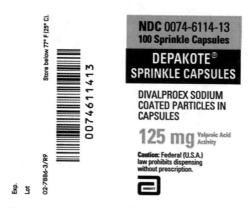

▶ FIGURE 12.21 Drug label for Depakote

7. The order reads: amrinone lactate 0.75 mg/kg IV bolus. How many milligrams will you prepare of this inotropic drug if the patient weighs 116 pounds? _____

8. The prescriber ordered 900 mL of 5% D/W IV in 5 h. Calculate the flow rate in drops per minute when the drop factor is 20 drops per milliliter.

_____

9. The order reads: cimetidine 300 mg IV in 50 mL of 5% D/W. Infuse in 20 minutes. Calculate the flow rate in milliliters per minute for this histamine receptor drug. _____

10. The prescriber ordered 1000 mL 5% D/W at 17 gtt/min IV. The infusion began at 9 P.M. At what time will this solution be completed? The drop factor is 15 drops per milliliter. _____

11. 0.002 g = gr _____

12. How many milligrams of cephalexin would you administer to an adult with a BSA of 1.9 square meters if the order is for 410 milligrams per square meter? _____

13. Describe how to prepare 100 milliliters of a $\frac{1}{4}$% solution from a $\frac{1}{2}$% solution. _____

14. The order is for 0.05 gram of nicardipine (Cardene) po. How many milligrams will you administer of this anti-anginal medication? _____

15. The order for a child with BSA of 1.2 square meters reads: Zithromax 175 mg/m² po. Read the label in Figure 12.22, and determine how many milliliters the child will receive. _____

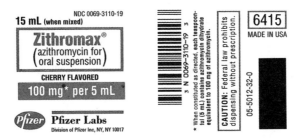

FOR ORAL USE ONLY.
Store dry powder below 86°F (30°C).
PROTECT FROM FREEZING.
DOSAGE AND USE
See accompanying prescribing information.
MIXING DIRECTIONS:
Tap bottle to loosen powder.
Add 9 mL of water to the bottle.
After mixing, store suspension at
41° to 86°F (5° to 30°C).
Oversized bottle provides extra space
for shaking.
After mixing, use within 10 days. Discard
after full dosing is completed.
SHAKE WELL BEFORE USING.
Contains 300 mg azithromycin.

NDC 0069-3110-19
15 mL (when mixed)

Zithromax®
(azithromycin for
oral suspension)

CHERRY FLAVORED

100 mg* per 5 mL

Pfizer **Pfizer Labs**
Division of Pfizer Inc, NY, NY 10017

* When constituted as directed, each teaspoonful (5 mL) contains azithromycin dihydrate equivalent to 100 mg of azithromycin.

CAUTION: Federal law prohibits dispensing without prescription.

05-5012-32-0

6415
MADE IN USA

▶ **FIGURE 12.22 Drug label for Zithromax**

Comprehensive
Self-Tests

Answers to *Comprehensive Self-Tests* 1–3 can be found in Appendix A at the back of the book. Your instructor has the answers to *Comprehensive Self-Tests* 4–6.

Comprehensive Self-Test 1

1. The prescriber has ordered ursodiol (Actigall), a drug for dissolving gall-stones, for Mr. Chang. The usual range for the dosage of this drug is 8–10 milligrams per kilogram per day in two or three divided doses. If the patient weighs 70 kilograms and the prescribed dose is 300 milligrams bid, is this a correct dose? _____

2. The nonsteroidal anti-inflammatory drug diclofenac sodium (Voltaren) is ordered for a patient with rheumatoid arthritis. The usual dose is 50 milligrams tid. Each enteric-coated tablet contains 50 milligrams of the drug. How many tablets should the patient receive each day? _____

3. An anti-infective medication, amoxicillin (Amoxil), has been ordered by the prescriber for Maria Hernandez, 0.25 gram q8h. How many capsules will you require for 24 hours if each capsule contains 250 milligrams?

_____

Read the information on the labels and medication administration record (MAR) in Figure S.1 to answer questions 4–9.

DAILY MEDICATION ADMINISTRATION RECORD

6056812
Marianne Doe
Rt 1, Box 456
Essex, Mt
60514

4/12/99
7/10/42
PROT
BCBS

Dr. A Giangrasso

PATIENT NAME _M. Doe_

ROOM # _22 B_

☐ IF ANOTHER RECORD IS IN USE

ALLERGIC TO (RECORD IN RED): _NKA_

DATES GIVEN ↓   DATE DISCHARGED:

RED CHECK INITIAL	ORDER DATE	INITIAL	EXP DATE	MEDICATION, DOSAGE, FREQUENCY AND ROUTE	HOURS	12	13	14	15	16	17	18	19	20	21	22	23	24	25
	4/12		4/17	Asulfidine 1.5 g q 12h po	9 AM	JO	JO	JO	JO	JO	JO								
					9 PM	HA	HA	HA	HA	HA	HA								
	4/12		4/19	Hytrin 0.004 g daily HS po	9 AM	HA	HA	HA	HA	HA	HA	HA	HA						
	4/12		4/19	Valproic acid 250 mg	9 AM	JO	JO	JO	JO	JO	JO	JO	HA						
				sprinkle capsules q8h	5 PM	HA	HA	HA	HA	HA	HA	HA	CC						
				po	1 AM	HA	HA	HA	HA	HA	HA	JO	JO						
	4/16		4/19	bromocriptine 5 mg daily po	9 AM	/	/	/	/	JO	JO	JO	HA						
	4/16		4/19	norvasc 10 mg qd h s po	9 PM	/	/	/	/	HA	HA	HA	HA						
	4/12		4/19	Penicillin G 15 million units															
				in 500mL D/5w IV	8 AM	CC	CC	CC	CC	CC	JO	JO	CC						
				AM															

SINGLE MEDICATION ORDERS, PRE-OPERATIVE MEDICATION ORDERS

RED CHECK & INT.	INT. DATE TO BE GIVEN	TIME TO BE GIVEN	SINGLE MEDICATION DOSAGE ROUTE OF ADMINISTRATION	ADMINISTERED DATE	TIME	INT.
CC			Connie Chun, RN			
HA			Holly Aciarino, RN			
JO			June Olsen, RN			

SINGLE MEDICATION ORDERS, PRE-OPERATIVE MEDICATION ORDERS

RED CHECK & INT.	INT. DATE TO BE GIVEN	TIME TO BE GIVEN	SINGLE MEDICATION DOSAGE ROUTE OF ADMINISTRATION	ADMINISTERED DATE	TIME	INT.

39171 (10/91)

▶ **FIGURE S.1 Medication administration record.**

See package insert for complete product information.

Dispense in a well-closed container.

Store at 25°C (77°F); excursions 15-30°C (59-86°F)

MADE IN SWEDEN
Mfd. by: Pharmacia & Upjohn AB
Stockholm, Sweden
For: **Pharmacia & Upjohn Co.**
Kalamazoo, MI 49001, USA
102041296   51-0052-89/03

Pharmacia&Upjohn

NDC 0013-0101-01

Azulfidine®
Tablets

sulfasalazine tablets, USP

500 mg

Caution: Federal law prohibits dispensing without prescription.

100 Tablets

Peel back for package insert

N 3 0013-0101-01 2

▶ **F I G U R E S.2 Drug label for Azulfidine.**

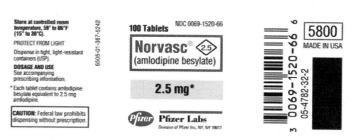

Store at controlled room temperature, 59° to 86°F (15° to 30°C).

PROTECT FROM LIGHT

Dispense in tight, light-resistant containers (USP).

DOSAGE AND USE
See accompanying prescribing information.

* Each tablet contains amlodipine besylate equivalent to 2.5 mg amlodipine.

CAUTION: Federal law prohibits dispensing without prescription.

6505-01-367-5242

100 Tablets   NDC 0069-1520-66

Norvasc® ⟨2.5⟩
(amlodipine besylate)

2.5 mg*

Pfizer **Pfizer Labs**
Division of Pfizer Inc, NY, NY 10017

3 0069-1520-66 6

05-4782-32-2

5800
MADE IN USA

▶ **F I G U R E S.3 Drug label for Norvasc.**

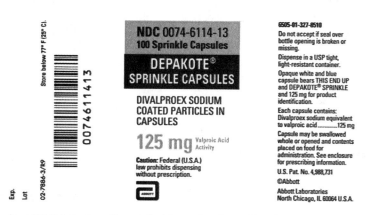

Store below 77° F (25° C).

0074611413

Exp.   Lot
02-7886-3/R9

NDC 0074-6114-13
100 Sprinkle Capsules

DEPAKOTE®
SPRINKLE CAPSULES

DIVALPROEX SODIUM
COATED PARTICLES IN
CAPSULES

125 mg Valproic Acid Activity

Caution: Federal (U.S.A.) law prohibits dispensing without prescription.

6505-01-327-0510

Do not accept if seal over bottle opening is broken or missing.

Dispense in a USP tight, light-resistant container.

Opaque white and blue capsule bears THIS END UP and DEPAKOTE® SPRINKLE and 125 mg for product identification.

Each capsule contains: Divalproex sodium equivalent to valproic acid............125 mg

Capsule may be swallowed whole or opened and contents placed on food for administration. See enclosure for prescribing information.

U.S. Pat. No. 4,988,731

©Abbott

Abbott Laboratories
North Chicago, IL 60064 U.S.A.

▶ **F I G U R E S.4 Drug label for valproic acid sodium.**

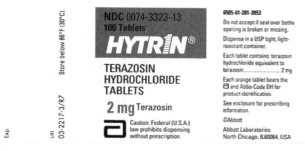

Store below 86°F (30°C).

Exp.   Lot
03-2217-3/R7

NDC 0074-3323-13
100 Tablets

HYTRIN®

TERAZOSIN
HYDROCHLORIDE
TABLETS

2 mg Terazosin

Caution: Federal (U.S.A.) law prohibits dispensing without prescription.

6505-01-281-2853

Do not accept if seal over bottle opening is broken or missing.

Dispense in a USP tight, light-resistant container.

Each tablet contains: terazosin hydrochloride equivalent to terazosin..................2 mg

Each orange tablet bears the ⊇ and Abbo-Code DH for product identification.

See enclosure for prescribing information.

©Abbott

Abbott Laboratories
North Chicago, IL60064, USA

▶ **F I G U R E S.5 Drug label for terazosin hydrochloride.**

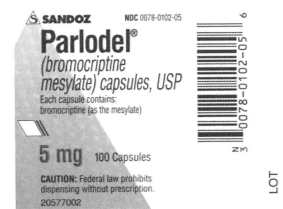

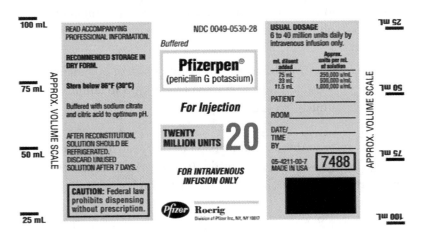

▶ F I G U R E S . 6 **Drug label for bromocriptine mesylate.**

▶ F I G U R E S . 7 **Drug label for Pfizerpen.**

4. Read the information for the first medication order in Figure S.1. How many tablets will you administer to Mrs. Doe? _____

5. Read the second order on the medication sheet in Figure S.1. How many tablets will Mrs. Doe receive? _____

6. The medication order for penicillin in Figure S.1 must be prepared.

   a. How many milliliters of diluent must be added to the vial so that 1 milliliter contains 1,000,000 units? _____

   b. How many milliliters of Pfizerpen will you add to 500 milliliters of 5% D/W? _____

7. The fourth order on the medication order sheet in Figure S.1 is for bromocriptine. Convert this order to grains. _____

8. Read the fifth order on the medication order sheet in Figure S.1, and calculate the number of tablets you will administer to the patient.

9. Read the third order in Figure S.1. How many capsules of the anticonvulsant drug Valproic Acid will you administer to this patient? _____

10. The injectable form of Zantac is labeled 25 milligrams per milliliter. If the order requires that 50 milligrams be diluted to 20 milliliters, how many milliliters of Zantac are required and how many milliliters of diluent?

_____

11. You are told to infuse 20 milliliters of a solution in 20 minutes. The drop factor is 60 microdrops per milliliter. Find the flow rate. _____

12. An infusion of 5% D/W has 800 milliliters left in bag (LIB). The flow rate is 31 drops per minute, and the drop factor is 15 drops per milliliter. How many hours will it take for this IV to infuse? _____

13. Calculate the number of milliliters per minute for an IV of 500 milliliters of 5% D/W with 0.5 gram of lidocaine when the order is to administer 2 milligrams per minute. _____

14. The patient has an order for 30 milliliters po of the laxative lactulose (Chronulac). The oral solution label reads 10 grams per 15 milliliters. How many grams of this drug is the patient receiving? _____

15. The patient requires 20 milligrams IV of labetalol (Normodyne, Trandate) in 3 minutes. The vial is labeled 5 milligrams per milliliter. How many milliliters of this antihypertensive drug will the patient receive?

_____

16. The order in Problem 15 has been changed to read:

Add 100 mg to 400 mL 5% D/W, infuse at rate of 2 mg/min

Calculate the flow rate in microdrops. _____

17. The prescriber has ordered 100 milligrams of bretylium tosylate (Bretylate, Bretylol), an adrenergic blocking agent, in 500 milliliters of normal saline solution, to be infused at a rate of 0.5 milligram per minute. The total amount of IV solution is 510 milliliters. Calculate the flow rate in milliliters per hour. _____

18. The patient was admitted with unstable ventricular tachycardia. The order reads:

500 mg bretylium tosylate (10 mL) to 50 mL 5% D/W IV

The total amount of solution is 60 milliliters; it is to be infused at a rate of 0.1 milligram per kilogram per minute. The patient weighs 180 pounds, and the drop factor is 15 drops per milliliter. Calculate the flow rate.

_____

19. The order reads: vitamin C 500 mg IV daily in 100 mL 5% D/W for 120 min. The vial is labeled 500 milligrams per milliliter. Calculate the flow rate when the drop factor is 15 drops per milliliter. _____

20. An IV solution of 5% D/W is started at 6:20 P.M. and is infusing at a rate of 8 drops per minute with a drop factor of 15 drops per milliliter, how many milliliters per hour is the patient receiving? _____

21. An IV solution of 0.9% NS has 120 milliliters LIB. If the infusion rate is 50 drops per minute and the drop factor is 15 drops per milliliter, how long will it take to complete this infusion? _____

22. Read the information on the label in Figure S.8. If the order is for 2000 micrograms of tolterodine tartrate, how many tablets will you prepare?

_____

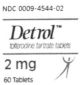

℞ only
See package insert for complete product information.
Dispense in tight container.
Store at controlled room temperature
20° to 25° C (68° to 77° F) [see USP].
817 373 000
MANUFACTURED IN ITALY
by Pharmacia & Upjohn S.p.A., Ascoli Piceno, Italy
For Pharmacia & Upjohn Company, Kalamazoo, MI 49001, USA

Lot
Exp

NDC 0009-4544-02

Detrol™
tolterodine tartrate tablets

2 mg
60 Tablets

▶ **FIGURE S.8 Drug label for tolterodine.**

23. A patient must have an IV infusion of 500 milliliters of 5% D/W with 50,000 units of heparin. Read the information in Figure S.9.

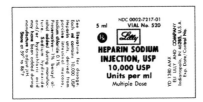

NDC 0002-7217-01
VIAL No. 520
5 ml
Lilly
HEPARIN SODIUM
INJECTION, USP
10,000 USP
Units per ml
Multiple Dose

▶ **FIGURE S.9 Drug label for heparin.**

a. How many milliliters of heparin must be added to the 5% D/W?

_____

b. Calculate the flow rate in milliliters per hour. The order is 1200 units per hour. _____

24. The patient must receive 150 milligrams per square meter of Depacon IV. Read the information on the label in Figure S.10, and calculate the number of milliliters you will administer to this patient if the patient's BSA is 1.8 square meters. _____

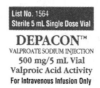

CONTAINS NO PRESERVATIVES:
Discard any unused solution.
Store at controlled room temperature 15° - 30°C (59° - 86°F).

Exp.

Lot

Each mL contains: valproate sodium equivalent to 100 mg valproic acid, edetate disodium 0.4 mg, and water for injection. pH adjusted with sodium hydroxide and/or hydrochloric acid.
See enclosure.
TM - Trademark

Abbott Laboratories
North Chicago, IL 60064, U.S.A.

06-8192-2/R1

List No. 1564
Sterile 5 mL Single Dose Vial

DEPACON™
VALPROATE SODIUM INJECTION
500 mg/5 mL Vial
Valproic Acid Activity
For Intravenous Infusion Only

▶ **FIGURE S.10 Drug label for Depacon.**

25. The prescriber ordered:

Trovan 300 mg in 100 mL 5% D/W IVPB in 30 min

Read the information on the label in Figure S.11, and calculate the total flow rate in drops per minute. The drop factor is 15 drops per milliliter.

_____

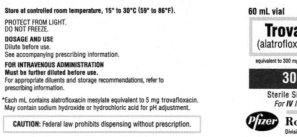
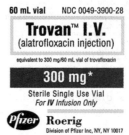

Store at controlled room temperature, 15° to 30°C (59° to 86°F).

PROTECT FROM LIGHT.
DO NOT FREEZE.

DOSAGE AND USE
Dilute before use.
See accompanying prescribing information.

FOR INTRAVENOUS ADMINISTRATION
Must be further diluted before use.
For appropriate diluents and storage recommendations, refer to prescribing information.

*Each mL contains alatrofloxacin mesylate equivalent to 5 mg trovafloxacin. May contain sodium hydroxide or hydrochloric acid for pH adjustment.

CAUTION: Federal law prohibits dispensing without prescription.

60 mL vial   NDC 0049-3900-28

Trovan™ I.V.
(alatrofloxacin injection)

equivalent to 300 mg/60 mL vial of trovafloxacin

300 mg*

Sterile Single Use Vial
For IV Infusion Only

Pfizer **Roerig**
Division of Pfizer Inc, NY, NY 10017

6204
MADE IN USA

05-5350-00-0

▶ **FIGURE S.11 Drug label for Trovan.**

Comprehensive Self-Test 2

1. The order is for 0.2 gram of sertraline (Zoloft). See Figure S.12, and determine how many tablets of this antidepressant drug equals 0.02 gram.

_____

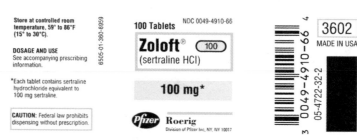

Store at controlled room temperature, 59° to 86°F (15° to 30°C).

DOSAGE AND USE
See accompanying prescribing information.

*Each tablet contains sertraline hydrochloride equivalent to 100 mg sertraline.

CAUTION: Federal law prohibits dispensing without prescription.

6505-01-360-8959

100 Tablets   NDC 0049-4910-66

Zoloft® (100)
(sertraline HCl)

100 mg*

Pfizer **Roerig**
Division of Pfizer Inc, NY, NY 10017

3602
MADE IN USA

0049-4910-66

05-4722-32-2

▶ **FIGURE S.12 Drug label for Zoloft.**

2. The prescriber's order reads:

> *Add 125 mg morphine SO$_4$ to 250 mL of 5% D/W; infuse at a rate of 5 mg/hr*

The drop factor is 60 microdrops per milliliter. How many microdrops per minute will the patient receive?

3. The patient is to receive 1 milligram per minute of a solution ordered by the prescriber, which is 1 gram of lidocaine added to 500 milliliters of 5% D/W. Calculate the flow rate in microdrops per minute. _____

Read the information on the medication order sheet in Figure S.13 to answer questions 4 through 8.

✚ GENERAL HOSPITAL ✚

Year 2001	Month December	Day	20	21	22	23	24	25
Medication Dosage and Interval			Initials* and Hours	Initials and Hours	Initials and Hours	Initials and Hours	Initials and Hours	Initials and Hours
Date started: 12/20/01 Feldene 20 mg po bid 10-6		I	AG	AG	AG	AG	AG	
		AM	10	10	10	10	10	
		I	JO	JO	JO	JO	JO	
Discontinued: 12/24/01		PM	6	6	6	6	6	
Date started: 12/20/01 Cytotec 200 mcg po bid 10-6		I	AG	AG	AG	AG		
		AM	10	10	10	10		
		I	JO	JO	JO	JO		
Discontinued: 12/24/01		PM	6	6	6	6		
Date started: 12/20/01 Carafate 1000 mg po ac meals and hs 8-12-5-10		I	AG	AG	AG	AG	AG	
		AM	8	8	8	8	8	
		I	AG JO JO	AG JO JO	AG JO JO	AG JO JO	AG JO JO	
Discontinued: 12/24/01		PM	12 5 10	12 5 10	12 5 10	12 5 10	12 5 10	
Date started: 12/20/01 prednisone 10 mg bid for 5 days po 10-6		I	AG	AG	AG	AG	AG	
		AM	10	10	10	10	10	
		I	JO	JO	JO	JO	JO	
Discontinued: 12/24/01		PM	6	6	6	6	6	
Date started: 12/20/01 digoxin 0.25 mg qd po 10 A.M.		I	AG	AG	AG	AG	AG	
		AM	10	10	10	10	10	
		I						
Discontinued: 12/24/01		PM						
Date started: 12/24/01 Cytotec 0.1 mg po bid 10-6		I					JO	JO
		AM					10	10
		I					AG	AG
Discontinued: 12/25/01		PM					6	6

Allergies: (Specify)

Init*	Signature
AG	Anthony Giangrasso
JO	Jane Oagers

MEDICATION ADMINISTRATION RECORD

PATIENT IDENTIFICATION

534011   12/20/01

June Jones   4/19/22
543 Main Street   RC
Hobbs, NM 102453   Aetna

Leon Ablon, MD

▶ **FIGURE S.13 Medication order sheet.**

4. The first order in Figure S.13 is for 20 milligrams bid of Feldene. If each tablet is labeled 0.02 gram, how many tablets would you administer to this patient? _____

5. The second order in Figure S.13 is changed to 0.1 milligram of Cytotec. How many micrograms would you administer to this patient? _____

6. Read the third order in Figure S.13. Each tablet is labeled 0.5 gram. How many tablets will the patient receive for each dose, and how many tablets will the patient receive in 7 days? _____

7. Prednisone tablets contain grain $\frac{1}{24}$. How many scored tablets are equal to the fourth order in Figure S.13? _____

8. Read the information in the fifth order in Figure S.13, and calculate the number of tablets you will give the patient if the label reads digoxin, 125 micrograms per tablet. _____

9. The order reads:

   vitamin B$_{12}$ 2 mcg/kg IM

   The patient weighs 114 pounds. How many milligrams of the vitamin equal this prescribed dose? _____

10. The order reads:

    cimetidine 10 mg/kg po

    The patient weighs 65 kilograms. The label on the bottle reads 300 mg/ 5 mL. How many milliliters contain the prescribed dose of this anti-ulcer agent? _____

11. The nonsteroidal anti-inflammatory drug ibuprofen (Motrin, Advil, Nuprin, Rufin) has been prescribed for Mr. James. He is to receive 900 milligrams per day in divided doses or tid. Each tablet contains 0.3 gram of medication. How many tablets will you need for the daily prescribed dose? _____

12. If a patient has an order for 0.075 gram of the tricyclic antidepressant imipramine pamoate (Tofranil) and each tablet contains 25 milligrams, how many tablets will you prepare for the patient? _____

13. A child has a BSA of 1.2 square meters. The order is for 30 milligrams per square meter IV of the antihypertensive drug methyldopa (Aldomet). The vial reads 250 milligrams per 5 milliliters. How many milliliters will equal this prescribed dose? _____

14. The antineoplastic drug lomustine (CeeNU) is ordered for a child with a BSA of 1 square meter. The prescribed dose is 0.1 gram per square meter, and each tablet is labeled 100 milligrams. How many tablets equal this prescribed dose? _____

15. The order reads:

liothyronine sodium 0.1 mg po

Each tablet is labeled 50 micrograms. How many tablets will you administer? _____

16. A child has an order for 1 milligram per kilogram of the diuretic furosemide (Lasix, Novosemide). The child weighs 40 kilograms. The tablets are 20 milligrams each. How many tablets will you prepare for this child? _____

17. The usual dose of the antiviral drug acyclovir (Zovirax) is 0.25 gram per square meter, and the child's BSA is 0.4 square meter. How many milliliters should you prepare for the child when the label on the vial reads 500 milligrams per 2 milliliters? _____

18. A child with a BSA of 1.04 square meters is to receive 175 milligrams per square meter po of the anticonvulsant drug Depakote. The label reads: 250 mg = 5 mL. How many milliliters equal the prescribed dose?

_____

19. Read the label in Figure S.14 and calculate the milliliters required for the order:

Timentin 3.1 g IVPB

_____

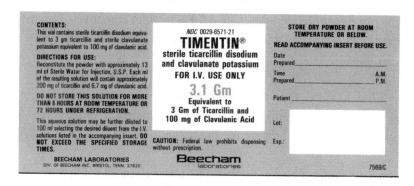

▶ **FIGURE S.14 Drug label for Timentin.**

20. The prescriber's order reads:

Add 275 u Humulin R insulin to 500 mL 0.9% NS; infuse at rate of 10 u/h

Determine the flow rate and the amount of insulin that must be added to the 500 milliliters of 0.9% NS solution. Read the information on the label in Figure S.15. _____

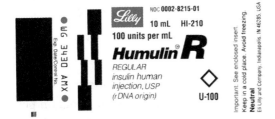

▶ **FIGURE S.15** Drug label for Humulin R.

21. The prescriber has written an order for 20,000,000 u of Pfizerpen to be added to 1,000 milliliters of 5% D/W and infused in 24 hours. The drop factor is 15 drops per milliliter. Read the label in Figure S.16. How many milliliters of Pfizerpen will you add to the 1000 milliliters of 5% D/W? Calculate the flow rate. _____

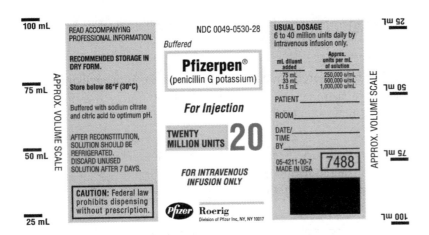

▶ **FIGURE S.16** Drug label for Pfizerpen.

22. The prescriber ordered:

   atropine sulfate 0.2 mg IV push stat

   Read the label in Figure S.17. How many milliliters will you administer to the patient? _____

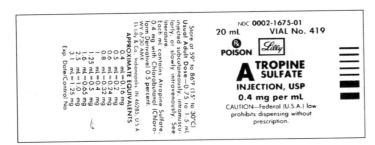

▶ **FIGURE S.17** Drug label for atropine sulfate.

23. The physician has ordered 0.15 gram po qid of aspirin. The scored tablets are 300 milligrams each. How many tablets equal 0.15 gram? _____

24. You have an order for 200 milligrams of chloroprocaine HCl (Nesacaine) and a 2% solution. How many milliliters equal 200 milligrams?

_____

25. An IV preparation of 500 milligrams of lidocaine HCl (Xylocaine) in 250 milliliters of 5% D/W has been ordered at 0.2 milligram per kilogram per minute for a patient weighing 66 kilograms. If the drop factor is 10 drops per milliliter, what will be the flow rate in drops per minute? _____

Comprehensive Self-Test 3

1. An IV solution of 1000 milliliters of Ringer's lactate in 12 hours is ordered. The drop factor is 10 drops per milliliter. What will be the flow rate in drops per minute? _____

2. How would you prepare 100 milliliters of a 2.5% solution from a 10% solution? _____

3. The prescriber has ordered 7500 units IV push of the anticoagulant heparin sodium (Liquaemin). The vial is labeled 10,000 units per milliliter. How many milliliters equal 7500 units? _____

4. Read the label in Figure S.18, and calculate the milliliters of Ceclor that should be administered if the order is for 250 milligrams per square meter and the patient's BSA is 1.7 square meters. _____

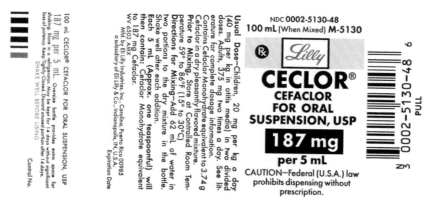

▶ **FIGURE S.18 Drug label for Ceclor.**

5. The order is 28.125 milligram per 35 kilograms of Cylert qd. Read the label in Figure S.19, and calculate the number of tablets you would administer to a patient who weighs 70 kilograms. _____

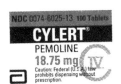

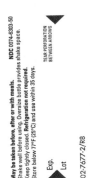

▶ **FIGURE S.19 Drug label for Cylert.**

6. The prescriber ordered:

EryPed 200 mg per m² po bid

Read the information on the label in Figure S.20, and determine the number of milliliters you will prepare for a patient with a BSA of 0.9 square meter. _____

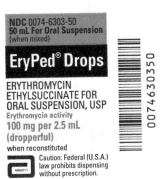

▶ **FIGURE S.20 Drug label for EryPed.**

7. The order reads:

Cardura 0.004g hs po

Read the information on the label in Figure S.21, and determine the amount of drug you will administer to this patient po. _____

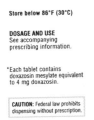
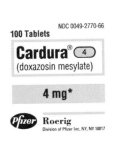
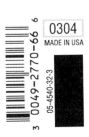

▶ **FIGURE S.21 Drug label for Cardura.**

8. Read the information in the label in Figure S.22, and calculate the strength of the lidocaine hydrochloride solution in grams per milliliter. Change this ratio to a percentage. _____

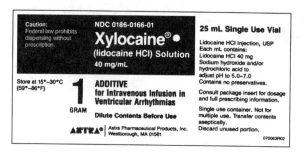

▶ **FIGURE S.22 Drug label for Xylocaine.**

9. An IV solution of 0.9% NS is infusing at a rate of 30 drops per minute. There are 360 milliliters LIB. The drop factor is 15 drops per milliliter. Calculate the number of hours this IV solution will infuse. _____

10. The order reads:

    Nembutal gr iss po

    Read the label in Figure S.23. How many capsules will you administer?

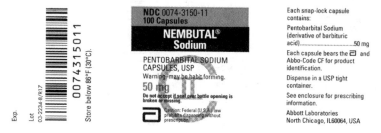

▶ **FIGURE S.23 Drug label for Nembutal.**

11. A 1-million-unit vial of penicillin G potassium powder has the following instructions for dilution: Add 9.6 mL of diluent, then 1 mL = 100,000 u. If the prescriber orders 250,000 units IM, how many milliliters will you prepare? _____

12. A child with a BSA of 0.8 square meter has an order for 100 milligrams per square meter po for the anti-arrhythmic agent amiodarone hydrochloride (Cordarone). How many milligrams equal the prescribed dose? _____

13. How would you prepare 1 pint (500 milliliters) of a 25% solution from a pure drug in powdered form? _____

14. The prescriber has ordered 10 micrograms per kilogram per minute IV of dobutamine (Dobutrex). Add 250 milligrams to 500 milliliters of 5% D/W. Each vial is labeled 12.5 milligrams per milliliter. The patient's weight is 70 kilograms.

a. How many milligrams per hour will the patient receive? _____

b. Calculate the flow rate in milliliters per hour. _____

Read the labels below to answer questions 15, 16.

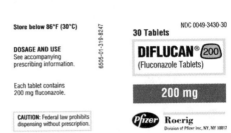

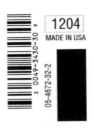

▶ **FIGURE S.24 Drug label for Diflucan.**

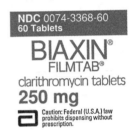

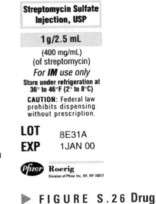

▶ **FIGURE S.26 Drug label for streptomycin.**

▶ **FIGURE S.25 Drug label for Biaxin.**

15. The prescriber has ordered grain 3 of fluconazole, po. Available tablets are 0.2 gram each. How many tablets of this antifungal drug equal the ordered dose? _____

16. The antibiotic clarithromycin has been ordered po for a patient. How many tablets will you administer if the order is 0.75 g? _____

17. A patient weighing 54 kilograms is to receive 4000 micrograms per kilogram per day IM of the antibiotic streptomycin. How many milliliters will you administer if the label reads 1 gram/2.5 mL? _____

18. The order is for 500 milliliters of an IV solution with 25 milligrams of a drug. The patient is to receive 0.05 milligram per minute. The drop factor is 60 microdrops per milliliter. What will the flow rate be in microdrops per minute? _____

Refer to the medication order sheet in Figure S.27 to answer questions 19 through 24.

☤ GENERAL HOSPITAL ☤

Year 2001 Month March	Day	12 Initials* and Hours	13 Initials and Hours	14 Initials and Hours	15 Initials and Hours	16 Initials and Hours	17 Initials and Hours
Medication Dosage and Interval							
Date started: 3/12/01 cefazolin 8 mg/kg IM q12h 10 A.M. 10 P.M. Discontinued: 3/13/01	I	LA	LA				
	AM	10	10				
	I	AG	AG				
	PM	10	10				
Date started: 3/12/01 Coumadin 2.5 mg qd po 10 A.M. Discontinued: 3/13/01	I	LA	LA				
	AM	10	10				
	I						
	PM						
Date started: 3/12/01 Quibron 300 mg po bid 10 A.M. 6 P.M. Discontinued: 3/13/01	I	LA	LA				
	AM	10	10				
	I	AG	AG				
	PM	6	6				
Date started: 3/12/01 prednisone 20mg po bid for 5 days 10 A.M. 6 P.M. Discontinued: 3/16/01	I	LA	LA	LA	LA	LA	
	AM	10	10	10	10	10	
	I	AG	AG	AG	AG	AG	
	PM	6	6	6	6	6	
Date started: 3/12/01 Diuril 0.5 g qd po 10 A.M. Discontinued: 3/13/01	I	LA	LA				
	AM	10	10				
	I						
	PM						
Date started: 3/12/01 Xanax 0.25 mg po tid 10 A.M. 2 P.M. 6 P.M. Discontinued: 3/13/01	I	LA	LA				
	AM	10	10				
	I	LA AG	LA AG				
	PM	2 6	2 6				

Allergies: (Specify)

Init*	Signature
LA	Leon Ablon
AG	Anthony Giangrasso

PATIENT IDENTIFICATION

```
7810056                          3/12/01

Melissa Dingmin                  6/6/41
451 Seaside Rd                   Buddhist
Tallahassee FL 10023             BCBS

Dr. Olsen
```

MEDICATION ADMINISTRATION RECORD

▶ FIGURE S.27 Medication order sheet.

19. The first order in Figure S.27 is for cefazolin. If the patient weighs 82 kilograms, how many milligrams will you prepare? Calculate the milliliters equivalent to this dose if the label reads 1 milliliter per 500 milligrams. _____

20. Read the second order in Figure S.27. If the medication is available in 5-mg scored tablets, how many Coumadin tablets will you administer to the patient? _____

21. The drug Quibron from the third order in Figure S.27 is available in an oral suspension labeled 0.3 gram per 10 milliliters. How many milliliters will you administer to the patient? _____

22. The fourth order in Figure S.27 is for 20 milligrams of prednisone. How many 10-mg tablets will you need for a 5-day supply? _____

23. If the medication in the fifth order in Figure S.27 for Diuril is changed to 1.5 grams po of Diuril, how many milligrams would you administer to the patient? _____

24. The drug available for the sixth medication order in Figure S.27 is 0.5-mg tablets of Xanax. How many scored tablets will you give this patient? _____

25. An initial dose (2 grams po) of sulfisoxazole suspension (Gantrisin) is ordered. The bottle is labeled 500 milligrams per 5 milliliters. How many milliliters of this antibiotic equal the prescribed dose? _____

Comprehensive Self-Test 4

1. The order is for 0.25 gram of ticlopidine (Ticlid). Calculate the number of tablets of this platelet aggregation inhibitor that you would administer if each tablet contains 250 milligrams. _____

2. A client has a history of migraine headaches, and the physician has ordered 0.006 g sc of sumatriptan (Imitrex). Each 0.5 milliliter contains 6 milligrams. How many milliliters will you administer to this patient?

   _____

3. A prescriber ordered 50 units per kilogram sc of epoetin alfa (Epogen). The label reads 2000 units per milliliter. The patient weighs 90 pounds. How many milliliters will you administer to this patient? _____

4. The antineoplastic drug cisplatin (Platinol) has been ordered IV for your patient, who is to receive 25 milligrams per square meter in 1000 milliliters of 0.9% NS, to be infused in 8 hours. The patient's BSA is 1.5 square meters, and the label reads 25 milligrams per 25 milliliters.

a. Calculate the total amount of solution with drug added. _____

b. Calculate the flow rate in milliliters per hour. _____

Refer to the medication order sheet in Figure S.28 to answer questions 5 through 9.

⊕ GENERAL HOSPITAL ⊕

Year 2001 Month October Day		14	15	16	17	18	19
Medication Dosage and Interval		Initials* and Hours	Initials and Hours	Initials and Hours	Initials and Hours	Initials and Hours	Initials and Hours
Date started: 10/14/01 colchicine gr $\frac{1}{50}$ po bid 10 A.M. 6 P.M.	I	AG	AG	AG	AG		
	AM	10	10	10	10		
	I	LA	LA	LA	LA		
Discontinued: 10/17/01	PM	6	6	6	6		
Date started: 10/14/01 Cardizem SR 120 mg po qd 10 A.M.	I	AG	AG	AG	AG		
	AM	10	10	10	10		
	I						
Discontinued: 10/17/01	PM						
Date started: 10/14/01 Aldactone 100 mg po bid 10 A.M. 6 P.M.	I	AG	AG	AG	AG		
	AM	10	10	10	10		
	I	LA	LA	LA	LA		
Discontinued: 10/17/01	PM	6	6	6	6		
Date started: 10/14/01 Estromed 0.625 mg po qd	I	AG	AG	AG	AG		
	AM	10	10	10	10		
	I						
Discontinued: 10/17/01	PM						
Date started: 10/14/01 famotidine 40 mg po hs 10 P.M.	I						
	AM						
	I	LA	LA	LA	LA		
Discontinued: 10/17/01	PM	10	10	10	10		

Allergies: (Specify)

PATIENT IDENTIFICATION

Init*	Signature
AG	Anthony Giangrasso
LA	Leon Ablon

9906431   9/14/01

Larissa Luby   7/7/40
93120 Second Ave S. E.   Prot
Detroit MI 60422   Medicare

June Olsen, MD

MEDICATION ADMINISTRATION RECORD

▶ **FIGURE S.28 Medication order sheet.**

5. If the drug available for the first order in Figure S.28 contains 1.2 milligrams of colchicine per tablet, how many tablets will you administer to the patient? _____

6. Read the second order in Figure S.28, and determine how many tablets you will administer to the patient if 0.12 g tablets of Cardizem SR is available. _____

7. Read the third order in Figure S.28, and calculate the number of tablets you will administer if each tablet contains grain $1\frac{1}{2}$. _____

8. If the Estromed in the fourth order in Figure S.28 is available in 325 μg tablets, how many tablets will you administer to this patient? _____

9. Read the fifth order in Figure S.28. How many milligrams of famotidine (Pepcid) will the patient receive in 7 days? _____

10. A child has been admitted to the hospital with a diagnosis of *Klebsiella* pneumonia. The prescriber orders:

    Cefamandole 25 mg/kg in 1000 mL 5% D/W

    The patient weighs 75 pounds. The label reads 1 g/100 mL. How many milliliters will you administer in 1 hour if the total solution must infuse in 24 hour? _____

11. A patient with AIDS has been diagnosed with CMV (cytomegalovirus). The prescriber has ordered the antiviral drug ganciclovir (Cytovene); the patient will receive 5 milligrams per kilogram IV in 100 milliliters of 5% D/W. Each vial reads 500 milligrams per 2 milliliters. The weight of the patient is 50 kilograms. Calculate the flow rate in drops per minute if the drop factor is 15 drops per milliliter. Infuse in 60 minutes. _____

12. Read the label in Figure S.29. A prescriber has ordered 764 mg po carbenicillin (Geocillin) for your patient. Each tablet contains 0.382 gram. How many tablets will you administer to this patient? _____

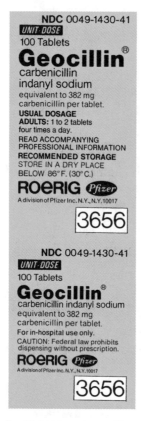

▶ **FIGURE S.29 Drug label for Geocillin.**

13. Read the label in Figure S.30. If the order is for 0.2 grams, how many milliliters will you administer to the patient? _____

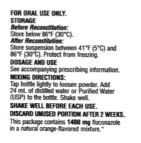 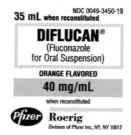 

▶ **FIGURE S.30 Drug label for Diflucan.**

14. The prescriber ordered:

7500 mcg clorazepate

Read the information in Figure S.31, and determine the number of tablets you will administer to the patient. _____

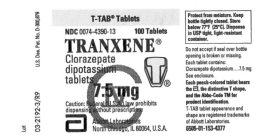

FIGURE S.31 Drug label for clorazepate.

15. Read the information on the label in Figure S.32. Determine the volume of Ceclor that you will administer to the patient if the order is for 7.5 milligrams per kilogram and the patient's weight is 60 kilograms.

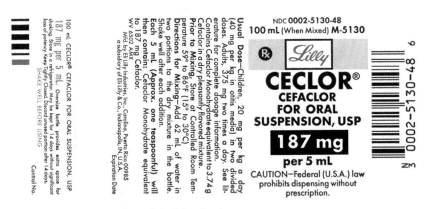

FIGURE S.32 Drug label for Ceclor.

16. Read the information on the label in Figure S.33. Calculate the number of tablets required if the order is for gr $\frac{1}{60}$ of cabergoline. _____

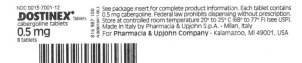

FIGURE S.33 Drug label for cabergoline.

17. Read the information on the label in Figure S.34. The prescriber's order is as follows:

Add 500 mg to 250 mL 0.9% NS; infuse at rate of 10 mg/h

How many milliliters of Depacon will you add to the 250 milliliters of 0.9% NS solution? Calculate the flow rate in milliliters per hour.

CONTAINS NO PRESERVATIVES:
Discard any unused solution.
Store at controlled room
temperature 15° - 30°C (59° -
86°F).

Exp.

Lot

Each mL contains: valproate
sodium equivalent to 100 mg
valproic acid, edetate disodium
0.4 mg, and water for injection. pH
adjusted with sodium hydroxide
and/or hydrochloric acid.
See enclosure.
TM - Trademark

Abbott Laboratories
North Chicago, IL 60064, U.S.A.

06-8192-2/R1

List No. 1564
Sterile 5 mL Single Dose Vial

DEPACON™
VALPROATE SODIUM INJECTION
500 mg/5 mL Vial
Valproic Acid Activity
For Intravenous Infusion Only

▶ FIGURE S.34 Drug label for Depacon.

18. 104F = _____ C   **19.** 36.4C = _____ F

For questions 20, 21, and 22, use the labels in Figures S.35, S.36, and S.37 to determine how many tablets to administer.

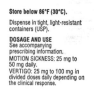

Store below 86°F (30°C)
Dispense in tight, light-resistant
containers (USP).
DOSAGE AND USE
See accompanying prescribing
information.
INITIAL THERAPY: 250 mg daily.
(Geriatric patients: 100-125 mg daily.)
MAINTENANCE THERAPY: 100-500 mg
daily, according to patient response.
Patients who do not respond to
500 mg daily will usually not respond
to higher doses.
Each tablet contains   MADE IN USA
100 mg chlorpropamide.

6505-01-153-2981

100 Tablets   NDC 0069-3930-66

Diabinese®
(chlorpropamide) 100

100 mg
Distributed by
Pfizer Pfizer Labs
Division of Pfizer Inc, NY, NY 10017

CAUTION: Federal law prohibits
dispensing without prescription.

1737

05-2141-32-9

▶ FIGURE S.35 Drug label for chlorpropamide.

Store below 86°F (30°C).

Dispense in tight, light-resistant
containers (USP).

DOSAGE AND USE
See accompanying
prescribing information.
MOTION SICKNESS: 25 mg to
50 mg daily.
VERTIGO: 25 mg to 100 mg in
divided doses daily depending on
the clinical response.

Each tablet contains
25 mg meclizine HCl.

CAUTION: Federal law prohibits
dispensing without prescription.

6505-01-051-5695

100 Tablets   NDC 0049-2110-66

Antivert® 25
(meclizine HCl)

25 mg
Distributed by
Pfizer Roerig
Division of Pfizer Inc, NY, NY 10017

4173
MADE IN USA

3 N 0049-2110-66 0

05-2150-32-6

▶ FIGURE S.36 Drug label for Antivert.

℞ only

See package insert
for complete product
information.
Dispense in tight, light-
resistant container.

Store at 25°C (77°F);
excursions permitted to
15°-30°C (59°-86°F)
[see USP Controlled
Room Temperature].

Pramipexole was jointly
developed by Pharmacia
& Upjohn Company and
Boehringer Ingelheim.
U.S. Pat. Nos. 4,886,812
and 4,843,086

817 044 001

Pharmacia & Upjohn Co.
Kalamazoo, MI 49001, USA

NDC 0009-0008-02

Mirapex®
pramipexole
dihydrochloride tablets

0.5 mg

90 Tablets

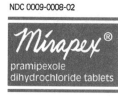

0009-0008-02 4

Lot
Exp

▶ FIGURE S.37 Drug label for Mirapex.

20. The order reads: chloropropamide 0.1 g po qd. How many tablets will you administer to the patient? _____

21. The order reads: Antivert 0.05 g. How many tablets will you prepare for the patient? _____

22. The order reads: Mirapex 1000 mcg po. Calculate the number of tablets you will prepare for your patient. _____

23. The prescriber ordered:

    digoxin 0.008 mg po

    The solution label reads 0.004 milligram per 5 milliliters. How many milliliters will you give to this patient? _____

24. A patient is to receive 0.5 milligram per kilogram per minute of cefuroxime (Ceftin). The order reads: Add 0.5 g to 100 mL 5% D/W. Calculate the flow rate in drops per minute. The patient weighs 60 kilograms, and the drop factor is 10 drops per milliliter. _____

25. The order reads:

    doxycycline 4.4 mg/kg po

    Each 5 mL = 50 mg. If the patient weighs 64 pounds, how many milliliters will you prepare of this antibiotic? _____

Comprehensive Self-Test 5

1. The antineoplastic drug bleomycin sulfate (Blenoxane) has been ordered for your patient, who will receive 4 units per square meter IV. Each vial is labeled 15 units per 2 milliliters. The patient's BSA is 1.4 square meters. How many milliliters will you prepare for your patient? _____

2. The prescriber has ordered 3 milligrams per square meter of the antineoplastic drug leucovorin calcium (Wellcovorin). The patient's BSA is 1.2 square meters. How many minims will you administer to this patient if the ampule reads 5 milligrams per milliliter? _____

3. Your patient has had an exacerbation of his rheumatoid arthritis symptoms, and the prescriber has ordered 10 milligrams per square meter IVPB of the antineoplastic drug methotrexate sodium in 50 milliliters of 0.9% NS. The patient's BSA is 1.7 square meters. The label on the vial reads 25 milligrams per milliliter.

    a. How many milliliters of this drug will you add to the 50 milliliters of 0.9% NS? _____

    b. Calculate the flow rate for the total amount of this solution, which must infuse in 30 minutes. The drop factor is 10 drops per milliliter.

    _____

4. The thrombolytic agent alteplase recombinant drug (t-PA, Activase) is to be prepared for a patient who will receive 1.25 milligrams per kilogram. This patient weighs 100 kilograms. The vial directions are as follows: Add 50 mL to vial and 1 mg/mL.

    a. How many milliliters will you prepare for this patient? _____

    b. Calculate the flow rate in milliliters per hour if the IV must infuse in 90 minutes. _____

5. The order reads:

    amikacin sulfate 7.5 mg/kg in 200 mL 5% D/W IVPB

    The label on the vial reads 250 milligrams per milliliter. The patient weighs 90 kilograms.

    a. How many milliliters of the antibiotic must be added to the 200 milliliters of 5% D/W? _____

    b. Calculate the flow rate in drops per minute if the drop factor is 10 drops per milliliter and the length of time for the infusion is 2 hours.

    _____

6. A corticosteroid, betamethasone sodium (Celestone), has been prescribed for its anti-inflammatory action. The patient is to receive 5 milligrams in an IV push. The label on the vial reads 4 milligrams per milliliter. How many milliliters will you prepare for this patient? _____

7. A child has had an acute onset of bronchial asthma. The prescriber ordered:

    aminophylline 0.3 mg/kg IV push stat

    The patient weighs 25 kilograms, and the label on the vial reads 4 milligrams per milliliter. How many milliliters will you prepare for this child? If there is an additional order of 0.125 milligram per kilogram per hour, how many milliliters per hour will you administer if the solution is labeled 100 milligrams per 100 milliliters? _____

8. Read the first order in Figure S.38 and calculate the number of tablets required if each tablet contains grain $\frac{1}{60}$. _____

⊕ GENERAL HOSPITAL ⊕

Year 2001 Month June Day		3	4	5	6	7	8
Medication Dosage and Interval		Initials* and Hours	Initials and Hours	Initials and Hours	Initials and Hours	Initials and Hours	Initials and Hours
Date started: 6/3/01 bumetanide 2 mg po qd 10 A.M.	I	LA	LA	LA			
	AM	10	10	10			
	I						
Discontinued: 6/5/01	PM						
Date started: 6/3/01 Procardia 20 mg po tid 10 A.M. 2 P.M. 6 P.M.	I	LA	LA	LA			
	AM	10	10	10			
	I	LA JO	LA JO	LA JO			
Discontinued: 6/5/01	PM	2 6	2 6	2 6			
Date started: 6/3/01 Elavil 0.05 g po bid 10 A.M. 6 P.M.	I	LA	LA	LA			
	AM	10	10	10			
	I	JO	JO	JO			
Discontinued: 6/5/01	PM	6	6	6			
Date started: 6/3/01 potassium chloride 20 mEq po bid 10 A.M. 6 P.M.	I	LA	LA	LA			
	AM	10	10	10			
	I	JO	JO	JO			
Discontinued: 6/5/01	PM	6	6	6			
Date started: 6/3/01 Paraflex 0.5 g po bid 10 A.M. 6 P.M.	I	LA	LA	LA			
	AM	10	10	10			
	I	JO	JO	JO			
Discontinued: 6/5/01	PM	6	6	6			

Allergies: (Specify)

PATIENT IDENTIFICATION

Init*	Signature
LA	Leon Ablon
JO	June Olsen

754886   6/3/01

John Petogna   4/12/52
451 Oceanside Blvd   Prot
Cayucas, CA 93041   Aetna

Anthony Giangrasso, MD

MEDICATION ADMINISTRATION RECORD

▶ **FIGURE S.38 Medication order sheet.**

9. A child with acute leukemia has been prescribed 3 milligrams per kilogram po of thioguanine (Lanvis). Each scored tablet contains 40 milligrams. Calculate the number of tablets required if the child weighs 20 kilograms. _____

10. The order reads:

antihemophilic factor (Factor VIII) 25 u/kg IV

The patient weighs 175 pounds. How many units will you prepare for this patient? _____

11. You have a 50 mL vial of 25% normal serum albumin.

  a. How many grams of serum albumin are contained in the vial?

  _____

  b. If the serum is to be infused at a rate of 3 milliliters per minute, how many minutes will it take to complete this infusion? _____

12. The prescriber ordered:

  Cortef 40 mg po q12h

The label on the vial reads 10 mg per 5 milliliters. How many milliliters will you administer to your patient? _____

13. You are to prepare 125 milligrams of methylprednisolone (Medrol) for IM injections. The label on the vial reads 80 milligrams per milliliter. How many milliliters will you administer to your patient? _____

14. The second order in Figure S.38 is for Procardia. If the available tablets are 0.01 gram each, how many tablets equal this order? _____

15. Determine the number of Elavil tablets you would administer to this patient according to the third order in Figure S.38 if each tablet contains 25 milligrams. _____

16. If 10 mEq of potassium chloride are equal to 750 milligrams of potassium chloride, how many milligrams would be equal to the medication in the fourth order of Figure S.38? _____

17. Read the fifth order in Figure S.38. If each Paraflex tablet contained grain VIISS, how many tablets would equal this ordered dose? _____

18. Read the label in Figure S.39. If the patient must receive 100 milligrams of Vibramycin po, how many milliliters will the patient receive?

  _____

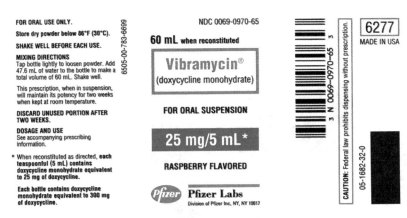

FIGURE S.39 Drug label for Vibramycin.

19. The prescriber's order reads:

Xylocaine 150 mg added to 250 mL 5% D/W, infuse in 4h

Read the label in Figure S.40, and calculate the milliliters of Xylocaine that you will add to the 250 milliliters of 5% D/W. What is the flow rate in milliliters per hour? _____

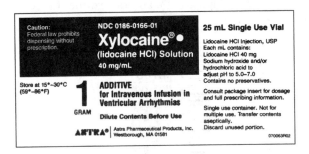

FIGURE S.40 Drug label for Xylocaine.

20. The order reads:

Zyflo 0.6 g bid

Read the information on the label in Figure S.41, and determine the number of tablets you will administer to the patient. _____

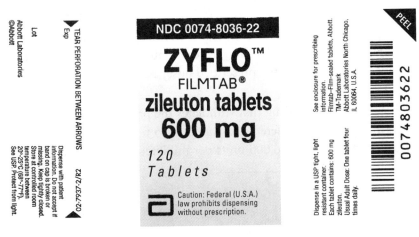

FIGURE S.41 Drug label for zileuton.

21. The patient must receive 0.8 g of E.E.S. 400. Read the information on the label in Figure S.42. How many tablets will you prepare for this patient? _____

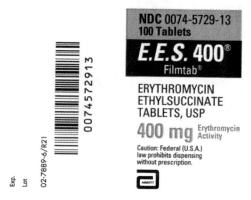

▶ FIGURE S.42 Drug label for E.E.S. 400.

22. The prescriber ordered:

cetirizine gr $\frac{1}{12}$ q12h

Read the information on the label in Figure S.43, and determine the number of tablets that contain gram $\frac{1}{12}$. _____

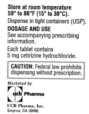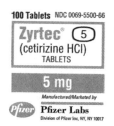

▶ FIGURE S.43 Drug label for Zyrtec.

23. The prescriber has ordered 0.7 milligram sc of epinephrine (Adrenalin) stat. The ampule reads 1:1000. How many milliliters equal the prescribed dose? _____

24. A PICC (peripherally inserted central catheter) must be irrigated with 5,000,000 units of urokinase. If the vial reads 250,000 units per milliliter, how many milliliters equal the prescribed dose? _____

25. Epoetin alfa (Epogen), a drug that stimulates the production of red blood cells (erythropoiesis), is ordered; the patient is to receive 7500 units sc. The label on the vial reads 6,000 units per milliliter. How many minims equal the prescribed dose? _____

1. The order reads:

   ceftazidime 2 g in 100 mL 5% D/W, IVPB

   The drop factor is 10 drops per milliliter, and the IVPB is to be infused in 2 hours. What is the flow rate in drops per minute? _____

2. The prescriber has ordered 400 milligrams of ciprofloxacin (Cipro) in 200 milliliters of 5% D/W. The patient is to receive 6 milligrams per kilogram per hour. The patient weighs 175 pounds, and the drop factor is 15 drops per milliliter. Calculate the flow rate in drops per minute.

   _____

3. The order reads: 1000 mL 5% D/W to infuse in 8 h, flow rate 41 gtt/min. After assessing the fluid intake, the nurse noted that 750 milliliters remained to be infused in 5 hours. The drop factor is 15 drops per milliliter. Recalculate the flow rate in drops per minute. _____

4. Read the information on the drug label for Zithromax in Figure S.44. If the prescriber ordered 3.2 milligrams per kilogram po daily and the child weighs 32 kilograms, how many milliliters would you prepare for this child? _____

   The above order has been changed to 110 milligrams per square meter, and the child's BSA is 0.9 square meter. How many milliliters will you prepare for this child now? _____

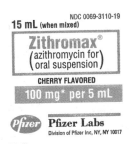 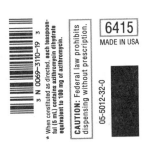

▶ **FIGURE S.44 Drug label for Zithromax.**

5. The order reads: Add 125 mg of morphine sulfate to 250 mL 5% D/W; infuse at rate 0.005 mg/kg/min. The patient weighs 95 kilograms. Calculate the flow rate in milliliters per hour. _____

6. The prescriber ordered:

   Streptomycin 20 mg/kg IM 7 A.M.

   The weight of the patient is 50 kilograms. Read the information on the label in Figure S.45. How many milliliters will you administer to this patient? _____

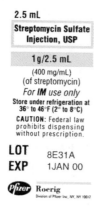

2.5 mL

Streptomycin Sulfate Injection, USP

1 g/2.5 mL

(400 mg/mL)
(of streptomycin)
For IM use only
Store under refrigeration at
36° to 46°F (2° to 8°C)
CAUTION: Federal law
prohibits dispensing
without prescription.

LOT 8E31A
EXP 1JAN 00

Pfizer Roerig
Division of Pfizer Inc., NY, NY 10017

▶ **FIGURE S.45** Drug label for streptomycin.

7. Read the information on the label in Figure S.46. How many tablets will you administer if the order is for 0.25 gram per 40 kilograms and the patient weighs 80 kilograms? _____

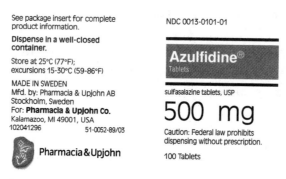

See package insert for complete
product information.

**Dispense in a well-closed
container.**

Store at 25°C (77°F);
excursions 15-30°C (59-86°F)

MADE IN SWEDEN
Mfd. by: Pharmacia & Upjohn AB
Stockholm, Sweden
For: **Pharmacia & Upjohn Co.**
Kalamazoo, MI 49001, USA
102041296   51-0052-89/03

Pharmacia & Upjohn

NDC 0013-0101-01

Azulfidine®
Tablets

sulfasalazine tablets, USP

500 mg

Caution: Federal law prohibits
dispensing without prescription.

100 Tablets

▶ **FIGURE S.46** Drug label for Azulfidine.

8. Your patient has an order for 1.7 milligrams per kilogram po of Vibramycin. Read the information on the label in Figure S.47. How many milliliters will you prepare for this patient if his weight is 60 kilograms? _____

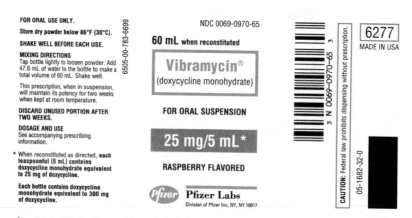

FOR ORAL USE ONLY.

Store dry powder below 86°F (30°C).

SHAKE WELL BEFORE EACH USE.

MIXING DIRECTIONS
Tap bottle lightly to loosen powder. Add
47.6 mL of water to the bottle to make a
total volume of 60 mL. Shake well.

This prescription, when in suspension,
will maintain its potency for two weeks
when kept at room temperature.

DISCARD UNUSED PORTION AFTER
TWO WEEKS.

DOSAGE AND USE
See accompanying prescribing
information.

* When reconstituted as directed, **each
teaspoonful (5 mL) contains
doxycycline monohydrate equivalent
to 25 mg of doxycycline.**

Each bottle contains doxycycline
monohydrate equivalent to 300 mg
of doxycycline.

6505-00-783-6699

NDC 0069-0970-65

60 mL when reconstituted

Vibramycin®
(doxycycline monohydrate)

FOR ORAL SUSPENSION

25 mg/5 mL*

RASPBERRY FLAVORED

Pfizer **Pfizer Labs**
Division of Pfizer Inc, NY, NY 10017

3 N 0069-0970-65 3

CAUTION: Federal law prohibits dispensing without prescription.

6277
MADE IN USA

05-1682-32-0

▶ **FIGURE S.47** Drug label for Vibramycin.

9. The label in Figure S.48 reads Ceclor, 125 milligrams per 5 milliliters. The order is for 250 milligrams bid po for 10 days.

   a. How many milliliters contain the prescribed dose? _____

   b. Calculate the amount of Ceclor you will need for 10 days. _____

   c. How many milligrams will the patient receive in 10 days? _____

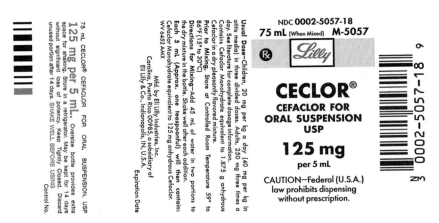

▶ FIGURE S.48 Drug label for Ceclor.

10. The order reads:

    verapamil HCl 0.075 mg/kg IV push over 2 min

    If the weight of the patient is 80 kilograms and the label on the vial reads 5 milligrams per 2 milliliters, how many milliliters will you prepare of this calcium channel blocker? _____

11. Read the first order in Figure S.49. How many tablets will you administer to the patient if each tablet contains 0.015 gram of Isordil? _____

12. Convert the second order in Figure S.49 to grams. _____

13. The prescriber has ordered 140 milligrams per kilogram stat of acetylcysteine as an antidote for acetaminophen toxicity. The patient weighs 70 kilograms. If you have a 20% solution, how many milliliters will you prepare? _____

14. If the third order in Figure S.49 were changed to 0.010 gram and each tablet of Reglan contained 5 milligrams, how many tablets would you administer to this patient? _____

15. How many tablets of Bentyl will you administer to the patient if each tablet contains grain $\frac{1}{6}$? (Refer to the fourth order in Figure S.49.)

_____

☩ GENERAL HOSPITAL ☩

Year 2001 Month November	Day	10	11	12	13	14	15
Medication Dosage and Interval		Initials* and Hours	Initials and Hours	Initials and Hours	Initials and Hours	Initials and Hours	Initials and Hours
Date started: 11/10/01 Isordil 15 mg po tid 10 A.M.	I	JO	JO	JO	JO	JO	
2 P.M.	AM	10	10	10	10	10	
6 P.M.	I	JO AG	JO AG	JO AG	JO AG	JO AG	
Discontinued: 11/14/01	PM	2 6	2 6	2 6	2 6	2 6	
Date started: 11/10/01 Inderal 40 mg po qid 10-2-6-10	I	JO	JO	JO	JO	JO	
	AM	10	10	10	10	10	
	I	JO AG AG	JO AG AG	JO AG AG	JO AG AG	JO AG AG	
Discontinued: 11/14/01	PM	2 6 10	2 6 10	2 6 10	2 6 10	2 6 10	
Date started: 11/10/01 Reglan 5 mg po hs 10 P.M.	I						
	AM						
	I	AG	AG	AG	AG	AG	
Discontinued: 11/14/01	PM	10	10	10	10	10	
Date started: 11/10/01 Bentyl 10 mg po ac dinner 6 P.M.	I						
	AM						
	I	AG	AG	AG	AG	AG	
Discontinued: 11/14/01	PM	6	6	6	6	6	
Date started: 11/10/01 digoxin 0.125 mg po qd 10 A.M.	I	JO	JO	JO	JO	JO	
	AM	10	10	10	10	10	
	I						
Discontinued: 11/14/01	PM						
Date started: 11/10/01 docusate sodium 200 mg po qd 10 A.M.	I	JO	JO	JO	JO	JO	
	AM	10	10	10	10	10	
	I						
Discontinued: 11/14/01	PM						

Allergies: (Specify)

Init*	Signature
JO	June Olsen
AG	Anthony Giangrasso

MEDICATION ADMINISTRATION RECORD

PATIENT IDENTIFICATION

5760030   11/10/01

Mark Patelro   1/31/40
1200 Seventh Ave #42   RC
Baltimore MD 400321   BCBS

Dr. Ablon

▶ **FIGURE S.49 Medication order sheet.**

16. If the available tablets of digoxin each contain 125 micrograms, how many tablets equal the fifth order in Figure S.49? _____

17. 102 F = _____ C

18. How many capsules of docusate sodium will be given to the patient for 30 days if each capsule contains 100 milligrams? (Refer to the sixth order in Figure S.49.) _____

19. The prescriber has written an order for the antineoplastic drug pentostatin (Nipent) for the treatment of hairy cell leukemia. The patient is to receive 4 milligrams per square meter in 50 milliliters of 5% D/W IVBP. The patient's BSA is 1.6 square meters. The medication label reads 10 milligrams per milliliter.

  a. How many milliliters of medication will you add to the 50 milliliters?

  _____

  b. Calculate the flow rate for this infusion in microdrops per minute when the total time for infusion is 90 minutes. _____

20. The order reads:

  phenobarbital 120 mg, added to 100 mL 5% D/W

  The label on the vial reads 60 milligrams per milliliter.

  a. How many milliliters of this drug must be added to this infusion?

  _____

  b. Calculate the flow rate in drops per minute when the drop factor is 10 drops per milliliter and the time for the infusion is 20 minutes.

  _____

21. The prescriber's order reads:

  ciprofloxacin 400 mg in 200 mL 5% D/W IVPB, infuse in 90 min

  The label on the vial reads 200 milligrams per 20 milliliters.

  a. How many milliliters of ciprofloxacin will you add to the infusion?

  _____

  b. Calculate the flow rate in drops per minute. The drop factor is 15 drops per milliliter. _____

22. Your patient is in diabetic ketoacidosis. Calculate the flow rate of her medication in milliliters per hour for a solution of 250 milliliters of 5% D/W with 2 grams of magnesium sulfate, to be infused in 6 hours.

———————

23. The order reads:

Add 2 g lidocaine to 1000 mL; 0.02 mg/kg/min

The patient weighs 206 pounds. Calculate the flow rate for this IV in milliliters per hour. —————

24. The order reads:

500 mL 5% D/W with 100 mg morphine sulfate IV

The patient is to receive 5 milligrams per hour. Calculate the flow rate in milliliters per hour. —————

25. The prescriber ordered:

1000 mL 0.9% NS IV 8h; flow rate 42 gtt/min

When the IV was reassessed, 150 milliliters had infused in 3 hours. The drop factor is 20 drops per milliliter. Recalculate the flow rate. —————

Answer Section

I Included in this section are answers to the *Case Studies, Exercises,* and *Cumulative Review Exercises* for all chapters. Also included are the answers to the *Practice Reading Labels* segments, which fall in Chapter 6, and *Comprehensive Self-Tests* 1 through 3. Your instructor has the answers for *Additional Exercises* and *Comprehensive Self-Tests* 4 through 6.

CHAPTER 1

Exercises

1. $\dfrac{24}{100} = \dfrac{6}{25}$

2. $3\dfrac{24}{100} = \dfrac{324}{100} = \dfrac{81}{25}$

3.
$$\begin{array}{r} .625 \\ 8\overline{)5.000} \\ \underline{4\,8} \\ 20 \\ \underline{16} \\ 40 \\ 40 \end{array}$$
so $\dfrac{5}{8} = 0.625$

4.
$$\begin{array}{r} .16 \\ 25\overline{)4.00} \\ \underline{2\,5} \\ 150 \\ 150 \end{array}$$
so $\dfrac{4}{25} = 0.16$

5. $\dfrac{1}{10} = 0.1$

6.
$$\begin{array}{r} .005 \\ 200\overline{)1.000} \\ 1\,000 \end{array}$$
so $\dfrac{1}{200} = 0.005$

7.
$$\begin{array}{r} .0033 \\ 300\overline{)1.0000} \\ \underline{900} \\ 1000 \\ 900 \end{array}$$
so $\dfrac{1}{300} = 0.003$ to the nearest thousandth

8. $45.\underset{\smile\smile}{0\,0}.$ so $\dfrac{4500}{100} = 45$

9. $\underset{\smile\smile\smile}{6.\,25}$ so $\dfrac{6.25}{1000} = 0.00625$

10.
$$\begin{array}{r} 20.37 \\ 7\overline{)142.60} \\ \underline{14} \\ 2\,6 \\ \underline{2\,1} \\ 5\,0 \\ 4\,9 \end{array}$$
so $\dfrac{142.6}{7} = 20.4$ to the nearest tenth

11.
$$\begin{array}{r} 120 \\ 0.\underset{\smile\smile}{0\,6}.\overline{)7.\underset{\smile\smile}{2\,0}.} \\ \underline{6} \\ 1\,2 \\ \underline{1\,2} \\ 00 \end{array}$$
so $\dfrac{7.2}{0.06} = 120$

12.

$$0.\underset{\smile}{0}\underset{\smile}{0}\underset{\smile}{6}\,)\overline{72.\underset{\smile}{0}\underset{\smile}{0}\underset{\smile}{0}.}$$ quotient $12\;0\;0\;0.$

so $\dfrac{72}{0.006} = 12{,}000$

13. $123\,\underset{\smile}{4}.$ so $123.4 \times 100 = 12{,}340$

$$\begin{array}{r} 6 \\ \hline 12 \\ 12 \\ \hline 0 \end{array}$$

14. 5.125 so $5.125 \times 1.3 = 6.6625$

$$\begin{array}{r} \times\,1.3 \\ \hline 15375 \\ 5125 \\ \hline 6.6625 \end{array}$$

15. $36.\underset{\smile}{4}\,\underset{\smile}{2}.$ so $36.42 \times 1000 = 36{,}420$

16.

$$0.\underset{\smile}{0}\underset{\smile}{5}\,)\overline{85.\underset{\smile}{0}\underset{\smile}{0}.}$$ quotient $17\;0\;0$

so $\dfrac{85}{0.05} = 1700$

$$\begin{array}{r} 5 \\ \hline 35 \\ 35 \\ \hline 0 \end{array}$$

17.

$$0.\underset{\smile}{5}\,)\overline{8.\underset{\smile}{5}.}$$ quotient $1\;7$

so $\dfrac{8.5}{0.5} = 17$

$$\begin{array}{r} 5 \\ \hline 3\;5 \\ 3\;5 \\ \hline 0 \end{array}$$

18. $\dfrac{\overset{2}{\cancel{4}}}{\underset{1}{\cancel{15}}} \div \dfrac{\overset{2}{\cancel{30}}}{1} \times \dfrac{1}{\underset{1}{\cancel{2}}} = 4$

19. $\dfrac{13}{2} \div \dfrac{3}{1} = \dfrac{13}{2} \times \dfrac{1}{3} = \dfrac{13}{6}$ or $2\dfrac{1}{6}$

20. $\dfrac{26}{1} \div \dfrac{13}{4} = \dfrac{26}{1} \times \dfrac{4}{13} = \dfrac{104}{13}$ or 8

21. $4.25 \times \dfrac{1}{5} = 4\dfrac{1}{4} \times \dfrac{1}{5} = \dfrac{17}{4} \times \dfrac{1}{5} = \dfrac{17}{20}$

22. $\dfrac{1}{\underset{2}{\cancel{250}}} \times \dfrac{\overset{1}{\cancel{125}}}{1} \times \dfrac{1}{0.5} = \dfrac{1}{1}$ or 1

23. $\dfrac{475}{100} \times \dfrac{1}{1.5} = \dfrac{475}{150} = \dfrac{19}{6} = 3\dfrac{1}{6}$ or $4.75 \times \dfrac{1}{1.5} = \dfrac{4.75}{1.5} = 3.2$ to the nearest tenth

24. $3 \div \dfrac{5}{10} = 3 \times \dfrac{\overset{2}{\cancel{10}}}{\underset{1}{\cancel{5}}} = 6$

25. $\left(\dfrac{1}{4} \div \dfrac{6}{1}\right) \times \dfrac{8}{1} = \dfrac{1}{\underset{1}{\cancel{4}}} \times \dfrac{1}{6} \times \dfrac{\overset{2}{\cancel{8}}}{1} = \dfrac{2}{6}$ or 0.3 to the nearest tenth

26. $\left(\dfrac{1}{4} \times \dfrac{160}{1}\right) \div \dfrac{5}{8} = \dfrac{1}{\underset{1}{\cancel{4}}} \times \dfrac{\overset{32}{\cancel{160}}}{1} \times \dfrac{\overset{2}{\cancel{8}}}{\underset{1}{\cancel{5}}} = 64$

27. $38\dfrac{2}{5}\% = 38.40\% = \underset{\smile}{3}\,\underset{\smile}{8}.40 = 0.384$

28. $35\% = 35 \div 100 = 0.35$

29. $6.75\% = 6\dfrac{3}{4}\% = 6\dfrac{3}{4} \div 100 = \dfrac{27}{4} \times \dfrac{1}{100} = \dfrac{27}{400}$

30. $1.5\% = 1\dfrac{1}{2} \div 100 = \dfrac{3}{2} \times \dfrac{1}{100} = \dfrac{3}{200}$

CHAPTER 2

Exercises

1. clomipramine hydrochloride
2. Voltaren
3. atropine sulfate
4. by mouth, po
5. Lotensin

6.

Name of Drug	Dose	Route of Administration	Time of Administration	Date Started	Date Discontinued
Isoproterenol	15 mg	sl	9 A.M. 1 P.M. 5 P.M.	7/18/01	7/21/01
Procardia	20 mg	po	9 A.M. 5 P.M.	7/18/01	7/21/01
indomethacin	25 mg	po	9 A.M. 5 P.M.	7/18/01	7/21/01
digoxin	0.25 mg	po	9 A.M.	7/18/01	7/23/01
Diuril	500 mg	po	9 A.M.	7/18/01	7/23/01
Carafate	1 gram	po	9 A.M. 1 P.M. 5 P.M. 9 P.M.	7/20/01	7/23/01

    a. Isoproterenol; Procardia; indomethacin; digoxin; Diuril

    b. Procardia; indomethacin; digoxin; Diuril and Carafate

    c. one drug, Carafate   d. digoxin and Diuril   e. Leon Ablon   f. digoxin   g. four

7. a. 300 mg   b. twice a day   c. 6 P.M.   d. 15 mL   e. 10/12/01

8. a. demeclocycline hydrochloride   b. four divided doses of 150 mg each or two divided doses of 300 mg each.   c. 600 mg   d. capsules

CHAPTER 3

Exercises

1. $2.5 \; \cancel{yr} \times \dfrac{12 \text{ mon.}}{1 \; \cancel{yr}} = 30 \text{ month}$

2. $7 \; \cancel{d} \times \dfrac{24 \text{ h}}{1 \; \cancel{d}} = 168 \text{ hours}$

3. $3 \; \cancel{lb} \times \dfrac{16 \text{ oz}}{1 \; \cancel{lb}} = 48 \text{ oz}$

4. $360 \; \cancel{sec} \times \dfrac{1 \text{ min}}{60 \; \cancel{sec}} = 6 \text{ minutes}$

5. $240 \; \cancel{in} \times \dfrac{1 \text{ ft}}{12 \; \cancel{in}} = 20 \text{ feet}$

6. $\overset{3}{\cancel{9}} \; \cancel{ft} \times \dfrac{1 \text{ yd}}{\underset{1}{\cancel{3}} \; \cancel{ft}} = 3 \text{ yd}$

7. $\overset{1}{\cancel{4}} \; \cancel{oz} \times \dfrac{1 \text{ lb}}{\underset{4}{\cancel{16}} \; \cancel{oz}} = \dfrac{1}{4} \text{ pound}$

8. $1\dfrac{1}{2} \; \cancel{yd} \times \dfrac{3 \text{ ft}}{1 \; \cancel{yd}} = \dfrac{3}{2} \times \dfrac{3}{1} = \dfrac{9 \text{ ft}}{2} = 4\dfrac{1}{2} \text{ feet}$

9. $1\dfrac{3}{4} \; \cancel{yr} \times \dfrac{12 \text{ mon}}{1 \; \cancel{yr}} = \dfrac{7}{4} \times \dfrac{12}{1} = \dfrac{84 \text{ mon}}{4} = 21 \text{ months}$

10. $\dfrac{1}{2} \; \cancel{min} \times \dfrac{60 \text{ sec}}{1 \; \cancel{min}} = 30 \text{ seconds}$

11. $6 \text{ ft} \times \dfrac{12 \text{ in}}{1 \text{ ft}} = 72$ inches

12. $5 \text{ min} \times \dfrac{60 \text{ sec}}{1 \text{ min}} = 300$ seconds

13. $3.75 \text{ h} \times \dfrac{60 \text{ min}}{1 \text{ h}} = 225$ minutes

14. $\overset{3}{18} \text{ mon} \times \dfrac{1 \text{ yr}}{\underset{2}{12} \text{ mon}} = \dfrac{3 \text{ yr}}{2} = 1\dfrac{1}{2}$ year

15. $\overset{3}{45} \text{ min} \times \dfrac{1 \text{ hr}}{\underset{4}{60} \text{ min}} = \dfrac{3}{4}$ hour

16. $66 \text{ in} \times \dfrac{1 \text{ ft}}{12 \text{ in}} = 5$ feet, 6 inches or $5\dfrac{1}{2}$ feet

17. $\overset{10}{80} \text{ hr} \times \dfrac{1 \text{ day}}{\underset{3}{24} \text{ hr}} = \dfrac{10 \text{ day}}{3} = 3\dfrac{1}{3}$ day

18. $6 \text{ lb} \times \dfrac{16 \text{ oz}}{1 \text{ lb}} = 96$ ounces

19. $5 \text{ ft} \times \dfrac{12 \text{ in}}{1 \text{ ft}} = 60 \text{ in} + 8 \text{ in} = 68$ inches

20. $7\dfrac{1}{2} \text{ lb} \times \dfrac{16 \text{ oz}}{1 \text{ lb}} = \dfrac{15}{\underset{1}{2}} \times \overset{8}{16} \text{ oz} = 120$ ounces

CHAPTER 4

Exercises

1. $2500 \text{ g} \times \dfrac{1 \text{ kg}}{1000 \text{ g}} = 2.5$ kg

2. $3.5 \text{ L} \times \dfrac{1000 \text{ cc}}{1 \text{ L}} = 3500$ cc

3. $\text{m} \, \overset{2}{120} \times \dfrac{\text{dram } 1}{\underset{1}{\text{m} \, 60}} = \mathfrak{z} \, 2$

4. $\mathfrak{z} \, \overset{4}{32} \times \dfrac{\mathfrak{z} \, 1}{\mathfrak{z} \, 8} = \mathfrak{z} \, 4$

5. $0.006 \text{ g} \times \dfrac{1000 \text{ mg}}{1 \text{ g}} = 6$ mg

6. $\mathfrak{z} \, 24 \times \dfrac{\mathfrak{z} \, 8}{\mathfrak{z} \, 1} = \mathfrak{z} \, 192$

7. $0.4 \text{ kg} \times \dfrac{1000 \text{ g}}{1 \text{ kg}} = 400$ g

8. $\text{qt } 4 \times \dfrac{\text{pt } 2}{\text{qt } 1} = \text{pt } 8$

9. $\mathfrak{z} \, 30 \times \dfrac{\text{m} \, 60}{\mathfrak{z} \, 1} = \text{m} \, 1800$

10. $3 \cancel{t} \times \dfrac{60 \text{ gtt}}{1 \cancel{t}} = 180$ gtt

11. $25\cancel{000} \cancel{\text{mcg}} \times \dfrac{1 \text{ mg}}{1\cancel{000} \cancel{\text{mcg}}} = 25$ mg

12. 50 mL = 50 cc   Remember mL and cc
    contain the same volume (are interchangeable)

13. $0.3 \cancel{\text{mg}} \times \dfrac{1 \text{ g}}{1000 \cancel{\text{mg}}} = 0.0003$ g

14. $0.075 \cancel{\text{g}} \times \dfrac{1000 \text{ mg}}{1 \cancel{\text{g}}} = 75$ mg

15. $\overset{1}{\cancel{\text{dr }4}} \times \dfrac{\text{oz } 1}{\underset{2}{\cancel{\text{dr }8}}} = \dfrac{1}{2}$ oz

16. $0.7 \cancel{\text{L}} \times \dfrac{1000 \text{ mL}}{1 \cancel{\text{L}}} = 700$ mL

17. $\dfrac{1}{\underset{1}{\cancel{4}}} \cancel{\text{pt}} \times \dfrac{\overset{4}{\cancel{16} \text{ oz}}}{1 \cancel{\text{pt}}} = 4$ oz q 1 hour

18. $0.75 \cancel{\text{mg}} \times \dfrac{1000 \text{ mcg}}{1 \cancel{\text{mg}}} = 750$ mcg

19. $\overset{1}{500} \cancel{\mu\text{g}} \times \dfrac{1 \text{ mg}}{\underset{2}{1000} \cancel{\mu\text{g}}} = 0.5$ mg

20. $1\cancel{00} \cancel{\text{mg}} \times \dfrac{1 \text{ g}}{1\cancel{000} \cancel{\text{mg}}} = 0.1$ g

Cumulative Review Exercises

1. 2500 mg
2. 0.2 mg
3. ℨ 3
4. ℨ 32
5. 25000 μg
6. 2 T
7. 1.2 L
8. 6 g
9. 2350 g
10. 3500 mg
11. $1\dfrac{1}{2}$ tsp
12. 3250 mL
13. $\dfrac{3}{4}$ oz
14. $\dfrac{1}{2}$ tsp
15. 0.24 L

CHAPTER 5

Exercises

1. $75 \cancel{\text{mcg}} \times \dfrac{1 \text{ mg}}{1000 \cancel{\text{mcg}}} = 0.075$ mg

2. $2.25 \cancel{\text{kg}} \times \dfrac{1000 \text{ g}}{1 \cancel{\text{kg}}} = 2250$ g

3. $0.003 \cancel{\text{g}} \times \dfrac{1000 \text{ mg}}{1 \cancel{\text{g}}} = 3$ mg

4. $0.005 \cancel{\text{mg}} \times \dfrac{1000 \text{ mcg}}{1 \cancel{\text{mg}}} = 5$ mcg

5. $6.25 \cancel{\text{L}} \times \dfrac{1000 \text{ mL}}{1 \cancel{\text{L}}} = 6250$ mL

6. $0.6 \text{ mg} \times \dfrac{\text{gr } 1}{60 \text{ mg}} = \dfrac{.6 \text{ gr}}{60} \times \dfrac{10}{10} = \dfrac{6 \text{ gr}}{600} = \dfrac{\text{gr } 1}{100}$

7. $0.4 \text{ mg} \times \dfrac{1 \text{ g}}{1000 \text{ mg}} = 0.0004 \text{ g}$

8. $0.2 \text{ mg} \times \dfrac{1000 \text{ mcg}}{1 \text{ mg}} = 200 \text{ mcg}$

9. $2400 \text{ mL} \times \dfrac{1 \text{ L}}{1000 \text{ mL}} = 2.4 \text{ L}$

10. $\text{gr } 3\dfrac{3}{4} \times \dfrac{60 \text{ mg}}{\text{gr } 1} = \dfrac{\text{gr } \overset{15}{\cancel{15}}}{\underset{1}{\cancel{4}}} \times \dfrac{\overset{15}{\cancel{60}} \text{ mg}}{\text{gr } 1} = 225 \text{ mg}$

11. $2\dfrac{1}{2} \text{ t} \times \dfrac{60 \text{ gtt}}{1 \text{ t}} = \dfrac{5}{\underset{1}{\cancel{2}}} \times \dfrac{\overset{30}{\cancel{60}} \text{ gtt}}{1} = 150 \text{ gtt}$

12. $\text{gr } \dfrac{1}{\underset{10}{\cancel{600}}} \times \dfrac{\overset{1}{\cancel{60}} \text{ mg}}{\text{gr } 1} = 0.1 \text{ mg}$

13. $0.2 \text{ mg} \times \dfrac{1000 \text{ mcg}}{\text{mg}} = 200 \text{ mcg}$

14. $\text{gr } 4 \times \dfrac{1 \text{ g}}{\text{gr } 15} = 0.27 \text{ g}$

15. $25 \text{ mg} \times \dfrac{1000 \text{ mcg}}{1 \text{ mg}} = 25000 \text{ mcg}$

16. $\text{gr } \dfrac{1}{\underset{1}{\cancel{3}}} \times \dfrac{\overset{20}{\cancel{60}} \text{ mg}}{\text{gr } 1} = 20 \text{ mg}$

17. $400 \text{ mg} \times \dfrac{1 \text{ g}}{1000 \text{ mg}} = 0.4 \text{ g}$

18. $250 \text{ mg} \times \dfrac{\text{gr } 1}{60 \text{ mg}} = \text{gr } 4\dfrac{1}{6}$

19. $250 \text{ mg} \times \dfrac{1 \text{ g}}{1000 \text{ mg}} = 0.25 \text{ g}$

20. $3730 \text{ mg} \times \dfrac{1 \text{ g}}{1000 \text{ mg}} = 3.73 \text{ g}$

Cumulative Review Exercises

1. 9000 mcg   **2.** ʒ 3   **3.** gr $3\dfrac{3}{4}$ **4.** 18 oz

5. 60 mg   **6.** drams $\dfrac{2}{3}$ **7.** gr $\dfrac{1}{2}$ **8.** 2 t

9. ʒ 2   **10.** 60 mL   **11.** 0.00225 g   **12.** 2750 mL

13. gr $\dfrac{5}{24}$ or gr $\dfrac{1}{5}$ **14.** 0.25 g   **15.** 0.1 g

CHAPTER 6

Case Study

1. 0.5 mg $\times$ 3/day = 1.5 mg digoxin received by the patient on 7/8/01

2. $250 \,\cancel{\mu g} \times \dfrac{1 \text{ mg}}{1000 \,\cancel{\mu g}} = 0.25$ mg of digoxin

3. $\overset{2}{\cancel{4}} \,\cancel{mg} \times \dfrac{1 \text{ tab}}{\underset{1}{\cancel{2} \,\cancel{mg}}} = 2$ tab

   The patient would receive two 2 tablets of Cardura (2 mg each)

4. $0.25 \,\cancel{mg} \times \dfrac{\overset{8}{\cancel{1000} \,\cancel{mcg}}}{1 \,\cancel{mg}} \times \dfrac{1 \text{ Tab}}{\underset{1}{\cancel{125} \,\cancel{mcg}}} = 2$ tab of digoxin on 7/9/01

5. $20 \,\cancel{mg} \times \dfrac{1 \,\cancel{g}}{1000 \,\cancel{mg}} \times \dfrac{1 \text{ Tab}}{0.02 \,\cancel{g}} \times \dfrac{3}{\text{d}} = 3$ tab of Inderal per day

6. $240 \text{ mL} \times \dfrac{\overset{6}{\cancel{24} \,\cancel{h}}}{\underset{1}{\cancel{4} \,\cancel{h}}} = 1440$ mL/day

   $\dfrac{1440 \text{ mL}}{\cancel{day}} \times \dfrac{7 \,\cancel{day}}{1} = 10{,}080$ mL of fluid in 7 days or 10.08 L

7. S/L indicates sublingual, under the tongue

8. $\overset{2}{\cancel{20}} \,\cancel{mEq} \times \dfrac{750 \text{ mg}}{\underset{1}{\cancel{10} \,\cancel{mEq}}} = 1500$ mg or 1.5 g

9. 6 A.M. and 2 P.M. would be the other times for administering Inderal.

Practice Reading Labels

1. $1 \,\cancel{g} \times \dfrac{1 \text{ cap}}{\underset{1}{\cancel{500} \,\cancel{mg}}} \times \dfrac{\overset{2}{\cancel{1000} \,\cancel{mg}}}{1 \,\cancel{g}} = 2$ capsule

2. $0.15 \,\cancel{g} \times \dfrac{\overset{40}{\cancel{1000} \,\cancel{mg}}}{1 \,\cancel{g}} \times \dfrac{1 \text{ Tab}}{\underset{3}{\cancel{75} \,\cancel{mg}}} = 2$ tab

3. $0.3 \,\cancel{g} \times \dfrac{1000 \,\cancel{mg}}{1 \,\cancel{g}} \times \dfrac{1 \text{ Tab}}{300 \,\cancel{mg}} = 1$ tab

4. $\overset{4}{\cancel{200}} \,\cancel{mg} \times \dfrac{1 \text{ cap}}{\underset{1}{\cancel{50} \,\cancel{mg}}} = 4$ capsule

5. $0.01 \,\cancel{g} \times \dfrac{1000 \,\cancel{mg}}{1 \,\cancel{g}} \times \dfrac{1 \text{ Tab}}{10 \,\cancel{mg}} = 1$ tab

6. $\overset{2}{\cancel{200}} \,\cancel{mg} \times \dfrac{1 \text{ cap}}{\underset{1}{\cancel{100} \,\cancel{mg}}} = 2$ capsules

7. $112 \,\cancel{mg} \times \dfrac{5 \text{ mL}}{187 \,\cancel{mg}} = 3$ mL

8. $\overset{2}{\cancel{50}} \text{ mg} \times \dfrac{1 \text{ tab}}{\underset{1}{\cancel{25} \text{ mg}}} = 2 \text{ tab}$

9. $\cancel{\text{gr}} \dfrac{1}{\underset{10}{\cancel{600}}} \times \dfrac{\overset{1}{\cancel{60} \text{ mg}}}{\cancel{\text{gr}} \, 1} \times \dfrac{1 \text{ Tab}}{0.1 \text{ mg}} = 1 \text{ tab}$

10. $\overset{5}{\cancel{5000}} \, \cancel{\mu g} \times \dfrac{1 \text{ mg}}{\underset{1}{\cancel{1000} \, \cancel{\mu g}}} \times \dfrac{1 \text{ Tab}}{5 \text{ mg}} = \dfrac{5 \text{ tab}}{5} = 1 \text{ Tab}$

11. $0.5 \text{ g} \times \dfrac{\overset{2}{\cancel{1000} \text{ mg}}}{1 \text{ g}} \times \dfrac{1 \text{ cap}}{\underset{1}{\cancel{500} \text{ mg}}} = 1 \text{ capsule}$

12. $0.1 \text{ g} \times \dfrac{\overset{20}{\cancel{1000} \text{ mg}}}{1 \text{ g}} \times \dfrac{1 \text{ Tab}}{\underset{1}{\cancel{50} \text{ mg}}} = 2 \text{ tab}$

13. $1.25 \text{ mg} \times \dfrac{1 \text{ Tab}}{2.5 \text{ mg}} = \dfrac{1}{2} \text{ tab}$

14. $0.4 \text{ g} \times \dfrac{\overset{5}{\cancel{1000} \text{ mg}}}{1 \text{ g}} \times \dfrac{1 \text{ Tab}}{\underset{1}{\cancel{200} \text{ mg}}} = 2 \text{ tab}$

15. $\overset{3}{\cancel{7.5}} \text{ mg} \times \dfrac{1 \text{ tab}}{\underset{1}{\cancel{2.5} \text{ mg}}} = 3 \text{ tab}$

16. $0.08 \text{ g} \times \dfrac{1000 \text{ mg}}{1 \text{ g}} \times \dfrac{1 \text{ cap}}{400 \text{ mg}} = 2 \text{ cap}$

17. $0.03 \text{ g} \times \dfrac{\overset{200}{\cancel{1000} \text{ mg}}}{1 \text{ g}} \times \dfrac{1 \text{ cap}}{\underset{3}{\cancel{15} \text{ mg}}} = 2 \text{ capsules}$

18. $0.1 \text{ g} \times \dfrac{\overset{20}{\cancel{1000} \text{ mg}}}{1 \text{ g}} \times \dfrac{1 \text{ cap}}{\underset{1}{\cancel{50} \text{ mg}}} = 2 \text{ capsules}$

19. $\cancel{400} \text{ mg} \times \dfrac{5 \text{ mL}}{\cancel{250} \text{ mg}} = 8 \text{ mL}$

20. $\overset{2}{\cancel{1000}} \text{ mg} \times \dfrac{1 \text{ cap}}{\underset{1}{\cancel{500} \text{ mg}}} = 2 \text{ capsules}$

21. $0.075 \text{ g} \times \dfrac{\overset{40}{\cancel{1000} \text{ mg}}}{1 \text{ g}} \times \dfrac{1 \text{ cap}}{\underset{3}{\cancel{75} \text{ mg}}} = 1 \text{ capsule}$

22. $0.03 \text{ g} \times \dfrac{1000 \text{ mg}}{1 \text{ g}} \times \dfrac{1 \text{ cap}}{30 \text{ mg}} = 1 \text{ capsule}$

23. $\cancel{\text{gr}} \dfrac{1}{120} \times \dfrac{60 \text{ mg}}{1 \, \cancel{\text{gr}}} \times \dfrac{1 \text{ Tab}}{0.5 \text{ mg}} = 1 \text{ tab}$

24. $0.005 \, \cancel{g} \times \dfrac{1000 \, \cancel{mg}}{1 \, \cancel{g}} \times \dfrac{1 \, cap}{5 \, \cancel{mg}} = 1$ capsule

25. $\overset{2}{\cancel{100}} \, \cancel{mg} \times \dfrac{1 \, cap}{\underset{1}{\cancel{50}} \, \cancel{mg}} = 2$ capsule

26. $0.01 \, \cancel{g} \times \dfrac{1000 \, \cancel{mg}}{1 \, \cancel{g}} \times \dfrac{1 \, Tab}{2.5 \, \cancel{mg}} = 4$ tab

27. $0.04 \, \cancel{g} \times \dfrac{\overset{50}{\cancel{1000}} \, \cancel{mg}}{1 \, \cancel{g}} \times \dfrac{1 \, Tab}{\underset{1}{\cancel{20}} \, \cancel{mg}} = 2$ tab

28. $0.5 \, \cancel{g} \times \dfrac{\overset{4}{\cancel{1000}} \, \cancel{mg}}{1 \, \cancel{g}} \times \dfrac{1 \, Tab}{\underset{1}{\cancel{250}} \, \cancel{mg}} = 2$ tab

29. $15 \, \cancel{mg} \times \dfrac{1 \, capsule}{7.5 \, \cancel{mg}} = 2$ capsules

30. $0.125 \, \cancel{g} \times \dfrac{\overset{2}{\cancel{1000}} \, \cancel{mg}}{1 \, \cancel{g}} \times \dfrac{5 \, mL}{\underset{1}{\cancel{500}} \, \cancel{mg}} = 1.25$ mL

Exercises

1. $0.2 \, \cancel{g} \times \dfrac{\cancel{1000} \, \cancel{mg}}{1 \, \cancel{g}} \times \dfrac{1 \, cap}{\cancel{100} \, \cancel{mg}} = 2$ capsule

2. $\overset{4}{\cancel{200}} \, \cancel{mg} \times \dfrac{5 \, mL}{\underset{1}{\cancel{50}} \, \cancel{mg}} = 20$ mL

3. $0.4 \, \cancel{g} \times \dfrac{\cancel{1000} \, \cancel{mg}}{1 \, \cancel{g}} \times \dfrac{1 \, cap}{\cancel{100} \, \cancel{mg}} = 4$ capsule

4. $0.01 \, \cancel{g} \times \dfrac{1000 \, \cancel{mg}}{1 \, g} \times \dfrac{1 \, tab}{\cancel{10} \, \cancel{mg}} = 1$ tab

5. $0.004 \, \cancel{g} \times \dfrac{\overset{250}{\cancel{1000}} \, \cancel{mg}}{1 \, \cancel{g}} \times \dfrac{1 \, patch}{\underset{1}{\cancel{4}} \, \cancel{mg}} = 1$ patch

6. $\cancel{10} \, \cancel{mg} \times \dfrac{1 \, \cancel{g}}{\cancel{1000} \, \cancel{mg}} \times \dfrac{1 \, Tab}{0.005 \, \cancel{g}} = 2$ tab

7. $5 \, \cancel{mg} \times \dfrac{1 \, \cancel{g}}{1000 \, \cancel{mg}} \times \dfrac{1 \, Tab}{0.005 \, \cancel{g}} = 1$ tab

8. Zoloft is the name of the drug.

$0.2 \, \cancel{g} \times \dfrac{\cancel{1000} \, \cancel{mg}}{1 \, \cancel{g}} \times \dfrac{1 \, Tab}{\cancel{100} \, \cancel{mg}} = 2$ tab

9. Dalmane is the name of the drug.

$15 \, \cancel{mg} \times \dfrac{1 \, \cancel{g}}{1000 \, \cancel{mg}} \times \dfrac{1 \, cap}{0.015 \, \cancel{g}} = 1$ capsule

10. $0.125 \text{ mg} \times \dfrac{1 \text{ tab}}{0.25 \text{ mg}} = \dfrac{1}{2} \text{ tab}$

11. $\overset{2}{50} \text{ mg} \times \dfrac{1 \text{ tab}}{\underset{1}{25} \text{ mg}} = 2 \text{ tab}$

12. $1.6 \text{ g} \times \dfrac{\overset{5}{1000} \text{ mg}}{1 \text{ g}} \times \dfrac{1 \text{ tab}}{\underset{2}{400} \text{ mg}} = 4 \text{ tab}$

13. $\overset{1}{20} \text{ mg} \times \dfrac{1 \text{ g}}{\underset{50}{1000} \text{ mg}} \times \dfrac{1 \text{ cap}}{0.01 \text{ g}} = 2 \text{ capsules}$

14. $0.375 \text{ g} \times \dfrac{\overset{4}{1000} \text{ mg}}{1 \text{ g}} \times \dfrac{1 \text{ tab}}{250 \text{ mg}} = 1.5 \text{ or } 1\dfrac{1}{2} \text{ tab}$

15. $46 \text{ kg} \times \dfrac{13 \text{ mg}}{\text{kg}} \times \dfrac{1 \text{ cap}}{300 \text{ mg}} = 2 \text{ capsules}$

16. $0.01 \text{ g} \times \dfrac{\overset{200}{1000} \text{ mg}}{1 \text{ g}} \times \dfrac{1 \text{ tab}}{\underset{2}{5} \text{ mg}} = 2 \text{ tablets}$

17. 1.75 m^2 is the BSA.

$1.75 \text{ m}^2 \times \dfrac{\overset{12}{60} \text{ mg}}{\text{m}^2} \times \dfrac{5 \text{ mL}}{\underset{5}{25} \text{ mg}} = 21 \text{ mL}$

18. $0.45 \text{ mg} \times \dfrac{1 \text{ Tab}}{0.3 \text{ mg}} = 1.5 \text{ or } 1\dfrac{1}{2} \text{ tab}$

19. $\sqrt{\dfrac{80 \text{ kg} \times 183 \text{ cm}}{3600}} = \sqrt{4.06} = 2.01 \text{ m}^2 \text{ BSA}$

$2.01 \text{ m}^2 \times \dfrac{\overset{1}{50} \text{ mg}}{\text{m}^2} \times \dfrac{1 \text{ tab}}{\underset{2}{100} \text{ mg}} = 1 \text{ tab}$

20. $154 \text{ lb} \times \dfrac{0.45 \text{ kg}}{1 \text{ lb}} \times \dfrac{7.2 \text{ mg}}{\text{kg}} \times \dfrac{1 \text{ cap}}{250 \text{ mg}} = 2 \text{ capsules}$

Cumulative Exercises

1. 15 mg   **2.** 1 tab   **3.** ℥ $1\dfrac{1}{4}$ **4.** grain 3

5. 0.04 g   **6.** gr $37\dfrac{1}{2}$ **7.** 500 mg   **8.** gr $3\dfrac{3}{4}$

9. 1 tab   **10.** 19.9 mL   **11.** 1 tab   **12.** 3 Tab

13. 10 mL   **14.** 1 cap   **15.** 1.25 mL

CHAPTER 7

1. Tuberculin syringe

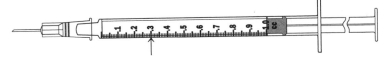

2. 10 cc syringe

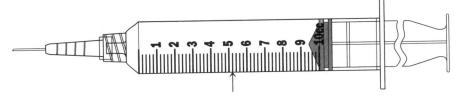

3. 50 unit insulin syringe

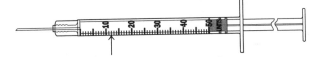

4. 100 unit insulin syringe

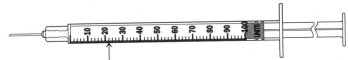

5. 3 cc syringe

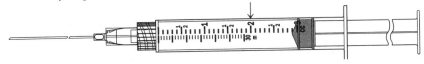

Exercises

1. 10 cc syringe

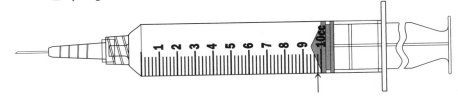

2. 3 cc syringe

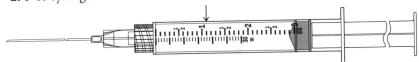

3. 3 cc syringe

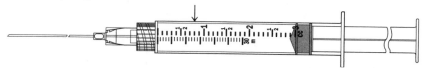

4. 100 insulin unit syringe

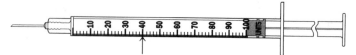

5. 100 unit insulin syringe

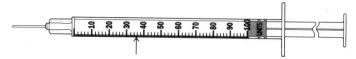

6. 3 cc syringe

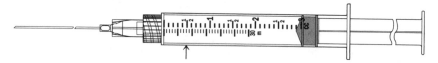

7. 10 cc syringe

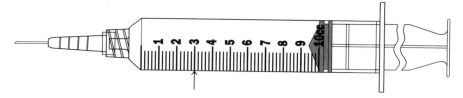

8. Insulin syringe

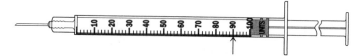

9. 3 cc syringe

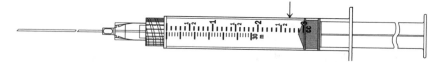

10. Tuberculin syringe

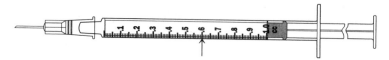

11. 50 unit insulin syringe

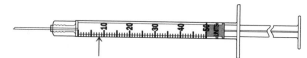

12. 10 cc syringe

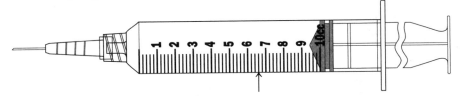

13. 100 unit insulin syringe

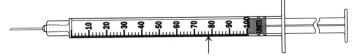

14. 100 unit insulin syringe

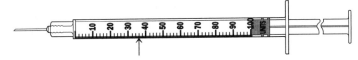

15. 5 cc syringe

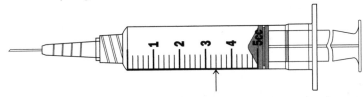

16. 100 unit insulin syringe

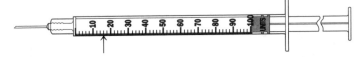

17. .75 cc

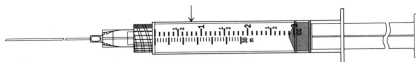

18. 42 units

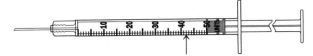

19. 1.5 cc

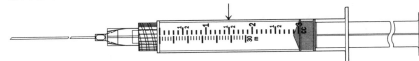

20. 2.5 cc

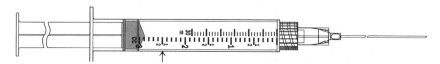

Cumulative Review Exercises

  1. 600 mg   **2.** 1.2 L   **3.** 1 cap   **4.** 10 mg

  5. 3.3 mL   **6.** 0.25 mg   **7.** 4 oz   **8.** oz 2

  9. gr $\dfrac{1}{100}$ **10.** gr $\dfrac{6}{100}$ or gr $\dfrac{3}{50}$ **11.** 1 cap

12. 3 tab   **13.** 1 tab   **14.** 2 tab   **15.** 2 mL

CHAPTER 8

Case Study

1. $40 \text{ mg} \times \dfrac{1 \text{ g}}{1000 \text{ mg}} \times \dfrac{1 \text{ tab}}{0.04 \text{ g}} = 1$ tab of Inderal three times a day

2. $20 \text{ mg} \times \dfrac{2 \text{ per}}{\text{day}} = 40$ mg/day which is 0.04 g

   $0.04 \text{ g} \times \dfrac{7}{\text{days}} = 0.28$ g in 7 days

3. $20 \text{ mEq} \times \dfrac{4 \text{ oz}}{40 \text{ mEq}} \times \dfrac{30 \text{ mL}}{\text{oz}} = \dfrac{120 \text{ mL}}{2} = 60$ mL will contain 20 mEq K-Lor

4. $600 \text{ mg} \times \dfrac{1 \text{ tab}}{600 \text{ mg}} = 1$ tab of azithromycin

5. $0.1 \text{ g} \times \dfrac{1000 \text{ mg}}{1 \text{ g}} \times \dfrac{1 \text{ tab}}{100 \text{ mg}} = 1$ tab of trovafloxacin

6. $0.01 \text{ g} \times \dfrac{1000 \text{ mg}}{1 \text{ g}} \times \dfrac{1 \text{ tab}}{10 \text{ mg}} = 1$ tab of glipizide

7. $0.05 \text{ g} \times \dfrac{1000 \text{ mg}}{1 \text{ g}} = 50$ mg., give one tablet of hydroxyzine to patient

Exercises

1. $\dfrac{2000 \text{ mL} \times \dfrac{2 \text{ mL}}{100 \text{ mL}}}{\dfrac{100 \text{ mL}}{100 \text{ mL}}} = 40$ mL of the 100% solution; dilute with H_2O to 2000 mL.

2. $\dfrac{500 \text{ mL} \times \dfrac{3 \text{ mL}}{100 \text{ mL}}}{\dfrac{15 \text{ mL}}{100 \text{ mL}}} = \dfrac{1500 \text{ mL}}{15 \text{ mL}} = 100$ mL of the 15% solution; dilute with H_2O to 500 mL.

3. $1000 \text{ mL} \times \dfrac{10 \text{ mL}}{100 \text{ mL}} = 100$ mL of pure drug, Weskodyne, and dilute with H_2O to 1000 mL.

4. $250 \text{ mL} \times \dfrac{0.45 \text{ g}}{100 \text{ mL}} = 1.1$ g of sodium crystals and dilute with H_2O to 250 mL.

5. $\overset{5}{2500} \text{ mL} \times \dfrac{1 \text{ g}}{\underset{2}{1000 \text{ mL}}} \times \dfrac{1 \text{ Tab}}{0.5 \text{ g}} = 5$ Tablets and dilute with H_2O to 2500 mL.

6. $\dfrac{2}{200 \text{ mL}} \times \dfrac{2 \text{ g}}{\underset{1}{100 \text{ mL}}} = 4$ g of boric acid crystals and dilute with H_2O to 200 mL.

7. $1000 \text{ mL} \times \dfrac{1 \text{ g}}{100 \text{ mL}} \times \dfrac{\text{Tab}}{1 \text{ g}} = 10$ tablets and dilute with H_2O to 1000 mL.

8. $5 \text{ mL} \times \dfrac{10 \text{ g}}{100 \text{ mL}} = 0.5$ g of calcium chloride in 5 milliliters

9. $\dfrac{600 \text{ mL} \times \dfrac{2.5 \text{ mL}}{100 \text{ mL}}}{\dfrac{3 \text{ mL}}{100 \text{ mL}}} = 500$ mL of the 3% solution, dilute with H_2O to 600 mL.

10. $0.005 \text{ g} \times \dfrac{10{,}000 \text{ mL}}{1 \text{ g}} = 50$ mL

11. $4000 \text{ mL} \times \dfrac{1 \text{ g}}{50 \text{ mL}} \times \dfrac{1 \text{ Tab}}{0.5 \text{ g}} = 160$ tablets and dilute with H_2O to 4000 mL.

12. $\dfrac{1000 \text{ mL} \times \dfrac{10 \text{ mL}}{100 \text{ mL}}}{\dfrac{25 \text{ mL}}{100 \text{ mL}}} = 400$ mL of the 25% solution, dilute with H_2O to 1000 mL.

13. $40 \text{ mL} \times \dfrac{25 \text{ g}}{100 \text{ mL}} = 10$ g of mannitol in 40 milliliter

14. $\dfrac{4000 \text{ mL} \times \dfrac{1 \text{ mL}}{40 \text{ mL}}}{\dfrac{1 \text{ mL}}{20 \text{ mL}}} = 2000$ mL of the 1:20 solution, dilute with H_2O to 4000 mL

15. $60 \text{ g} \times \dfrac{\overset{5}{100} \text{ mL}}{\underset{1}{20 \text{ g}}} = 300$ mL of serum albumin solution will contain 60 g of serum albumin.

16. $\dfrac{500 \text{ mL} \times \dfrac{0.025 \text{ mL}}{100 \text{ mL}}}{\dfrac{1 \text{ mL}}{\underset{1}{100 \text{ mL}}}^{1}} = 12.5$ mL of the 1% solution and dilute with H_2O to 500 mL.

17. 3 g:1000 mL so the strength of the solution is 3:1000

18. $1250 \text{ mL} \times \dfrac{10 \text{ g}}{100 \text{ mL}} \times \dfrac{1 \text{ tab}}{1 \text{ g}} = 125$ tablets diluted with H_2O to 1250 mL.

19. $\dfrac{500 \text{ mL} \times \dfrac{1 \text{ mL}}{1000 \text{ mL}}}{\dfrac{2 \text{ mL}}{100 \text{ mL}}} = 25$ mL of the 2% solution; dilute with H_2O to 500 mL.

20. $\dfrac{250 \ \cancel{mL} \times \dfrac{0.05 \ \cancel{mL}}{\cancel{100 \ mL}}}{\dfrac{1 \ \cancel{mL}}{\cancel{100 \ mL}}} = 12.5$ mL of the 1% solution; dilute with H_2O to 250 mL.

Cumulative Review Exercises

1. 62.5 mL of 10% solution dilute with H_2O to 250 mL
2. 2.5 g of magnesium sulfate
3. 50 mL of the 2% solution would be added
4. $\dfrac{1}{2}$ tablet   5. 6 tablets   6. 1 tab
7. ℥ 60 or ℥ 75   8. 250 mg
9. 0.4 g   10. 1.5 g   11. gr $1\dfrac{1}{3}$ 12. 8 tab
13. 0.6 mg   14. 240 mg   15. 7 pt

CHAPTER 9

Case Study

1.

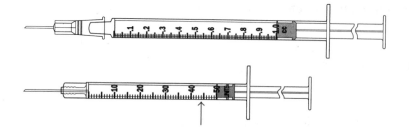

2. Lasix can be administered in two ways, for example, three 20 mg tab = 60 mg or one 20 mg and one 40 mg tablet = 60 mg

3. $\overset{3}{\cancel{30}} \ \cancel{mEq} \times \dfrac{1 \ tab}{\underset{1}{\cancel{10} \ \cancel{mEq}}} = 3$ tablets of K-Lor

4. $0.2 \ \cancel{g} \times \dfrac{1000 \ \cancel{mg}}{1 \ \cancel{g}} \times \dfrac{1 \ tab}{100 \ \cancel{mg}} = 2$ tab of chlorpropamide

5. $0.004 \ \cancel{g} \times \dfrac{1000 \ \cancel{mg}}{1 \ \cancel{g}} \times \dfrac{1 \ tab}{4 \ \cancel{mg}} = 1$ tab of Cardura

6. $20 \ \cancel{mg} \times \dfrac{5 \ mL}{25 \ \cancel{mg}} = 4$ mL of hydroxyzine

7. $0.025 \ \cancel{g} \times \dfrac{1000 \ \cancel{mg}}{1 \ \cancel{g}} \times \dfrac{1 \ tab}{25 \ \cancel{mg}} \times \dfrac{\overset{6}{\cancel{24}} \ \cancel{h}}{\underset{1}{\cancel{4} \ \cancel{h}}} = 6$ tab could be administered per day

8. $0.1 \text{ g} \times \dfrac{1000 \text{ mg}}{1 \text{ g}} \times \dfrac{1 \text{ tab}}{100 \text{ mg}} = 1 \text{ tab of sertraline}$

Exercises

1. $\overset{1}{25} \text{ units} \times \dfrac{2 \text{ mL}}{\underset{2}{50} \text{ units}} = 1 \text{ mL}$

2. $\overset{31}{62} \text{ kg} \times \dfrac{2.5 \text{ units}}{\text{kg}} \times \dfrac{1 \text{ mL}}{\underset{50}{100} \text{ units}} = 1.55 \text{ or } 1.6 \text{ mL}$

3. $0.025 \text{ g} \times \dfrac{1000 \text{ mg}}{1 \text{ g}} \times \dfrac{1 \text{ mL}}{10 \text{ mg}} = 2.5 \text{ mL}$

4. $200 \text{ mg} \times \dfrac{1 \text{ mL}}{150 \text{ mg}} = 1.3 \text{ mL}$

5. $45 \text{ kg} \times \dfrac{0.1 \text{ mg}}{\text{kg}} \times \dfrac{1 \text{ mL}}{10 \text{ mg}} = \dfrac{4.5}{10} = 0.45 \text{ or } 0.5 \text{ mL}$

6. $0.05 \text{ g} \times \dfrac{\overset{20}{1000} \text{ mg}}{1 \text{ g}} \times \dfrac{1 \text{ mL}}{\underset{1}{50} \text{ mg}} = 1 \text{ mL}$

7. $0.25 \text{ mg} \times \dfrac{1 \text{ g}}{1000 \text{ mg}} \times \dfrac{5 \text{ mL}}{0.025 \text{ g}} = 0.05 \text{ mL}$

8. $75 \text{ kg} \times \dfrac{100 \text{ mEq}}{\text{kg}} \times \dfrac{1 \text{ mg}}{1000 \text{ mEq}} \times \dfrac{1 \text{ mL}}{12.5 \text{ mg}} = \dfrac{75 \text{ mL}}{125} = 0.6 \text{ mL}$

9. $0.3 \text{ mg} \times \dfrac{\overset{1}{10} \text{ mL}}{\underset{5}{50} \text{ mg}} = 0.06 \text{ mL}$

10. $2.5 \text{ mg} \times \dfrac{\overset{2}{4} \text{ mL}}{\underset{5}{10} \text{ mg}} = 1 \text{ mL}$

11. $100,000 \text{ units} \times \dfrac{1 \text{ mL}}{50,000 \text{ units}} = 2 \text{ mL}$

12. $0.015 \text{ g} \times \dfrac{1000 \text{ mg}}{1 \text{ g}} \times \dfrac{1 \text{ mL}}{10 \text{ mg}} = 1.5 \text{ mL}$

13. $\overset{4}{40} \text{ units} \times \dfrac{1 \text{ mL}}{\underset{10}{100} \text{ units}} = 0.4 \text{ mL}$

14. $\overset{1}{25} \text{ kg} \times \dfrac{10 \text{ mg}}{\text{kg}} \times \dfrac{1 \text{ mL}}{\underset{2}{50} \text{ mg}} = 5 \text{ mL}$

15. $\overset{2}{190} \text{ mg} \times \dfrac{1 \text{ mL}}{\underset{1}{95} \text{ mg}} \times \dfrac{\text{m} 15}{1 \text{ mL}} = \text{m} 30$

16. $75 \text{ mg} \times \dfrac{1 \text{ mL}}{20 \text{ mg}} = 3.75 \text{ mL}$

17. $0.2 \text{ g} \times \dfrac{\overset{5}{1000} \text{ mg}}{1 \text{ g}} \times \dfrac{2 \text{ mL}}{\underset{1}{200} \text{ mg}} = 2 \text{ mL}$

18. $1.42 \text{ m}^2 \times \dfrac{3.3 \text{ mg}}{\text{m}^2} \times \dfrac{1 \text{ mL}}{25 \text{ mg}} = 0.18$ or 0.2 mL; the prescribed dose is inappropriate.

19. $1550 \text{ mg} \times \dfrac{1 \text{ mL}}{200 \text{ mg}} = 7.75$ mL or 7.8 mL

20. $0.0002 \text{ g} \times \dfrac{1000 \text{ mg}}{1 \text{ g}} \times \dfrac{1 \text{ mL}}{0.2 \text{ mg}} = 1$ mL

$\dfrac{0.2 \text{ mg}}{1 \text{ mL}} \times 3 \text{ mL} = 0.6$ mg

Cumulative Review Exercises

1. 3 mL   **2.** 2 tab   **3.** 2 capsules   **4.** 1 tab

5. ℥ 4   **6.** 3 packets, 12 oz   **7.** 1 tab   **8.** 1 mL

9. 2 capsules   **10.** 0.5 mL   **11.** 0.0003 g   **12.** 3 mg

13. gr $1\dfrac{1}{2}$ **14.** 150 gtt   **15.** gr $\dfrac{1}{1000}$

CHAPTER 10

Case Study

1. $\dfrac{240 \text{ mL}}{\underset{10}{180} \text{ min}} \times \dfrac{18 \text{ gtt}}{\text{mL}} = 24$ drops per minute of Sustacol

2. a. $\dfrac{400 \text{ mL}}{\underset{6}{360} \text{ min}} \times \dfrac{\overset{1}{60} \ \mu\text{gtt}}{\text{mL}} = 67$ microdrops per minute of 5% D/$\frac{1}{2}$ ns

3. $\overset{2}{100} \text{ mg} \times \dfrac{15 \text{ mL}}{\underset{3}{150} \text{ mg}} = 10$ milliliters of Colace

4. $\overset{6}{750} \text{ mg} \times \dfrac{5 \text{ mL}}{\underset{1}{125} \text{ mg}} = 30$ milliliters of Azithromycin

5. $\overset{}{40} \text{ mg} \times \dfrac{1 \text{ g}}{1000 \text{ mg}} \times \dfrac{5 \text{ ml}}{0.04 \text{ g}} = 5$ milliliters of Lasix

6. $\overset{6}{600} \text{ mg} \times \dfrac{1 \text{ mL}}{\underset{1}{100} \text{ mg}} = 6$ milliliters of Tylenol

7. Tube feeding

Sustacal 240 mL $\times \dfrac{\overset{8}{24} \text{ h}}{3 \text{ h}} = 1920$ mL

Sterile H_2O 50 mL $\times \dfrac{\overset{8}{24} \text{ h}}{\underset{1}{3} \text{ h}} = 400$ mL

$$5\% \ D/\frac{1}{2 \ ns} \ 400 \ mL \ \frac{\overset{4}{\cancel{24 \ h}}}{\underset{1}{\cancel{6 \ h}}} = 1600 \ mL$$

Total fluid intake = 3920 milliliters

Exercises

1. $\dfrac{560 \ \cancel{mL}}{12 \ \cancel{h}} \times \dfrac{1 \ \cancel{h}}{\underset{1}{\cancel{60} \ min}} \times \dfrac{\overset{1}{\cancel{60}} \ \mu gtt}{\cancel{mL}} = \dfrac{560 \ \mu gtt}{12 \ min} = 46.6 \ \text{or} \ \dfrac{47 \ \mu gtt}{min}$

2. $\dfrac{1 \ mL}{\underset{1}{\cancel{10} \ \cancel{gtt}}} \times \dfrac{42 \ \cancel{gtt}}{\cancel{min}} \times \dfrac{\overset{6}{\cancel{60} \ \cancel{min}}}{1 \ hr} = 252 \ mL/hr$

3. $\dfrac{1 \ mL}{\underset{1}{\cancel{15} \ \cancel{gtt}}} \times \dfrac{16 \ \cancel{gtt}}{\cancel{min}} \times \dfrac{\overset{4}{\cancel{60} \ \cancel{min}}}{1 \ hr} = 64 \ mL/hr$

4. $\dfrac{400 \ \cancel{mL}}{6 \ \cancel{hr}} \times \dfrac{1 \ \cancel{hr}}{\underset{6}{\cancel{60} \ min}} \times \dfrac{\overset{1}{\cancel{10} \ gtt}}{\cancel{mL}} = \dfrac{400 \ gtt}{36 \ min} \ \text{or} \ 11 \ gtt/min$

5. $\dfrac{1 \ mL}{\underset{1}{\cancel{15} \ \cancel{gtt}}} \times \dfrac{36 \ \cancel{gtt}}{\cancel{min}} \times \dfrac{\overset{4}{\cancel{60} \ \cancel{min}}}{1 \ hr} = 144 \ mL/hr$

6. $\dfrac{1 \ mL}{\underset{1}{\cancel{20} \ \cancel{gtt}}} \times \dfrac{31 \ \cancel{gtt}}{\cancel{min}} \times \dfrac{\overset{3}{\cancel{60} \ \cancel{min}}}{1 \ hr} = 93 \ mL/hr$

7. $40 \ mL/h = 40 \ \mu gtt/min$

8. $\dfrac{250 \ \cancel{mL}}{2.5 \ \cancel{hr}} \times \dfrac{1 \ \cancel{hr}}{\underset{4}{\cancel{60} \ min}} \times \dfrac{\overset{1}{\cancel{15} \ gtt}}{\cancel{mL}} = \dfrac{250 \ gtt}{10 \ min} = \dfrac{25 \ gtt}{min}$

9. $240 \ mL/4 \ h = 60 \ mL \ \text{per hour}$

10. $\dfrac{\overset{4}{\cancel{480} \ \cancel{mL}}}{\underset{1}{\cancel{120} \ min}} \times \dfrac{20 \ gtt}{\cancel{mL}} = 80 \ gtt/min$

11. $\dfrac{3000 \ mL}{24 \ H} = 125 \ mL/H$

12. $\dfrac{2500 \ \cancel{mL}}{\underset{12}{\cancel{24} \ \cancel{hr}}} \times \dfrac{\overset{5}{\cancel{10} \ gtt}}{\cancel{mL}} \times \dfrac{1 \ \cancel{hr}}{60 \ min} = \dfrac{12500}{720} = 17.4 \ \text{or} \ 17 \ gtt/min$

13. $125 \ \mu gtt/min = 125 \ mL/hr$

14. $\dfrac{400 \ mL}{4.4 \ hr} = \dfrac{90.9 \ mL}{hr}$

15. percutaneous endoscopic gastrotomy

16. $\dfrac{1 \text{ mL}}{\underset{1}{\cancel{15} \text{ gtt}}} \times \dfrac{25 \cancel{\text{ gtt}}}{\cancel{\text{min}}} \times \dfrac{\overset{4}{\cancel{60} \cancel{\text{ min}}}}{1 \text{ hr}} = \dfrac{100 \text{ mL}}{\text{hr}}$

17. $\dfrac{1 \text{ mL}}{\underset{1}{\cancel{15} \text{ gtt}}} \times \dfrac{26 \cancel{\text{ gtt}}}{\cancel{\text{min}}} \times \dfrac{\overset{4}{\cancel{60} \cancel{\text{ min}}}}{\text{hr}} = 104 \text{ mL/hr}$

18. $\dfrac{\overset{180}{\cancel{900} \text{ mL}}}{\underset{1}{\cancel{5} \cancel{\text{ H}}}} \times \dfrac{1 \cancel{\text{ H}}}{\underset{6}{\cancel{60} \text{ min}}} \times \dfrac{\overset{1}{\cancel{10} \text{ gtt}}}{\cancel{\text{mL}}} = \dfrac{180 \text{ gtt}}{6 \text{ min}} = \dfrac{30 \text{ gtt}}{\text{min}}$

19. $\dfrac{1 \text{ mL}}{\underset{1}{\cancel{10} \cancel{\text{ gtt}}}} \times \dfrac{30 \cancel{\text{ gtt}}}{\cancel{\text{min}}} \times \dfrac{\overset{6}{\cancel{60} \cancel{\text{ min}}}}{1 \text{ hr}} = \dfrac{180 \text{ mL}}{\text{hr}}$

20. $\dfrac{80 \ \mu\text{gtt}}{\text{min}} = 80 \text{ mL/hr}$

Cumulative Review Exercises

  1. 40 mL/hr   **2.** 166.7 mL/hr   **3.** 156 μgtt/min   **4.** 17 gtt/min

  5. 0.4 mg   **6.** 1 cap   **7.** 234 mg/mL   **8.** 0.5 mL

  9. 2 cap.   **10.** 2.4 mL   **11.** 6 tsp   **12.** gr $\dfrac{2}{15}$ or gr $\dfrac{1}{8}$

  13. 75 gtt   **24.** 0.0007 g   **15.** 30 mL

CHAPTER 11

Case Study

1. Unasyn:

$$\dfrac{100 \cancel{\text{ mL}}}{\underset{6}{\cancel{60} \text{ min}}} \times \dfrac{\cancel{10} \text{ gtt}}{1 \cancel{\text{ mL}}} = 17 \text{ gtt/min}$$

Pepcid:

$$\dfrac{100 \cancel{\text{ mL}}}{\underset{3}{\cancel{30} \text{ min}}} \times \dfrac{\cancel{10} \text{ gtt}}{1 \cancel{\text{ mL}}} = 33 \text{ gtt/min}$$

2. $\cancel{\text{gr}} \ \dfrac{1}{100} \times \dfrac{60 \cancel{\text{ mg}}}{\cancel{\text{gr}} 1} \times \dfrac{1 \text{ mL}}{0.4 \cancel{\text{ mg}}} = 1.5 \text{ mL of atropine sulfate}$

3. 1 mL of Demerol and 1 mL of Versed

4. Unasyn: 100 mL $\times$ 3 (q8h) =   300 mL

    Pepcid: 100 mL $\times$ 3 (q8h) =   <u>300 mL</u>

                           Total   600 mL

    Unasyn: 100 mL in 1 hr $\times$ 3 =   3 hr

    Pepcid: 100 mL in $\frac{1}{2}$ hr $\times$ 3 = $1\frac{1}{2}$ hr

                           Total   600 mL in $4\frac{1}{2}$ h

$24 \text{ hr} - 4\frac{1}{2} \text{ hr} = 19\frac{1}{2} \text{ hr}$ (time that the patient is receiving 5% D/0.45% NS)

$$19\frac{1}{2} \,\cancel{\text{h}} \times \frac{125 \text{ mL}}{1 \,\cancel{\text{h}}} = 2437.5 \text{ mL of } 5\% \text{ D/}0.45\% \text{ NS}$$

2437.5 mL + 600 mL = 3037.5 or 3038 mL of IV fluid in 24 hr

5. $0.005 \,\cancel{\text{g}} \times \dfrac{1000 \,\cancel{\text{mg}}}{\cancel{\text{g}}} \times \dfrac{1 \text{ ml}}{1 \,\cancel{\text{mg}}} = 5$ milliliters of Versed

6. $25 \,\cancel{\text{mg}} \times \dfrac{1 \text{ tab}}{12.5 \,\cancel{\text{mg}}} = 2$ tab of Antivert

7. $0.5 \,\cancel{\text{hr}} \times \dfrac{100 \,\cancel{\text{mL}}}{1 \,\cancel{\text{hr}}} \times \dfrac{1.5 \,\cancel{\text{g}}}{100 \,\cancel{\text{mL}}} \times \dfrac{1000 \text{ mg}}{1 \,\cancel{\text{g}}} = 750$ mg in 30 minutes

Exercises

1. $\dfrac{250 \,\cancel{\text{mL}}}{1 \,\cancel{\text{g}}} \times \dfrac{0.15 \,\cancel{\text{g}}}{\cancel{\text{hr}}} \times \dfrac{\overset{1}{\cancel{10}} \text{ gtt}}{\cancel{\text{mL}}} \times \dfrac{1 \,\cancel{\text{hr}}}{\underset{6}{\cancel{60}} \text{ min}} = 6.25$ or 6 gtt/min

2. $\dfrac{115 \,\cancel{\text{mL}}}{\underset{4}{\cancel{60}} \text{ min}} \times \dfrac{\overset{1}{\cancel{15}} \text{ gtt}}{1 \,\cancel{\text{mL}}} = \dfrac{115 \text{ gtt}}{4 \text{ min}} = 28.75$ or 29 gtt/min

3. $\dfrac{500 \text{ mL}}{\underset{1}{\cancel{20}} \,\cancel{\text{units}}} \times \dfrac{0.002 \,\cancel{\text{unit}}}{\cancel{\text{min}}} \times \dfrac{\overset{3}{\cancel{60}} \,\cancel{\text{min}}}{1 \text{ hr}} = 3$ mL/hr

4. $120 \,\cancel{\text{lb}} \times \dfrac{0.45 \,\cancel{\text{kg}}}{1 \,\cancel{\text{lb}}} \times \dfrac{18 \text{ mg}}{\cancel{\text{kg}}} = 972$ mg

$972 \,\cancel{\text{mg}} \times \dfrac{100 \text{ mL}}{1000 \,\cancel{\text{mg}}} = 97.2$ mL

5. a. $500 \,\cancel{\text{mg}} \times \dfrac{1 \text{ mL}}{200 \,\cancel{\text{mg}}} = 2.5$ milliliters of lidocaine

   b. 25 μgtt/min = 25 mL/hr

   c. $\dfrac{252.5 \text{ mL}}{5 \text{ hr}} = \dfrac{50.5 \text{ mL}}{\text{hr}}$

6. a. $1.7 \,\cancel{\text{m}^2} \times \dfrac{20 \text{ mg}}{\cancel{\text{m}^2}} = 34$ mg   b. $34 \,\cancel{\text{mg}} \times \dfrac{1 \text{ mL}}{1 \,\cancel{\text{mg}}} = 34$ mL

   c. $\dfrac{1034 \text{ mL}}{8 \text{ h}} = 129.3$ mL/hr

7. $\dfrac{\overset{1}{\cancel{250}} \text{ mL}}{\underset{1}{\cancel{250}} \,\cancel{\text{mg}}} \times \dfrac{0.006 \,\cancel{\text{mg}}}{\cancel{\text{kg}} \times \cancel{\text{min}}} \times \dfrac{60 \,\cancel{\text{min}}}{1 \text{ hr}} \times 66 \,\cancel{\text{kg}} = 23.76$ or 23.8 mL/hr

8. $\dfrac{50 \,\cancel{\text{mL}}}{\text{H}} \times \dfrac{\overset{10}{\cancel{2500}} \text{ units}}{\underset{1}{\cancel{250}} \,\cancel{\text{mL}}} = 500$ units/hour

9. $\dfrac{\overset{5}{\cancel{250}} \text{ mL}}{\underset{4}{\cancel{200}} \,\cancel{\text{mg}}} \times \dfrac{10 \,\cancel{\text{mg}}}{\text{hr}} = \dfrac{50 \text{ mL}}{4 \text{ hr}} = \dfrac{12.5 \text{ mL}}{\text{hr}}$

10. $100 \ \cancel{lb} \times \dfrac{0.45 \ \cancel{kg}}{1 \ \cancel{lb}} \times \dfrac{250 \ mL}{180 \ \cancel{mg}} \times \dfrac{0.005 \ \cancel{mg}}{\cancel{kg} \times \cancel{min}} \times \dfrac{60 \ \cancel{min}}{1 \ hr} = \dfrac{18.8 \ mL}{hr}$

11. $70 \ \cancel{kg} \times \dfrac{4.8 \ \cancel{mcg}}{\cancel{kg/min}} \times \dfrac{100 \ mL}{200 \ \cancel{mg}} \times \dfrac{1 \ \cancel{mg}}{1000 \ \cancel{mcg}} \times \dfrac{60 \ \cancel{min}}{1 \ hr} = \dfrac{10.8 \ mL}{hr}$

12. $122 \ \cancel{lb} \times \dfrac{0.45 \ \cancel{kg}}{1 \ \cancel{lb}} \times \dfrac{0.003 \ \cancel{mg}}{\cancel{kg} \times \cancel{min}} \times \dfrac{250 \ mL}{\underset{8}{\cancel{160}} \ \cancel{mg}} \times \dfrac{\overset{3}{\cancel{60}} \ \cancel{min}}{1 \ hr} = 15.5 \ mL/hr$

13. $60 \ \cancel{kg} \times \dfrac{1 \ \cancel{mL}}{\cancel{kg} \times \cancel{hr}} \times \dfrac{\overset{1}{\cancel{60}} \ \mu gtt}{\cancel{mL}} \times \dfrac{1 \ \cancel{hr}}{\underset{1}{\cancel{60}} \ min} = 60 \ \mu gtt/min$

14. $\overset{25}{\cancel{500}} \ \cancel{mL} \times \dfrac{1 \ \cancel{min}}{0.7 \ \cancel{mL}} \times \dfrac{1 \ hr}{\underset{3}{\cancel{60}} \ \cancel{min}} = \dfrac{25 \ hr}{2.1} = 11.9 \ hr$ or $11 \ hr \ 54 \ min$

15. $\dfrac{\overset{4}{\cancel{2000}} \ mg}{\underset{1}{\cancel{500}} \ \cancel{mL}} \times \dfrac{\overset{1}{\cancel{15}} \ \cancel{mL}}{\cancel{hr}} \times \dfrac{1 \ \cancel{hr}}{\underset{4}{\cancel{60}} \ min} = \dfrac{1 \ mg}{min}$

16. $\overset{50}{\cancel{1000}} \ \cancel{mL} \times \dfrac{\overset{1}{\cancel{20}} \ \cancel{gtt}}{\cancel{mL}} \times \dfrac{1 \ min}{\underset{1}{\cancel{20}} \ \cancel{gtt}} \times \dfrac{1 \ hr}{\underset{3}{\cancel{60}} \ \cancel{min}} = \dfrac{50 \ hr}{3} = 16.7 \ hr$ or $16 \ hr \ 42 \ min.$

The infusion will finish at 3:40 A.M.

17. $74 \ \cancel{kg} \times \dfrac{0.08 \ \cancel{mg}}{\cancel{kg} \times min} \times \dfrac{\overset{1}{\cancel{50}} \ \cancel{mL}}{\underset{4}{\cancel{200}} \ \cancel{mg}} \times \dfrac{10 \ gtt}{\cancel{mL}} = 14.8$ or $15 \ gtt/min$

18. $200 \ \cancel{lb} \times \dfrac{0.45 \ \cancel{kg}}{1 \ \cancel{lb}} \times \dfrac{0.005 \ \cancel{mg}}{\cancel{kg} \times \cancel{min}} \times \dfrac{\overset{5}{\cancel{250}} \ mL}{\underset{4}{\cancel{200}} \ \cancel{mg}} \times \dfrac{60 \ \cancel{min}}{1 \ hr} = 33.8 \ mL/hr$

19. $\dfrac{\overset{1}{\cancel{1200}} \ \cancel{units}}{hr} \times \dfrac{250 \ mL}{\underset{1}{\cancel{12000}} \ \cancel{units}} = 25 \ mL/hr$

20. $0.9 \ \cancel{m^2} \times \dfrac{120 \ \cancel{mg}}{\cancel{m^2} \times hr} \times \dfrac{\overset{4}{\cancel{100}} \ mL}{\underset{10}{\cancel{250}} \ \cancel{mg}} = 43.2 \ mL/hr$

Cumulative Review Exercises

1. 5.9 mL   2. 2 mL   3. 3 mL   4. m 13

5. 12 mL   6. 1 mL   7. 2 tab   8. 10 mL

9. 0.02 mg   10. gr $\dfrac{1}{150}$ 11. $187\dfrac{1}{2}$ gr

12. 0.0004 g   13. 15 gtt   14. 3 tsp   15. oz 1

CHAPTER 12

1. $\dfrac{50 \text{ mL}}{\text{hr}} \times 12 \text{ hr} = 600$ milliliter of 5% D/W

2. a. BSA is 1 m^2 (weight 35 kg and height 112 cm) so patient will receive 2 mg of vincristine/week for 4 weeks

2. b. Patient will need 2 mL of vincristine added to 50 mL 5% D/W (total 52 mL)

$\dfrac{52 \text{ mL}}{15 \text{ min}} = \dfrac{3.5 \text{ mL}}{\text{min}}$ of the vincristine solution

3. a. $35 \text{ kg} \times \dfrac{1000 \text{ IU}}{\text{kg}} = 35000$ IU of asparaginase

b. $35{,}000 \text{ IU} \times \dfrac{5 \text{ mL}}{10{,}000 \text{ IU}} = \dfrac{175}{10} = 17.5$ mL of asparaginase

add 17.5 mL of asparaginase to 50 mL 5% D/W = 67.5 mL

c. $\dfrac{67.5 \text{ mL}}{30 \text{ min}} = \dfrac{2.3 \text{ mL}}{\text{min}}$ asparaginase solution

4. a. 40 mg/m^2; patient has a BSA of 1 m^2, so patient would receive a total of 40 mg/day of prednisone

b. 13.4 mg per dose

c. $13.4 \text{ mg} \times \dfrac{5 \text{ mL}}{5 \text{ mg}} = 13.4$ mL per dose po

d. $21 \text{ days} \times 40 \text{ mg} = 840 \text{ mg} \left(\dfrac{40 \text{ mg}}{\text{day}} \times \dfrac{21 \text{ days}}{1} = 840 \text{ mg} \right)$

5. The BSA is 1m.^{2} Because the order is 3.3 mg and the vial is labeled 2.5 mg/mL, the patient will receive

a. $3.3 \text{ mg} \times \dfrac{1 \text{ mL}}{2.5 \text{ mg}} = 1.32$ mL of methotrexate + 25 mL 0.9% NS

b. $\dfrac{26.32 \text{ mL}}{20 \text{ min}} = \dfrac{1.3 \text{ mL}}{\text{min}}$ of methotrexate

c. $\dfrac{3.3 \text{ mg}}{\text{day}} \times 42 \text{ days} = 138.6$ mg of methotrexate in 42 days (6 wk.)

6. The IV solution of vincristine infuses in 15 minutes.

The IV solution of methotrexate infuses in 20 minutes.

35 minutes or 0.6 h

The patient has the primary IV infusing for 24 hours (1440 minutes) − 0.6 h (55 min) = 1405 min or 23 hr and 25 min; so the primary IV actually infuses in 1405 min (23 h + 25 min)

$\dfrac{50 \text{ mL}}{\text{hr}} \times 23.4 \text{ hr} = 1170$ mL IV

vincristine   52 mL

methotrexate   26.3 mL

(78.3 mL)

1170 mL   5% D/W

$\underline{ 78.3 \text{ mL}}$ medication

1248.3 mL (vincristine and methotrexate)

total IV fluid on Monday

7. $650 \text{ mg} \times \dfrac{1 \text{ g}}{1000 \text{ mg}} = 0.65$ g of Tylenol

8. $35 \text{ kg} \times 2.5 \text{ mg/kg} = 87.5$ mg of Benadryl

$87.5 \text{ mg} \times \dfrac{1 \text{ mL}}{50 \text{ mg}} = 1.8$ mL of Benadryl added to 200 mL 5% D/W

$\dfrac{201.8 \text{ mL}}{6 \text{ hr}} \times \dfrac{1 \text{ hr}}{60 \text{ min}} \times \dfrac{\overset{1}{10} \text{ gtt}}{1 \text{ mL}} = 6$ gtt/minute of Benadryl solution

Exercises

1. $0.025 \; \cancel{g} \times \dfrac{\overset{40}{\cancel{1000 \; mg}}}{\cancel{g}} \times \dfrac{5 \; mL}{\underset{1}{\cancel{25 \; mg}}} = 5$ mL or 1 tsp

2. $\overset{2}{\cancel{162 \; mg}} \times \dfrac{1 \; Tab}{\underset{1}{\cancel{81 \; mg}}} = 2$ tab

3. $40 \; \cancel{kg} \times \dfrac{6.25 \; \cancel{mg}}{\cancel{kg}} \times \dfrac{\overset{1}{\cancel{5 \; mL}}}{\underset{25}{\cancel{125 \; mg}}} = 10$ mL

4. $\overset{3}{\cancel{30 \; kg}} \times \dfrac{3.3 \; \cancel{mg}}{\cancel{kg}} \times \dfrac{1 \; mL}{\underset{5}{\cancel{50 \; mg}}} = 1.98$ or 2 mL

5. $0.6 \; \cancel{m^2} \times \dfrac{0.3 \; mg}{\cancel{m^2}} = 0.18$ mg

6. $0.93 \; \cancel{m^2} \times \dfrac{100 \; mg}{\cancel{m^2}} = 93$ mg

7. $1.1 \; \cancel{m^2} \times \dfrac{45 \; mg}{\cancel{m^2}} = 49.5$ mg

8. $1.04 \; \cancel{m^2} \times \dfrac{50 \; mg}{\cancel{m^2}} = 52$ mg

9. $0.8 \; \cancel{m^2} \times \dfrac{\overset{1}{\cancel{0.2 \; mg}}}{\cancel{m^2}} \times \dfrac{1 \; mL}{\underset{1}{\cancel{0.2 \; mg}}} = 0.8$ mL

10. $35 \; \cancel{kg} \times \dfrac{0.01 \; \cancel{mg}}{\cancel{kg}} \times \dfrac{1 \; mL}{0.4 \; \cancel{mg}} = \dfrac{0.35 \; mL}{0.4} = 0.9$ mL

11. $1.25 \; \cancel{m^2} \times \dfrac{\overset{2}{\cancel{250 \; mg}}}{\cancel{m^2}} \times \dfrac{1 \; mL}{\underset{1}{\cancel{125 \; mg}}} = 2.5$ mL

12. $45 \; \cancel{kg} \times \dfrac{0.5 \; \cancel{mg}}{\cancel{kg}} \times \dfrac{100 \; mL}{1 \; \cancel{g}} \times \dfrac{1 \; \cancel{g}}{1000 \; \cancel{mg}} = \dfrac{22.5}{10} = 2.25$ mL

13. $\overset{22}{\cancel{44 \; kg}} \times \dfrac{0.54 \; \cancel{unit}}{\cancel{kg}} \times \dfrac{1 \; mL}{\underset{50}{\cancel{100 \; unit}}} = \dfrac{11.88 \; unit}{50} = 0.23$ or 0.2 mL

14. $42 \; \cancel{kg} \times \dfrac{\overset{1}{\cancel{2 \; mg}}}{\cancel{kg}} \times \dfrac{1 \; mL}{\underset{5}{\cancel{10 \; mg}}} = \dfrac{42}{5} = 8.4$ mL

15. $0.4 \; \cancel{g} \times \dfrac{1000 \; \cancel{mg}}{1 \; \cancel{g}} \times \dfrac{\overset{1}{\cancel{5 \; mL}}}{160 \; \cancel{mg}} \times \dfrac{1 \; tsp}{\underset{1}{\cancel{5 \; mL}}} = \dfrac{40 \; tsp}{16} = 2.5$ or $2\dfrac{1}{2}$ tsp

16. $50 \; \cancel{kg} \times \dfrac{1 \; \cancel{mg}}{\cancel{kg}} \times \dfrac{100 \; mL}{2 \; \cancel{g}} \times \dfrac{1 \; \cancel{g}}{1000 \; \cancel{mg}} = 2.5$ mL

17. $42 \; \cancel{kg} \times \dfrac{1.2 \; \cancel{mg}}{\cancel{kg}} \times \dfrac{1 \; mL}{50 \; \cancel{mg}} = 1$ mL

18. $38 \; \cancel{kg} \times \dfrac{0.1 \; \cancel{mg}}{\cancel{kg}} \times \dfrac{1 \; mL}{5 \; \cancel{mg}} = \dfrac{3.8 \; mL}{5} = 0.76$ or 0.8 mL

19. $75 \, \overset{3}{\cancel{lb}} \times \dfrac{0.45 \, \cancel{kg}}{\cancel{lb}} \times \dfrac{1 \, mL}{\underset{4}{\cancel{100 \, mg}}} \times \dfrac{1.04 \, \cancel{mg}}{\cancel{kg}} = \dfrac{1.404 \, mL}{4}$ or 0.4 mL

20. $1.02 \, \cancel{m^2} \times \dfrac{3 \, \cancel{mg}}{\cancel{m^2}} \times \dfrac{tab}{2 \, \cancel{mg}} = 1.53$ tab or $1\frac{1}{2}$ tab

Cumulative Review Exercises

1. 525 mg   **2.** 300 mg

3. 160 mg   **4.** m 8   **5.** 2.4 ml

6. 1 capsule   **7.** 39.15 or 39.2 mg

8. 60 gtt/min

9. 2.5 mL/min   **10.** 14.7 hr or 14 hr 42 min The infusion will end at 11:42 A.M.

11. gr $\dfrac{3}{100}$ **12.** 779 mg   **13.** Take 50 mL of the $\frac{1}{2}$% solution and dilute to 100 mL

14. 50 mg   **15.** 10.5 mL

Comprehensive Self-Test 1

1. Prescribed is $\dfrac{300 \, mg \times 2}{1 \, day} = \dfrac{600 \, mg}{day}$

usual dosage $70 \, \cancel{kg} \times \dfrac{8 \, mg}{1 \, \cancel{kg} \times 1 \, day} = \dfrac{560 \, mg}{day}$

$70 \, \cancel{kg} \times \dfrac{10 \, mg}{1 \, \cancel{kg} \times 1 \, day} = \dfrac{700 \, mg}{day}$

The prescribed dose is within the usual range, so the dose is correct.

2. $\overset{1}{\cancel{50 \, mg}} \times \dfrac{3}{d} \times \dfrac{1 \, Tab}{\underset{1}{\cancel{50 \, mg}}} = 3$ tab/day

3. $\dfrac{0.25 \, \cancel{g}}{\underset{1}{\cancel{8 \, hr}}} \times \overset{3}{\cancel{24 \, hr}} \times \dfrac{\overset{4}{\cancel{1000 \, mg}}}{1 \, \cancel{g}} \times \dfrac{1 \, cap}{\underset{1}{\cancel{250 \, mg}}} = 3$ cap/24 hr

4. $1.5 \, \cancel{g} \times \dfrac{\overset{2}{\cancel{1000 \, mg}}}{1 \, \cancel{g}} \times \dfrac{1 \, Tab}{\underset{1}{\cancel{500 \, mg}}} = 3$ tablets

5. $0.004 \, \cancel{g} \times \dfrac{1000 \, \cancel{mg}}{\cancel{g}} \times \dfrac{1 \, tab}{2 \, \cancel{mg}} = \dfrac{4 \, tab}{2} = 2$ tablets

6. a. Add 11.5 mL of diluent to the vial of Pfizerpen

b. $15{,}000{,}000 \, \cancel{units} \times \dfrac{1 \, mL}{1{,}000{,}000 \, \cancel{units}} = 15$ mL of Pfizerpen must be added to 500 mL of 5% D/W

7. $\overset{1}{\cancel{5 \, mg}} \times \dfrac{1 \, grain}{\underset{12}{\cancel{60 \, mg}}} = $ grain $\dfrac{1}{12}$

8. $10 \, \cancel{mg} \times \dfrac{1 \, Tab}{2.5 \, \cancel{mg}} = 4$ tab

9. $\overset{2}{\cancel{250 \, mg}} \times \dfrac{1 \, cap}{\underset{1}{\cancel{125 \, mg}}} = 2$ capsules

10. $\overset{2}{5\!\!\!/0} \text{ mg} \times \dfrac{1 \text{ mL}}{\underset{1}{2\!\!\!/5 \text{ mg}}} = 2 \text{ mL of Zantac required and}$ 18 mL of diluent

11. $\dfrac{\overset{1}{2\!\!\!/0 \text{ mL}}}{\underset{1}{2\!\!\!/0 \text{ min}}} \times \dfrac{60 \ \mu\text{gtt}}{1 \text{ mL}} = \dfrac{60 \ \mu\text{gtt}}{\text{min}}$

12. $\overset{40}{8\!\!\!/0\!\!\!/0 \text{ mL}} \times \dfrac{15 \text{ gtt}}{\text{mL}} \times \dfrac{1 \text{ min}}{31 \text{ gtt}} \times \dfrac{1 \text{ h}}{\underset{3}{6\!\!\!/0 \text{ min}}} = 6.45 \text{ hr}$

$0.45 \text{ hr} \times \dfrac{60 \text{ min}}{1 \text{ hr}} = 27 \text{ minutes}$

It will take 6 hours and 27 minutes for this infusion to be completed.

13. $\dfrac{2 \text{ mg}}{\text{min}} \times \dfrac{1 \text{ g}}{\underset{2}{1000 \text{ mg}}} \times \dfrac{\overset{1}{5\!\!\!/0\!\!\!/0 \text{ mL}}}{0.5 \text{ g}} = 2 \text{ mL/min}$

14. $\overset{2}{3\!\!\!/0 \text{ mL}} \times \dfrac{10 \text{ g}}{\underset{1}{1\!\!\!/5 \text{ mL}}} = 20 \text{ g}$

15. $\overset{4}{2\!\!\!/0 \text{ mg}} \times \dfrac{1 \text{ mL}}{\underset{1}{5 \text{ mg}}} = 4 \text{ mL}$

16. $\dfrac{2 \text{ mg}}{\text{min}} \times \dfrac{100 \text{ mL}}{100 \text{ mg}} \times \dfrac{\overset{3}{6\!\!\!/0 \ \mu\text{gtt}}}{\text{mL}} = \dfrac{120 \ \mu\text{gtt}}{\text{min}}$

17. $\dfrac{\overset{5}{5\!\!\!/1\!\!\!/0 \text{ mL}}}{5\!\!\!/0\!\!\!/0 \text{ mg}} \times \dfrac{0.5 \text{ mg}}{\text{min}} \times \dfrac{60 \text{ min}}{1 \text{ hr}} = \dfrac{30.6 \text{ mL}}{\text{hr}}$

18. $180 \text{ lb} \times \dfrac{0.45 \text{ kg}}{1 \text{ lb}} \times \dfrac{0.1 \text{ mg}}{\text{kg/min}} \times \dfrac{60 \text{ mL}}{500 \text{ mg}} \times$

$\dfrac{15 \text{ gtt}}{\text{mL}} = 15 \text{ gtt/min}$

or

$180 \text{ lb} \times \dfrac{1 \text{ kg}}{2.2 \text{ lb}} \times \dfrac{0.1 \text{ mg}}{\text{kg/min}} \times \dfrac{60 \text{ mL}}{500 \text{ mg}} \times$

$\dfrac{15 \text{ gtt}}{\text{mL}} = \dfrac{162 \text{ gtt}}{11 \text{ min}} = 15 \text{ gtt/min}$

19. $\dfrac{100 \text{ mL}}{120 \text{ min}} \times \dfrac{15 \text{ gtt}}{1 \text{ mL}} = 13 \text{ gtt/min}$

20. $\dfrac{8 \text{ gtt}}{\text{min}} \times \dfrac{1 \text{ mL}}{15 \text{ gtt}} \times \dfrac{60 \text{ min}}{1 \text{ hr}} = 32 \text{ mL/hr}$

21. $120 \text{ mL} \times \dfrac{\overset{1}{1\!\!\!/5 \text{ gtt}}}{1 \text{ mL}} \times \dfrac{1 \text{ min}}{5\!\!\!/0 \text{ gtt}} \times \dfrac{1 \text{ hr}}{\underset{4}{6\!\!\!/0 \text{ min}}} =$

$\dfrac{12}{20} \text{ hr or 36 min}$

22. $\overset{2}{2\!\!\!/0\!\!\!/0\!\!\!/0 \text{ mcg}} \times \dfrac{1 \text{ mg}}{\underset{1}{1000 \text{ mcg}}} \times \dfrac{1 \text{ tab}}{2 \text{ mg}} = 1 \text{ tab}$

23. a. $50000 \text{ units} \times \dfrac{1 \text{ mL}}{10,000 \text{ units}} = 5 \text{ mL}$

b. $\dfrac{505 \text{ mL}}{50000 \text{ units}} \times \dfrac{1200 \text{ units}}{\text{hr}} = \dfrac{12.12 \text{ mL}}{\text{hr}}$

24. $1.8 \text{ m}^2 \times \dfrac{\overset{3}{150 \text{ mg}}}{\text{m}^2} \times \dfrac{5 \text{ mL}}{\underset{10}{500 \text{ mg}}} = 2.7 \text{ mL}$

25. $60 \text{ mL of Trovan} + 100 \text{ mL 5\% D/W} = 160 \text{ mL}$

$\dfrac{160 \text{ mL}}{\underset{2}{3\!\!\!/0 \text{ min}}} \times \dfrac{\overset{1}{1\!\!\!/5 \text{ gtt}}}{\text{mL}} = 80 \text{gtt/min}$

Comprehensive Self-Test 2

1. $0.2 \text{ g} \times \dfrac{1000 \text{ mg}}{1 \text{ g}} \times \dfrac{1 \text{ Tab}}{100 \text{ mg}} = 2 \text{ tab sertraline}$

2. $\dfrac{\overset{2}{2\!\!\!/5\!\!\!/0 \text{ mL}}}{\underset{1}{1\!\!\!/2\!\!\!/5 \text{ mg}}} \times \dfrac{5 \text{ mg}}{\text{hr}} \times \dfrac{\overset{1}{6\!\!\!/0 \ \mu\text{gtt}}}{\text{mL}} \times \dfrac{1 \text{ hr}}{\underset{1}{6\!\!\!/0 \text{ min}}} =$

$\dfrac{10 \ \mu\text{gtt}}{\text{min}}$

3. $\dfrac{\overset{1}{5\!\!\!/0\!\!\!/0 \text{ mL}}}{1 \text{ g}} \times \dfrac{1 \text{ g}}{1000 \text{ mg}} \times \dfrac{1 \text{ mg}}{\text{min}} \times \dfrac{60 \ \mu\text{gtt}}{\text{mL}} =$

$30 \ \mu\text{gtt/minute}$

4. $20 \text{ mg} \times \dfrac{1 \text{ g}}{1000 \text{ mg}} \times \dfrac{1 \text{ Tab}}{0.02 \text{ g}} = \dfrac{20}{20} = 2 \text{ tab of}$ Feldene

5. $0.1 \text{ mg} \times \dfrac{1000 \text{ mcg}}{1 \text{ mg}} = 100 \text{ microgram of}$ Cytotec

6. $\overset{1}{1000 \text{ mg}} \times \dfrac{1 \text{ g}}{\underset{1}{1000 \text{ mg}}} \times \dfrac{1 \text{ Tab}}{0.5 \text{ g}} = 2 \text{ tab for each}$

dose of Carafate

$$2 \text{ Tab} \times \frac{4}{\text{day}} \times \frac{7 \text{ day}}{1} = 56 \text{ tablets of Carafate}$$

in seven days

7. $10 \text{ mg} \times \frac{\text{gr } 1}{60 \text{ mg}} \times \frac{1 \text{ tab}}{\text{gr } \frac{1}{24}} = \frac{10 \text{ tab}}{2.5} = 4 \text{ tab}$

of prednisone

8. $0.25 \text{ mg} \times \frac{\overset{8}{1000} \text{ mcg}}{\text{mg}} \times \frac{1 \text{ tab}}{\underset{1}{125} \text{ mcg}} = 2 \text{ Tab of}$

digoxin

9. $114 \text{ lb} \times \frac{0.45 \text{ kg}}{1 \text{ lb}} \times \frac{2 \text{ mcg}}{\text{kg}} \times \frac{1 \text{ mg}}{1000 \text{ mcg}} =$

$\frac{102.6 \text{ mg}}{1000} = 0.1 \text{ mg of vitamin } B_{12}$

or

$114 \text{ lb} \times \frac{1 \text{ kg}}{2.2 \text{ lb}} \times \frac{2 \text{ mcg}}{\text{kg}} \times \frac{1 \text{ mg}}{1000 \text{ mcg}} =$

$\frac{228 \text{ mg}}{2200} = 0.1 \text{ mg of vitamin } B_{12}$

10. $65 \text{ kg} \times \frac{10 \text{ mg}}{\text{kg}} \times \frac{5 \text{ mL}}{300 \text{ mg}} = \frac{325 \text{ mL}}{30} =$

10.8 mL of cimetidine

11. $900 \text{ mg} \times \frac{1 \text{ g}}{1000 \text{ mg}} \times \frac{1 \text{ tab}}{0.3 \text{ g}} = 3 \text{ tab of ibuprofen}$

12. $0.075 \text{ g} \times \frac{1000 \text{ mg}}{1 \text{ g}} \times \frac{1 \text{ tab}}{25 \text{ mg}} = 3 \text{ tab of Tofranil}$

13. $1.2 \text{ m}^2 \times \frac{30 \text{ mg}}{\text{m}^2} \times \frac{5 \text{ mL}}{250 \text{ mg}} = 0.7 \text{ mL of}$

methyldopa

14. $1 \text{ m}^2 \times \frac{0.1 \text{ g}}{\text{m}^2} \times \frac{1000 \text{ mg}}{\text{g}} \times \frac{1 \text{ tab}}{100 \text{ mg}} = 1 \text{ tab of}$

lomustine

15. $0.1 \text{ mg} \times \frac{1000 \text{ mcg}}{1 \text{ mg}} \times \frac{1 \text{ tab}}{50 \text{ mcg}} = 2 \text{ tab of}$

liothyronine sodium

16. $\overset{2}{40} \text{ kg} \times \frac{1 \text{ mg}}{\text{kg}} \times \frac{1 \text{ tab}}{\underset{1}{20} \text{ mg}} = 2 \text{ tablets of furosemide}$

17. $0.4 \text{ m}^2 \times \frac{0.25 \text{ g}}{\text{m}^2} \times \frac{\overset{}{1000} \text{ mg}}{1 \text{ g}} \times \frac{2 \text{ mL}}{\underset{1}{500} \text{ mg}} = 0.4 \text{ mL}$

of acyclovir

18. $1.04 \text{ m}^2 \times \frac{\overset{7}{175} \text{ mg}}{\text{m}^2} \times \frac{5 \text{ mL}}{\underset{10}{250} \text{ mg}} = 3.7 \text{ mL of}$

Depokote

19. Add 13 mL to vial and 1 mL = 200 mg

$3.1 \text{ g} \times \frac{\overset{1}{1000} \text{ mg}}{\text{g}} \times \frac{1 \text{ mL}}{\underset{1}{200} \text{ mg}} = 15.5 \text{ mL will}$

contain 3.1 g of Timentin

20. $275 \text{ units} \times \frac{1 \text{ mL}}{100 \text{ units}} = 2.75 \text{ mL of Hamulin R}$

insulin add 2.75 mL to the 500 mL of 0.9% NS =

$502.75 \text{ mL} \frac{502.75 \text{ mL}}{275 \text{ units}} \times \frac{10 \text{ units}}{\text{hour}} = 18.3 \text{ mL/hour}$

21. a. If 1 mL contains 1,000,000 u, then 20,000,000 u would be contained in a total of 20 mL; so, you would add 20 mL of Pfizerpen to 1000 mL = 1020 mL

b. $\frac{1020 \text{ mL}}{24 \text{ hr}} \times \frac{1 \text{ hr}}{\underset{4}{60} \text{ min}} \times \frac{\overset{1}{75} \text{ gtt}}{1 \text{ mL}} = \frac{1020 \text{ gtt}}{96 \text{ min}} =$

11 gtt/minute

22. $0.2 \text{ mg} \times \frac{1 \text{ mL}}{0.4 \text{ mg}} = \frac{0.2 \text{ mL}}{0.4} = 0.5 \text{ mL of}$

atropine sulfate

23. $0.15 \text{ g} \times \frac{\overset{10}{1000} \text{ mg}}{1 \text{ g}} \times \frac{1 \text{ Tab}}{\underset{3}{300} \text{ mg}} = \frac{1}{2} \text{ tab of aspirin}$

24. $200 \text{ mg} \times \frac{1 \text{ g}}{1000 \text{ mg}} \times \frac{100 \text{ mL}}{2 \text{ g}} = 10 \text{ mL of}$

Nesacaine

25. $66 \text{ kg} \times \frac{0.2 \text{ mg}}{1 \text{ kg} \times 1 \text{ min}} \times \frac{\overset{1}{250} \text{ mL}}{\underset{2}{500} \text{ mg}} \times \frac{10 \text{ gtt}}{\text{mL}} =$

66 gtt/minute

Comprehensive Self-Test 3

1. $\frac{1000 \text{ mL}}{12 \text{ hr}} \times \frac{1 \text{ hr}}{\underset{6}{60} \text{ min}} \times \frac{\overset{1}{10} \text{ gtt}}{\text{mL}} = \frac{1000 \text{ gtt}}{72 \text{ min}} =$

14 gtt/min

2. $\overset{1}{\cancel{100\ \text{mL}}} \times \dfrac{2.5\ \text{mL}}{\cancel{100\ \text{mL}}} \Big/ \dfrac{\overset{1}{\cancel{10\ \text{mL}}}}{\cancel{100\ \text{mL}}} = 25\ \text{mL of the 10\%}$

solution and dilute with water to make 100 mL

3. $7500\ \cancel{\text{units}} \times \dfrac{1\ \text{mL}}{10000\ \cancel{\text{units}}} = 0.75\ \text{mL of heparin}$

4. $1.7\ \cancel{\text{m}^2} \times \dfrac{250\ \cancel{\text{mg}}}{\cancel{\text{m}^2}} \times \dfrac{5\ \text{mL}}{187\ \cancel{\text{mg}}} = \dfrac{2125\ \text{mL}}{187} =$

11.4 mL of Ceclor

5. $70\ \cancel{\text{kg}} \times \dfrac{28.125\ \cancel{\text{mg}}}{35\ \cancel{\text{kg}}} \times \dfrac{1\ \text{Tab}}{18.75\ \cancel{\text{mg}}} = 3\ \text{tab of Cylert}$

6. $0.9\ \cancel{\text{m}^2} \times \dfrac{\overset{2}{\cancel{200\ \text{mg}}}}{\cancel{\text{m}^2}} \times \dfrac{2.5\ \text{mL}}{\underset{1}{\cancel{100\ \text{mg}}}} = 4.5\ \text{mL of}$

erythromycin

7. $0.004\ \cancel{\text{g}} \times \dfrac{\overset{250}{\cancel{1000\ \text{mg}}}}{\cancel{\text{g}}} \times \dfrac{1\ \text{Tab}}{\underset{1}{\cancel{4\ \text{mg}}}} = 1\ \text{Tab of Cardura}$

8. $\dfrac{40\ \text{mg}}{\text{mL}} \times \dfrac{1\ \text{g}}{1000\ \text{mg}} = 40\ \text{g} : 1000\ \text{mL} = 1 : 25,$

or 1 g in 25 mL of the lidocaine solution, or 4%

9. $\overset{6}{\cancel{360\ \text{mL}}} \times \dfrac{\overset{1}{\cancel{15\ \text{gtt}}}}{\cancel{\text{mL}}} \times \dfrac{1\ \text{min}}{\underset{2}{\cancel{30\ \text{gtt}}}} \times \dfrac{1\ \text{hr}}{\underset{1}{\cancel{60\ \text{min}}}} = 3\ \text{hr}$

10. Nembutal gr $1\dfrac{1}{2} \times \dfrac{1\ \text{cap}}{50\ \text{mg}} \times \dfrac{60\ \cancel{\text{mg}}}{\cancel{\text{gr}}\ 1} = 2\ \text{capsule}$

of Nembutal

11. $250,000\ \cancel{\text{units}} \times \dfrac{1\ \text{mL}}{100000\ \cancel{\text{units}}} = 2.5\ \text{mL of}$

penicillin G

12. $0.8\ \cancel{\text{m}^2} \times \dfrac{100\ \text{mg}}{\cancel{\text{m}^2}} = 80\ \text{mg of Cordarone}$

13. $\overset{5}{\cancel{500\ \text{mL}}} \times \dfrac{25\ \text{g}}{\underset{1}{\cancel{100\ \text{mL}}}} = 125\ \text{g. Take 125 g of the}$

pure drug and dilute with H_2O to make 500 mL

14. $70\ \cancel{\text{kg}} \times \dfrac{10\ \cancel{\text{mcg}}}{1\ \cancel{\text{kg}} \times 1\ \cancel{\text{min}}} \times \dfrac{1\ \text{mg}}{1000\ \cancel{\text{mcg}}} \times \dfrac{60\ \cancel{\text{min}}}{1\ \text{hr}} =$

42 mg/hr of the Dobutrex $250\ \text{mg} \times \dfrac{1\ \text{mL}}{12.5\ \text{mg}} =$

20 mL. Add this to the 500 mL.

$\dfrac{520\ \cancel{\text{mL}}}{250\ \cancel{\text{mg}}} \times \dfrac{42\ \cancel{\text{mg}}}{\text{hr}} = 87.4\ \text{mL/hr}$

15. $\cancel{\text{grain}}\ 3 \times \dfrac{1\ \cancel{\text{g}}}{15\ \cancel{\text{gr}}} \times \dfrac{1\ \text{Tab}}{0.2\ \cancel{\text{g}}} = \dfrac{3\ \text{tab}}{3} = 1\ \text{tab of}$

fluconazole

16. $0.75\ \cancel{\text{g}} \times \dfrac{\overset{4}{\cancel{1000\ \text{mg}}}}{1\ \cancel{\text{g}}} \times \dfrac{1\ \text{tab}}{\underset{1}{\cancel{250\ \text{mg}}}} = 3\ \text{tab of}$

clarithromycin

17. $54\ \cancel{\text{kg}} \times \dfrac{4000\ \cancel{\text{mcg}}}{\cancel{\text{kg}}} \times \dfrac{1\ \cancel{\text{mg}}}{1000\ \cancel{\text{mcg}}} \times \dfrac{1\ \cancel{\text{g}}}{1000\ \cancel{\text{mg}}} \times$

$\dfrac{2.5\ \text{mL}}{1\ \cancel{\text{g}}} = 0.5\ \text{mL of streptomycin}$

18. $\dfrac{0.05\ \cancel{\text{mg}}}{\text{min}} \times \dfrac{\overset{20}{\cancel{500\ \text{mL}}}}{\underset{1}{\cancel{25\ \text{mg}}}} \times \dfrac{60\ \mu\text{gtt}}{\cancel{\text{mL}}} = 60\ \mu\text{gtt/min}$

19. $82\ \cancel{\text{kg}} \times \dfrac{8\ \text{mg}}{\cancel{\text{kg}}} = 656\ \text{mg}$

$656\ \cancel{\text{mg}} \times \dfrac{1\ \text{mL}}{500\ \cancel{\text{mg}}} = 1.3\ \text{mL of cefazolin}$

20. $2.5\ \cancel{\text{mg}} \times \dfrac{1\ \text{tab}}{5\ \cancel{\text{mg}}} = \dfrac{1}{2}\ \text{tab of Coumadin}$

21. $\overset{3}{\cancel{300\ \text{mg}}} \times \dfrac{1\ \cancel{\text{g}}}{\underset{10}{\cancel{1000\ \text{mg}}}} \times \dfrac{10\ \text{mL}}{0.3\ \cancel{\text{g}}} = 10\ \text{mL of}$

Quibron

22. $\overset{2}{\cancel{20\ \text{mg}}} \times \dfrac{1\ \text{tab}}{\underset{1}{\cancel{10\ \text{mg}}}} \times \dfrac{2}{\cancel{\text{d}}} \times \dfrac{5\ \cancel{\text{d}}}{1} = 20\ \text{tab of}$

prednisone

23. $1.5\ \cancel{\text{g}} \times \dfrac{1000\ \text{mg}}{1\ \cancel{\text{g}}} = 1500\ \text{mg of Diuril}$

24. $0.25\ \cancel{\text{mg}} \times \dfrac{1\ \text{tab}}{0.5\ \cancel{\text{mg}}} = \dfrac{0.25}{0.5} = \dfrac{1}{2}\ \text{tablet of Xanax}$

25. $2\ \cancel{\text{g}} \times \dfrac{\overset{2}{\cancel{1000\ \text{mg}}}}{1\ \cancel{\text{g}}} \times \dfrac{5\ \text{ml}}{\underset{1}{\cancel{500\ \text{mg}}}} = 20\ \text{mL of Gantrisin}$

Common Abbreviations on Medication Orders

To someone unfamiliar with prescriptive abbreviations, medication orders may look like a foreign language. To interpret prescriptive orders accurately and to administer drugs safely, a qualified person must have a thorough knowledge of common abbreviations. For instance, when the prescriber writes, **"Hydromorphone 1.5 mL IM q4h pc & hs,"** the administrator knows how to interpret it as "Hydromorphone, 1.5 milliliters, intramuscular, every four hours, after meals and at hour of sleep." Study the following list of common abbreviations for smooth navigation through the medication orders in this book. For measurement abbreviations, refer to Appendix H.

Abbreviation	Meaning	Abbreviation	Meaning
$\bar{a}$	before (*abante*)	IV	intravenous
$\overline{aa}$	of each	IVP	intravenous push
ac	before meals (*ante cibium*)	IVPB	intravenous piggy-back
ad	up to (*ad*)		
ad lib	as desired (*ad libitum*)	KVO	keep vein open
A.M., am	morning	LA	long acting
amp	ampule	LIB	left in bag, left in bottle
aq	aqueous water		
bi	two	min	minute
bid, BID	two times a day	mU	milliunit
$\bar{c}$	with	n	night
C	Celsius; centigrade	NPO	nothing by mouth (*per ora*)
cap	capsule		
CVP	central venous pressure	NS	normal saline
		NSAID	nonsteroidal anti-inflammatory drug
d	day		
DC, dc	discontinue		
D/W	dextrose in water	od	every day (*omni die*)
D5W	5% dextrose in water	OD	right eye (*oculus dexter*)
Dx	diagnosis	OS	left eye (*oculus sinister*)
elix	elixir	OU	both eyes
F	Fahrenheit	$\bar{p}$	after
		pc	after meals (*post cibum*)
h, hr, H	hour		
hs, HS	hour of sleep; bedtime (*hora somni*)	PICC	peripherally inserted central catheter
		P.M., pm	afternoon, evening
IC	intracardia	po, PO	by mouth (*per os*)
ID	intradermal	postop	after surgery
IM	intramuscular	preop	before surgery

Abbreviation	Meaning	Abbreviation	Meaning
prn	when required or whenever necessary	R/O	rule out
		R	respiration
Pt	patient	$\bar{s}$	without (*sine*)
P	pulse	sc, SC, SQ	subcutaneous
		sl, sL	under the tongue (sublingual)
q	every (*quaque*)		
qd	every day (*quaque die*)	SR	sustained release
		$\overline{ss}$, ss	one-half
qh	every hour (*quaque hora*)	stat	immediately (*statum*)
		supp	suppository
q2h	every two hours	susp	suspension
q3h	every three hours		
q4h	every four hours	tid, TID	three times a day (*ter in die*)
qid, QID	four times a day (*quarter in die*)	TPN	total parenteral nutrition
qod	every other day		
qn	every night (*quaque noct*)	T	temperature
qs	quantitiy sufficient or sufficient amount (*quantitas sufficiens*)	wt	weight
		>	greater than
		<	less than

Dosage Preparation Forms and Packaging

PREPARATION FORMS

Medications are manufactured in many preparation forms. Each form serves a distinct purpose. One form might release medication into the body at a slower rate than another. One form might be manufactured to facilitate swallowing. Use the following definitions of preparation forms as a reference for understanding medication orders.

Aqueous solution   One or more medications completely dissolved in water.

Capsule   Gelatinous container enclosing a powder, a liquid, or time-release granules of medication.

Elixir   Medication dissolved in a mixture of water, alcohol, sweeteners, and flavoring.

Metered-dose inhaler   Aerosol device containing multiple doses of medication for inhalation.

Ointment   Semisolid preparation of medication to be applied to the skin.

Suppository   Mixture of medication with a firm base that melts at body temperature and is molded into a shape suitable for insertion into body cavities.

Suspension   Finely divided particles of medication undissolved in water.

Syrup   Medication in water and sugar solution.

Tablet   Powdered medication compressed or molded into a small disk.

Transdermal patch   Adhesive disk that attaches to the skin with a center reservoir containing medication to be slowly absorbed through the skin.

PARENTERAL PACKAGING

There are three common types of parenteral medication containers for sterile solutions.

Ampule   Sealed glass container with only one dose of powdered or liquid medication.

Prefilled cartridge   Small, slender single-dose vial with an attached needle. A metal or plastic holder is used to inject the medication.

Vial   Sealed glass container of a liquid or powdered medication with a rubber stopper, allowing multiple-dose use.

APPENDIX D

Celsius and Fahrenheit Temperature Conversions

Reading and recording a temperature is a crucial step in assessing a patient's health. Temperatures can be measured using either the Fahrenheit (F) scale or the Celsius or centrigrade (C) scale. Most health-care settings use Fahrenheit, but some are switching to Celsius. Celsius/Fahrenheit equivalency tables make it easy to convert Celsius to Fahrenheit, or vice versa. Still, it is useful to be able to make this conversion yourself.

You can use the following rules to convert from one temperature scale to the other

NOTE

$$F = \tfrac{9}{5}C + 32 \qquad \text{or} \qquad C = \tfrac{5}{9}(F - 32)$$

For those unfamiliar with algebra, the following rules are equivalent to the algebraic formulas.

First rule: To convert to Celsius.   Subtract 32 and then divide by 1.8.

Second rule: To convert to Fahrenheit.   Multiply by 1.8 and then add 32.

NOTE

Temperatures are rounded to the nearest tenth.

> **EXAMPLE D.1**

Convert 102.5°F to Celsius.

Using the first rule, we subtract 32.

$$
\begin{array}{r}
102.5 \\
-32.0 \\
\hline
70.5
\end{array}
$$

Then we divide by 1.8.

$$1.8\,)\overline{70.5\,000} \quad 39.17$$

So, 102.5°F equals about 39.2°C.

350

Convert 3°C to Fahrenheit.

Using the second rule, we first multiply by 1.8.

$$\begin{array}{r} 1.8 \\ \times 3 \\ \hline 5.4 \end{array}$$

Then we add 32.

$$\begin{array}{r} 5.4 \\ +32.0 \\ \hline 37.4 \end{array}$$

So, 3°C equals about 37.4°F.

Tables of Weight Conversions

Use the following tables to convert between the metric kilogram and the household pound.

▶ TABLE E.1

Pounds to Kilograms

lb	kg	lb	kg	lb	kg
2.2	1.0	120	54.5	240	109.1
5	2.3	125	56.8	245	111.4
10	4.5	130	59.1	250	113.6
15	6.8	135	61.4	255	115.9
20	9.1	140	63.6	260	118.2
25	11.4	145	65.9	265	120.5
30	13.6	150	68.2	270	122.7
35	15.9	155	70.5	275	125
40	18.2	160	72.7	280	127.3
45	20.5	165	75	285	129.5
50	22.7	170	77.3	290	131.8
55	25	175	79.5	295	134.1
60	27.3	180	81.8	300	136.4
65	29.5	185	84.1	305	138.6
70	31.8	190	86.4	310	140.9
75	34.1	195	88.6	315	143.2
80	36.4	200	90.9	320	145.5
85	38.6	205	93.2	325	147.7
90	40.9	210	95.5	330	150
95	43.2	215	97.7	335	152.3
100	45.5	220	100	340	154.5
105	47.7	225	102.3	345	156.8
110	50	230	104.5	350	159.1
115	52.3	235	106.8	355	161.4

▶ TABLE E.2

Kilograms to Pounds

kg	lb	kg	lb	kg	lb
2	4.4	56	123.2	110	242
4	8.8	58	127.6	112	246.4
6	13.2	60	132	114	250.8
8	17.6	62	136.4	116	255.2
10	22	64	140.8	118	259.6
12	26.4	66	145.2	120	264
14	30.8	68	149.6	122	268.4
16	35.2	70	154	124	272.8
18	39.6	72	158.4	126	277.2
20	44	74	162.8	128	281.6
22	48.4	76	167.2	130	286
24	52.8	78	171.6	132	290.4
26	57.2	80	176	134	294.8
28	61.6	82	180.4	136	299.2
30	66	84	184.8	138	303.6
32	70.4	86	189.2	140	308
34	74.8	88	193.6	142	312.4
36	79.2	90	198	144	316.8
38	83.6	92	202.4	146	321.2
40	88	94	206.8	148	325.6
42	92.4	96	211.2	150	330
44	96.8	98	215.6	152	334.4
46	101.2	100	220	154	338.8
48	105.6	102	224.4	156	343.2
50	110	104	228.8	158	347.6
52	114.4	106	233.2	160	352
54	118.8	108	237.6	162	356.4

APPENDIX F

Nomograms

Dosages are sometimes based on a patient's body surface area (BSA), and nomograms are the equivalency charts used to determine the patient's BSA.

PEDIATRIC NOMOGRAM

The boxed column listing weight on the left and surface in square meters on the right can be used when a child is of normal height for his or her weight.

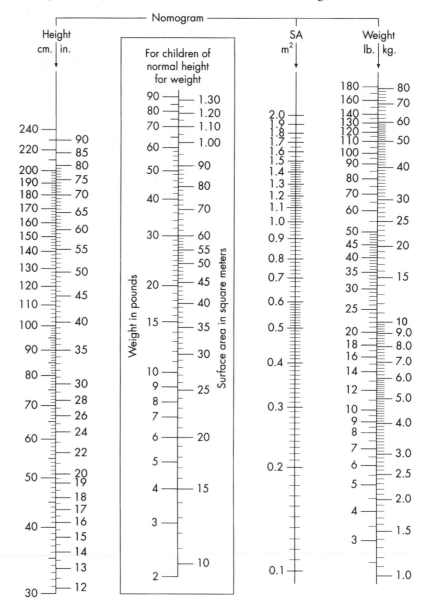

Courtesy of R.E. Behrman and V.C. Vaughn, (eds.), *Nelson Textbook of Pediatrics*, 13th ed., Philadelphia: W.B. Saunders Co., 1987. Reprinted with permission

ADULT NOMOGRAM

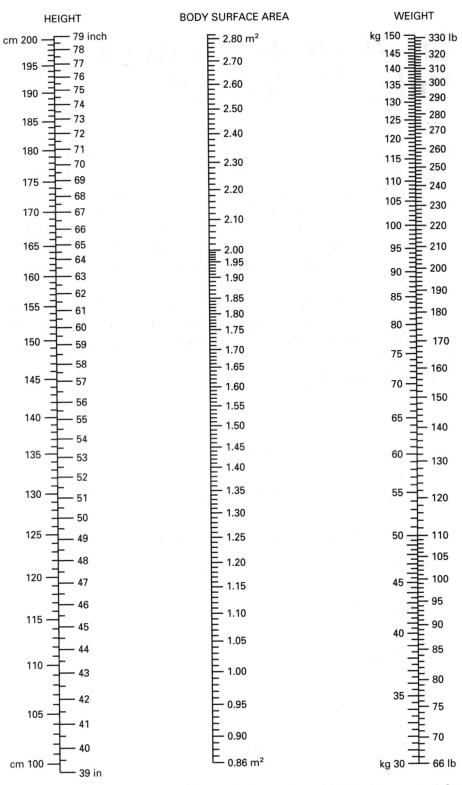

HEIGHT	BODY SURFACE AREA	WEIGHT

To use the nomogram, you need the patient's weight and height. Draw a straight line between the patient's height (first column) and the patient's weight (last column). The point at which the line crosses the SA column is the estimated *BSA in square meters.*

Fried's Rule, Young's Rule, Clark's Rule

Pediatric dosages for children are primarily based on body surface area (BSA), weight, and/or age. Currently the preferred method is the amount of medication per kilogram of body weight or BSA. However, children's dosages can also be determined by relating the child's age in months or the child's weight in pounds to adult dosages. The formulas used to do this are known as **Fried's Rule** and **Young's Rule,** both of which use the patient's age to determine the correct pediatric dose, and **Clark's Rule,** which uses the patient's weight to determine the correct pediatric dose.

If you used **Fried's Rule** to determine a safe dose of ampicillin (Omnipen) for a 5-month-old infant, for example, you would have to know that the usual recommended adult dose of this drug is 500 milligrams and that the adult age is 150 months.

This is the formula for Fried's Rule:

$$\frac{\text{Age of infant (months)}}{\text{Adult age (months)}} \times \text{adult dose} = \text{safe dose for an infant}$$

So, for the 5-month-old infant, the dose would be calculated as follows:

$$\frac{5 \cancel{\text{ mon}}}{\underset{3}{\cancel{150 \text{ mon}}}} \times \overset{10}{\cancel{500}} \text{ mg} = \frac{50}{3} \text{ mg or } 16.6 \text{ mg}$$

So, 16.6 or 17 milligrams is a safe dose for a 5-month-old infant.

Young's Rule is used for the calculation of pediatric dosages for children between the ages of 1 and 12.

$$\frac{\text{Age of child (years)}}{\text{Age of child} + 12 \text{ (years)}} \times \text{adult dose} = \text{safe dose for a child}$$

So, for a 5-year-old child and an adult dose of 500 milligrams. Young's Rule would yield the following result:

$$\frac{5 \cancel{\text{ yr}}}{(5 + 12) \cancel{\text{ yr}}} \times 500 \text{ mg} = \frac{2500}{17} \text{ mg or } 147.05 \text{ mg}$$

So, 147.05 or 147 milligrams would be a safe dose for a 5-year-old child.

Clark's Rule uses the child's weight to calculate pediatric dosages. The formula is

$$\frac{\text{Child's weight (lb)}}{\text{Adult weight (lb)}} \times \text{adult dose} = \text{safe dose for child}$$

So if a child weighs 30 pounds and the adult dose is 500 milligrams, Clark's Rule would be

$$\frac{\overset{1}{\cancel{30 \text{ lb}}}}{\underset{5}{\cancel{150 \text{ lb}}}} \times 500 \text{ mg} = 100 \text{ mg}$$

NOTE

The weight used here is the average adult weight in pounds—that is, 150 pounds.

So, 100 milligrams is a safe dose for a 30-pound child.

As you can see, it is very similar to dimensional analysis; for example, you can use Clark's Rule with kilograms. For a child weighing 15 kilograms, the formula is

$$\frac{15 \cancel{\text{ kg}}}{70 \cancel{\text{ kg}}} \times 500 \text{ mg} = \frac{7500 \text{ mg}}{70} = 107 \text{ mg}$$

NOTE

The weight used here is the average adult weight in kilograms—that is, 70 kilograms.

So, 107 milligrams is a safe dose for a 15-kilogram child.

While most prescribers today base medication orders on weight or BSA, Clark's Rule, Fried's Rule, and Young's Rule are still used by some pediatricians, advanced nurse practitioners, and physician's assistants.

APPENDIX H

Abbreviations

Volume	Metric	Household	
milliliter	mL	microdrop	μgtt or mcgtt
liter	L	drop	gtt
cubic centimeter	cc	teaspoon	t or tsp
		tablespoon	T or tbs
Apothecary		fluid ounce	ʒ
minim	ℳ	pint	pt
fluid dram	ʒ	quart	qt
		gallon	gal

Weight	Metric		Household
microgram	μg or mcg	ounces	ʒ or oz
milligram	mg	pound	lb
gram	g		
kilogram	kg		
Apothecary			
grain	gr		
dram	ʒ		

Length	Metric		Household
centimeter	cm	inch	in
meter	m	foot	ft
		yard	yd

Area	Metric
square meter	m^2

Numeric	Apothecary		Other
$\frac{1}{2}$	ss	milliunit	mU
		unit	u or U
$1\frac{1}{2}$	iss	milliequivalent	mEq
		tablet	tab
$2\frac{1}{2}$	iiss		
		Roman	
$7\frac{1}{2}$	viiss	1 I	7 VII
		2 II	10 X
		3 III	15 XV
		4 IV	20 XX
		5 V	25 XXV
		6 VI	30 XXX